PRAISE
HEAL ENDO

"It is rare to find a single resource that is as comprehensive and user-friendly as this book, especially for such a common, widely misunderstood, and under-studied condition as endometriosis. *Heal Endo* manages to cover what could take months or years in 1-1 work with an empowering root cause approach. This book has the potential to help countless people break the cycle of painkillers and surgery and find lasting relief from endo."

—Ayla Barmmer, MS, Registered Dietitian, Co-Founder of Women's Health Nutrition Academy, CEO FullWell

"Whether you're newly diagnosed with endometriosis or have been living with it for years, *Heal Endo* will deepen your understanding of this disease and clear the confusion. By reframing endometriosis from a "women's issue" - relegated to the realms of gynecology - to instead a body-wise disease fraught with immune dysregulation, we can change our current mainstream approach to addressing this complex disease."

—Dr. Jolene Brighten, Bestselling author of *Beyond the Pill*

"Katie Edmonds has written a truly comprehensive and compassionate guide to endometriosis. *Heal Endo* provides readers with a revolutionary approach to understanding and treating this condition. It includes the latest research on how endometriosis develops, effective treatment protocols, and how to live an endo-healing life. This book is definitely one to have on your shelf!"

—Nicole Jardim, Certified Women's Health Coach, Author of *Fix Your Period*

"Something unusual happened to me while I was reading *Heal Endo* . . . I started to experience hope. As someone who has personally battled with the most invasive form of endometriosis, enduring excruciating pain, three surgeries, and the loss of organs and fertility over the course of several decades, and someone who has professionally supported others on their endo journeys as their health coach & nutritional therapist, I can honestly say that Katie's book is a very rare glimpse of hope for the treatment of endometriosis. Such a complex disease requires a nuanced approach and Katie has successfully woven all the threads together."

   –Angie Alt, CHC, NTP, co-author of *The Autoimmune Wellness Handbook*

"In this beautifully illustrated book, Katie Edmonds, an endo warrior herself, offers easy-to-follow recommendations for supporting women with endometriosis to reduce the chronic and systemic inflammation that often amplifies endometriosis symptoms. She helpfully explains how endometriosis is a systemic disease and must be approached with integrative and systemic healing strategies. Of course, I am in strong agreement. I especially enjoyed her detailed recommendations on stress buffering and management which is a huge part of living healthfully with endometriosis but is not discussed often enough."

   –Dr. Jessica Drummond, DCN, CNS, PT, Founder and CEO of The Integrative Women's Health Institute and author of *Outsmart Endometriosis.*

"It's about time we approached endometriosis from an inflammatory perspective. The combination of a one, two punch for endometriosis — 1) decrease inflammation and immune upregulation and 2) excision of endometriosis — in combination, are the ideal approach to 'beat' and 'heal' endo. Kudos to Katie!"

   –Dr. Iris Kerin Orbuch, Director of the Advanced Gynecologic Laparoscopy Center in Los Angeles, Author of *Beating Endo: How to Reclaim Your Life From Endometriosis.*

"What an amazing book!!! This book will be the 'gold standard' resource for patients with endometriosis. Outstanding!!! *Heal Endo* will certainly help save many women with endometriosis unnecessary pain and suffering. It has been an honor to work with you and help with this project."

—Dr. Andrew Cook, Founder and Medical Director of the Vital Health Endometriosis Center

"This book is a gift to the endo community at large. Truly, the depth and breadth of research that went into making this book is astounding, and the way Katie is able to break down the science in interesting and understandable language is simply invaluable. I expect that it will become a widely circulating book among both those living with endo and those who treat it."

—Merritt Jones, DAIM, LAc, CNC, Clinical Director at Natural Harmony Reproductive Health

"For ten years I have read *all the* books, articles, and been down hundreds of rabbit holes about my endometriosis diagnosis. But after reading *Heal Endo*, for the first time in my life I felt like I could understand this beast of a disease. *Heal Endo* will help you answer so many of the questions that have left you feeling hopeless and, for possibly the first time, give you a sense of optimism for the future. No matter where you are in your endo journey, whether you've just been diagnosed or have had multiple surgeries, *Heal Endo* will help you connect the dots of YOUR endometriosis and give you direction and hope. Not only will this book help you understand your body so much better, but Katie clearly lays out every step you can take to give your body the best chance of finding remission."

—Roxanne van Zyl, Endometriosis Health Coach

heal ENDO

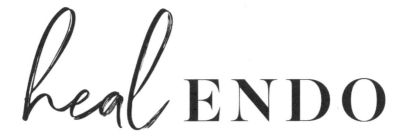

heal ENDO

An Anti-inflammatory Approach to Healing
from Endometriosis

Katie Edmonds, (F)NTP

To everyone who's suffered from endometriosis.

And to my daughter, Nola, may your journey be different.

Table of Contents

PART IV: BEYOND NUTRITION – AN ENDO-HEALING LIFE

FOREWORD

by Dan C. Martin, M.D., Scientific and
  Medical Director of the Endometriosis
  Foundation of America

Katie Edmonds is a force of nature in birthing an amazing and wonderful book covering the spectrum of endometriosis. Throughout *Heal Endo* she not only presents the modern understanding of endometriosis but also integrates contemporary therapy, complementary methods, alternative medicine, and body ecology in an easy-to-read style that makes this book useful to beginners and experts alike.

Katie has avoided the tendency of social and mass media to focus on one aspect of endometriosis development and/or treatment at a time, and instead offers suggestions on how to integrate multiple healing possibilities into individual care. She understands that all women are different and need individualized approaches to their care—that's why we need better answers for the care of those with endometriosis, and this book is one of them.

As with much of my life that has benefited from serendipitous events (as predicted by Louis Pasteur's "chance favors the prepared mind"), I was invited to write this foreword at a time when I myself was reviewing a theoretical plan to proactively decrease the inflammatory responses of endometriosis and endometriotic progression so that women can avoid surgery and chronic morbidity, including pain and infertility. This plan was based on a variety of research documenting women with endometriosis that is either not active, not causing problems, or not progressing—endometriosis that had been "stopped" in some way without surgical intervention.

To understand why, we need look no further than the immune system. When the immune system works, it is capable of inactivating, stabilizing, and clearing endometriosis. If we can harness the innate ability of the immune system, we may improve the lives of women and transgender men. While we of course must be diligent in seeking earlier and better treatment for those with endometriosis, we can remember that endometriosis is not always a devastating disease, especially if we can approach it with a modern understanding of the immune system, and a unique care plan for those suffering.

This book does exactly that, making a case for additional, complementary, and alternative medicine with compelling logic. Katie's suggestions have stood the test of time and have helped give women control over their illness. As she points out, endometriosis is only one of many inflammatory triggers that can cause disease. Others include lethargy, loss of sleep, decreased activities, and many other daily problems. Because no single approach will be helpful for all sufferers, and because no one treatment works for everyone, understanding what has helped others gives important guidance for what to try. What has worked for one may work for others, so the numerous approaches presented within may offer useful new opportunities for treatment.

Heal Endo covers the basics of what I learned in medical training. The sections on the endocrinologic and immunologic concepts of endometriosis could be a primer in college or medical school or in a postgraduate course for older physicians who were not trained in these concepts. It's a $200 medical textbook on immunology written in plain English for the price of a consumer text. It also includes alternative treatments that sufferers and their friends, families, and providers need to know about but can be difficult to find. There are very few providers who will understand all of them. I have studied endometriosis for more than 50 years but did not know, much less understand all the available treatment options. I doubt there are many people, including providers, who do.

This comprehensive volume covers systemic inflammation, regulation of the immune system, cellular clearance, immune dysfunction, autoimmunity, environmental factors, epigenetic alterations, anti-inflammatory diets, the role of a properly done excision surgery, complementary and alternative methods, triggers, healing the gut, mucosal immunity, and decreased oxygenation. As Katie points out, this research is available despite the underfunding of endometriosis research compared to other medical issues, showing there is still much that is being done. (Note that PubMed has added almost 2,000 papers on endometriosis in 2021, with more than 1,000 on treatment).

Yet, as a researcher, academic, and former surgeon, I intimately understand the divide between what research has uncovered and what the average sufferer (or doctor) knows about this disease, a divide this book aims to address.

Perhaps the most important takeaway is this: the care of endometriosis is more than the care of the individual lesions; it is the care of the entire body. The more we can remember that endometriosis is a full-body issue and commit to taking full-body care, the better these sufferer's immune systems will function, leading to better management of their endometriosis.

Dr. Martin is the Scientific and Medical Director for the Endometriosis Foundation of America. He has studied endometriosis since 1970 and to date has 443 publications, with most on endometriosis. He's taught in full-time and clinical academia for 44 years with 27 of those from a private practice offering professional excision surgery. Dr. Martin is on the editorial boards of four medical journals. He is the past President of the AAGL (formerly the American Association of Gynecologic Laparoscopists) and the Gynecologic Laser Society. You can find him at www.danmartinmd.com

PREFACE

Endometriosis really knocked me sideways. It came on hard and fast; one moment I was a healthy, athletic young woman, and the next I was rolling on the floor with an astounding level of pain. During the years after my diagnosis, I unraveled, becoming sicker, enduring chronic pain, and feeling more exhausted. My hair broke off and my belly bloated. Doctors didn't give me much hope that I could turn it around. When I wanted babies and conception eluded us for years, I was told I would have to resort to IVF... or just have a hysterectomy and adopt.

There was nothing like being sick and tired of being sick and tired to motivate me to question everything I had been told about this disease. I was in my late twenties, with a deep desire to have children. Yet I was terrified of coming off the birth control pills that were supposed to alleviate my endo symptoms, even though they weren't helping very much.

I kept wondering, why was I slowly getting worse if I was diligently following the commonly prescribed path of hormonal birth control pills, painkillers, food restriction, and multiple rounds of surgeries? If estrogen was my problem, why was nothing helping when I did everything possible to lower estrogen? Why was I suffering body-wide issues if endo was relegated to my pelvis? Having had two surgeries previously—which showed there was no physical impediment preventing pregnancy—why was I still infertile? Anger and frustration at the unfairness of the situation fueled my research.

My journey of discovery uncovered new truths about endo, although these truths (shockingly) weren't new discoveries. Researchers have long known that endometriosis is an inflammatory disease and that there are multiple factors that drive the inflammation—and multiple ways we can heal from it. But this information was brand new to me, and it changed the entire way I approached healing.

Instead of my laser focus on "problematic estrogen," I suddenly understood how I could incorporate many diet and lifestyle changes to help re-regulate my immune system, quell chronic inflammation, and heal from within. It helped me understand that while birth control was helping suppress the symptoms, it wasn't fixing the problem. It allowed me to realize that a holistic approach wasn't just helpful for endo, but necessary.

While it was surprising to discover the disease I was suffering from was, in actuality, quite different from the disease I had thought it was, it was not nearly as shocking as finding my endometriosis slowly fade into full clinical remission. *I had never been told this was possible.* Yet here I was, a few years into new holistic healing therapies, discovering my chronic fatigue had dissolved, my digestive woes had healed, my chronic pelvic pain had vanished. Even more, I found my body capable of healing from three years of infertility and it has since blessed me with two children (cue happy tears).

This discovery that endo doesn't have to be a life sentence led me on the path I'm on today. I went back to school to become a Functional Nutritional Therapy Practitioner (FNTP) in order to work exclusively with endo sufferers. I also started a successful website about holistic ways to approach this disease (www. healendo.com) and published *The 4-Week Endometriosis Diet Plan* to help sufferers create a new type of roadmap to healing.

But after years of connecting with so many sufferers around the world, it became more and more apparent just how much frustration remains around the lack of understanding about this disease, and how that's hurting treatment options. We hear that we need more research and, yes, we do—funding for endo research is pitifully low. Yet, science knows a lot more about endo than you may realize. A search for scientific publications in early 2021 listed approximately 30,000 endo-related scientific articles on PubMed, and 425,000 on Google Scholar—with an increase of about 5 new papers *daily* during 2020. That means there has been really *quite a bit of new research* released in the past few years.

I no longer believe that getting a diagnosis should feel like the beginning of the end. Neither should you. That's why I wrote this book.

The question I kept coming back to in my research was whether I was an outlier or anomaly as someone who was able to put her endometriosis into "magical" remission. After extensively researching endometriosis both in the literature and in patients' personal journeys, I have found the answer to be: no. There are many sufferers who have curtailed their disease through diet and lifestyle, Western medicine, complementary and alternative medicine, a properly done surgery—or any combination of these. They may have been able to achieve full clinical remission like me, or have found a place on the partial remission spectrum where they have symptoms that are manageable rather than life-destroying.

It's clear that endometriosis, a disease that radically and terribly affects the quality of life of *tens of millions* of women, shouldn't have to be devastating. It shouldn't lead a 23-year-old to thinking her life is totally over; a 35-year-old being told her endo damage is too far progressed to maintain a pregnancy; or a 16-year-old in pain being told not to seek a diagnosis for endo, since "nothing can be done about it anyway." It shouldn't mean that you, as a patient, need to know more than your doctor to advocate for your health, while facing doctors who don't take your symptoms seriously and friends and family who just don't understand what you're going through. It should *never* equate to a lifetime of sadness, pain, stress, infertility, sickness, misdiagnosis, or dare I say thoughts of suicide.

So while, yes, we need more research, the goal of this book is to help deliver what we've already uncovered about the disease and how to heal from it. Here I hope to offer a bridge of understanding from endo researchers to you, including how endo is an inflammatory condition, how it may be stabilized or perhaps even regress, diet and lifestyle support mechanisms that help, and why the type of surgery you select matters. It's information the average endo patient has never been updated on—nor many general doctors.

This book will teach you how to better understand your endo and know what steps to take today to start healing from it. Part I will re-introduce you to our disease, what it is, how to get a diagnosis, and working with doctors. Part II will unravel the deeper story of endo, such as how you develop endo and how it's truly an inflammatory disease, rooted in immune dysfunction. Part III and IV will unlock the keys to healing, addressing everything from nutrition to movement, bacteria to chemicals, surgery and more.

I believe knowledge is power, and we together need to make sure this information is better disseminated. We *need* to know what endo is, *need* fast and accurate diagnosis to prevent irreversible damage, and *need* to be offered proper treatment options that have been proven to help. We should be able to have babies (if we want them), and we certainly deserve a life without chronic, unrelenting pain due to an obscure notion that endo is some mysterious "women's condition."

If our own endo story is already written in irreversible ways, we need to make sure our daughters have a chance to avoid the hell we've been through without being told to accept that "it runs in families." We deserve better, all of us, and my hope is that this book helps shift the conversation around endo from one of darkness to one of hope.

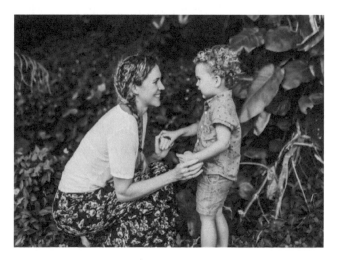

Me with my miracle son, and newly pregnant with my miracle daughter

Part I:

Endometriosis 2.0: A Modern Understanding

In this section you will be re-introduced to endo as you've never been before; you'll learn what endometriosis really is, the basics of how it's treated, and how to create a new path forward.

Chapter 1:

What Is Endometriosis, Really?

When I was 23, I had a sudden burst of pelvic pain so intense I thought an organ had ruptured. Within a day the acute pain had minimized, only to be replaced by a deep, chronic pain that needled my every move. I was terrified that I had cancer.

I was "lucky" to be diagnosed with suspected endo within three months of the onset of pain (the average wait time for an endo diagnosis can be up to a decade), thanks to a wonderful doctor who took my pain seriously. However, being told that the pain could be mitigated only through synthetic hormones, painkillers, chemical menopause, or eventually a hysterectomy, isn't what a 23-year-old hopes to hear at a doctor's appointment. I was devastated.

I remember my body-racking sobs that day because I had researched endometriosis, and I'd discovered that its informal tagline is "there's no cure." Sufferers online documented decades of pain, infertility, and health crises. In my mind, I could have done *something* with even a cancer diagnosis, but now my deep, chronic pelvic pain was stamped as "incurable" endometriosis. And it appeared that I couldn't do much about it.

Like the sufferers I'd read about online, I too witnessed a rapid decline in health over the next few years. I had two surgeries recommended and performed by general OB-GYNs. I stayed on the recommended oral contraceptives. I tried cutting out many different foods. While some days were better than others, nothing really helped. Living on the North Shore of Kaua`i, I had formerly been very athletic, but slowly my everyday joys of running, surfing, and active island life faded into chronic fatigue, joint pain, digestive issues, and chronic pelvic pain—maybe we could call it "unraveling by endo" and I absolutely know most of you reading this can relate.

While miserable, I certainly wasn't alone. Endometriosis is a disease that affects an estimated 1 in 10 women, which is roughly 390 million across the globe. That's a lot of women! One-third of us suffer under a crushing tide of pain, one-third struggle with infertility, and many, many have digestive woes. And yet... up to half of us may have little to no symptoms.[1] It's confusing at first glance, that's for sure.

To cut through the confusion, I started to research the basics. I found that, with endometriosis, abnormal cells that are *similar to* the lining of the uterus (called the endometrium) are found outside of the uterus. These cells develop into endometriotic lesions (i.e., endometriosis), which grow and bleed in response to hormonal fluctuations throughout the menstrual cycle. This is probably why the lesions of endometriosis are so often confused with the endometrium, although they are quite different.

These lesions commonly affect the pelvic organs, including the uterus, fallopian tubes, and ovaries. But endo is not limited to the reproductive organs or pelvis. It's not uncommon for patients to have extra pelvic and distal endo, meaning endo found on other abdominal organs and even outside of the abdomen in places such as the skin, heart, lungs, or the brain.

Although not always, endometriosis can also be progressive. This means, if left untreated, it may advance into worse forms of the disease, along with potentially irreversible scar tissue and adhesions (when scar tissue adheres tissue or organs together). While symptoms of endo are often related to the menstrual cycle, they may also be related to urination or defection, or sometimes seemingly not related to much at all. In my case, I had pelvic pain nearly all the time *except* at menses. Some sufferers never have pelvic pain, but instead have terrible digestive symptoms, maybe joint pain, back pain, unexplained infertility, or chronic fatigue. Yes, endo can be so much more than a painful period, and that's why treating periods alone hasn't been able to offer many of us the vibrant quality of life we deserve.

Yet, as I was learning the basics, I also learned that things I'd been told about the disease weren't exactly accurate. For example, I had heard that endometriosis is caused by too much estrogen coursing through my body. I'd heard it was some sort of "menstrual disorder", relegated solely to the pelvis. I'd heard that there's really nothing that can be done except for diligently managing symptoms and hoping for the best. If you've Googled endo over the years, you've probably read the same information, leaving you feeling the same despair that I felt. That's why I'm happy to tell you that none of this is entirely accurate.

Here's the truth: endometriosis is an inflammatory condition, rooted in immune dysfunction. Although endo is affected by estrogen, it's not caused by estrogen. And while symptoms are often related to the menstrual cycle and reproduction, endometriosis is really a full-body disease—it's systemic.

Understanding that inflammation was at the heart of endo helped answer questions plaguing me for years: if estrogen is to blame then why is lowering my estrogen not helping? Why is stopping my periods not helping? Why am I so chronically fatigued if endo only affects my pelvis? Why am I dealing with infertility if I only have moderate endo? Moreover, by learning what endo really is, I was finally able to understand what healing I needed to do.

No matter who you are and what your symptoms are, treating the inflammation behind endo is the foundation from which we all can heal anew.

ENDO, CHRONIC INFLAMMATION, AND IMMUNE DYSFUNCTION

To understand an inflammatory condition, you first have to understand *inflammation*, a bodily process that is often misunderstood. Inflammation is actually something the immune system *does*. It's your body's fire-breathing dragon protecting you from harm anytime there is an injury or invader. Inflammation should also be short-lived. When there is cellular damage triggered by a cut, scrape, virus, bacteria, or anything foreign, inflammation comes in a burst, sanitizes the scene, and leaves without much fuss while your body heals. Think of all the fevers you've had over the years—body-wide inflammation to protect you from bacteria or viruses that might otherwise have killed you. All those cuts and scrapes you've had? Thank inflammation for keeping infection at bay. So yes, while it can be irritating and painful, you want that immune-based inflammation to protect you. Without it, you would die.

Chronic inflammation is different. If the damaging trigger is never removed, your body is left in that fire-breathing-dragon mode, which will begin to damage surrounding cells, tissues, or organs. That's right, chronic inflammation *creates* more damage. It's why you need the triggers leading to your inflammation to be removed, just like you'd need to remove a fallen eyelash from the eye, or poison ivy from your skin, otherwise they'd continue to do harm.

Not only will chronic inflammation create chronic damage, but it will also start to trigger the immune system as a whole to go a bit haywire, doing things it shouldn't while not doing things it should. This is called *immune dysfunction*, a hallmark of autoimmune disorders, cancers, and endo. Activities that shouldn't be happening inside your body are actually *fueled* by your immune system's confused behavior. In the case of endo, an inflammatory cycle like this is exactly what helps your endometriosis develop into something sinister.

In fact, it's your confused immune system that is responsible for "rooting down" an endometriosis-like cell into your tissue, connecting it to your blood and oxygen supply, to establish a full-blown endometriosis lesion. Yes, you can thank your immune system for this. Moreover, your immune system's defense mechanisms aren't behaving as they should, letting the endo lesions stay rather than clearing them from the body as they should. Once endo is established, the lesions make their own inflammatory immune factors, while the repeated injury from all that chronic inflammation creates scar tissue and adhesions. This is how inflammation—and the wayward immune response fostering it—becomes the driving force behind endo.

And even though we most often experience issues associated with the pelvis and reproductive organs, endo is actually a body-wide disease. No matter where your endometriosis lesions are, endometriosis actually *affects* and is *affected by* the whole body. It's systemic.

THERE'S EVEN MORE TO THE STORY

Because this is such a big transition away from what many of us think endometriosis is (i.e., some sort of period problem), I reached out to Dr. Dan Martin to ask how we should start re-imagining endo in an understandable way. As the Scientific and Medical Director of one of the largest endo nonprofits in the world—The Endometriosis Foundation of America—Dr. Martin suggests thinking about endometriosis in a similar way to another inflammatory issue we're better familiar with...acne.

First of all, acne is *heterogeneous*, meaning there are different types of acne (seven to be exact). You may be surprised to know there are different types of endo too, currently four, although this list will likely expand.[2] Research has already isolated up to 65 different endo phenotypes with potential differences in behavior, physical form, and biochemical properties![3] This means one day your endo diagnosis may not just include stage and location. It may also describe your type (or types) of endo, which could be more aggressive or stubborn, or perhaps more associated with pain or infertility. Just as some small pimples hurt terribly while some large pimples can be ugly with no pain at all, different types of endo can behave in different ways. The fact that there are so many different types and behaviors of endometriosis is one reason that it is so complex to diagnose and treat.

Secondly, acne is *multifactorial*, meaning there are many factors that contribute to disease development, such as bacteria, hormones, irritating chemicals from skincare, stress, or food intolerances. Endo too is multifactorial, with different factors that drive the making and progression of (different types of) endo. And the factors don't line up the same with every patient. No, you didn't just "catch" endo, even if you were like me and felt symptoms come on fast and strong. And yes, other sufferers may have had their own endo develop from circumstances different than yours. Endo develops through a complex symphony of factors that together create the chronic condition you're facing today.

Third, certain types of acne are affected by *estrogen*, a potent trigger of inflammation and increased zit formation for some, yet acne is not a "hormonal disease." Rather, hormones become one trigger of many. Endo too is estrogen-sensitive, but it is not caused by estrogen either.

Of course, endometriosis isn't *exactly* like acne, so please don't be offended by my likening your level 10/10 pain, or the adherence of your ovaries to your bowel, with a bad zit outbreak. Yet, understanding endo as a heterogeneous, multifactorial disease of inflammation—like acne—*is* the cornerstone of this book. By viewing endo in a similar way to this well-known condition which can progress or *regress*, sometimes with lots of intervention and sometimes without, that can be painful or not, cause scarring or not, and which develops from different factors into different types of disease depending on the sufferer, we can begin to re-imagine endo in new ways.

THE ECOLOGY OF ENDOMETRIOSIS

This idea that endometriosis can stabilize without progression or scarring, regress in size and volume, or simply continue to exist without causing problems, may be news to many, but it's well-documented. One review found that while 29 percent of those with endo had disease that ended up progressing, 42 percent actually showed disease *regression* and 29 percent remained stable.[4] Another review of healthy, fertile women having their "tubes tied" to prevent pregnancy found asymptomatic endo in nearly 6 percent of these women at the time of surgery—with lesions that were established but not causing problems.[5]

Endo (verb)

The many ways endo can behave when exposed to, or sheltered from, inflammatory triggers.

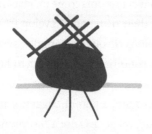

Progress

Growth in lesion size or area affected, turn into worse forms of endo, develop scar tissue/adhesions.

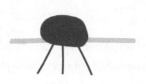

Stabilize

Still active, but no growth or progression.

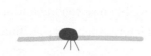

Regress or de-activate

Shrink, or still be there but not causing problems.

Understanding that endo lesions can grow *or* shrink, and be active or not, highlights the important point that endo is not so much a noun (something static and unchanging) as it is a verb (a process unfolding that can change over time). In other words, if we have active endo we are *endo-ing*. This shift in perspective gives us back control in many ways over our disease. We can't do much if we believe we just *get* endo, but we can seek real solutions if we understand that many elements go into endo-ing.

Endo (verb): To endo; endo-ing. The many processes that spur the development and progression of endometriosis. New Goal: To stop endo-ing

---

To better understand how this is possible, I'd like to introduce the concept of *whole-body ecology*. Ecology itself is the scientific study of the interconnected relationship between living organisms and their environment. For example, when studying the health of a tree you must also look at the bugs, grass, rainfall, animals, and even wind patterns the tree is in contact with. Each contributes to overall tree health, and the forest ecology at large. Using this example, we can use the term "whole-body ecology" to describe the same type of interwoven relationship between the eleven main systems within their environment, the human body:

- Immune system
- Endocrine (hormonal) system
- Circulatory system
- Digestive system
- Exocrine (skin, hair, nails, and sweat) system
- Muscular system
- Nervous system
- Urinary system
- Reproductive system
- Respiratory system
- Skeletal system

Like forest ecosystems, our bodily systems respond to information they pick up from our environment, our everyday living, to operate. And the operations of each system affect other systems. This is how stress can affect the muscular system, how immune health affects the reproductive system, or how our breathing affects the digestive system. They're all connected through vast networks of communication channels. You could imagine extensive text threads between these systems that, quite literally, never stop.

To properly function, these systems *all* rely on a continuous stream of healthy, soothing inputs. This includes proper nutrition, hydration, a calm and loving mental/emotional state, proper breathing patterns, adequate sleep, few toxins, and so much more. When most inputs are beneficial like this, these systems will communicate properly, working in harmony to maintain balance in the body.

The problem begins when modern-day living slaps our body ecology with so many negative inputs that our systems respond in more problematic than beneficial ways. Too much battery from negative inputs will, over the years, start to create dysfunction within these systems and the communication between them. What emerges is an inflammatory body ecology that benefits endometriosis—development, progression, or even just symptoms. It's how pathogenic bacteria from the digestive or reproductive tract may stimulate lesions to grow, while removing bacterial overgrowths may support the regression of lesions; how nutrient deficiencies may foster endo progression, whereas nutrient infusion may help curtail disease; how high levels of stress hormones may increase lesion size and volume, whereas the elimination of stress hormones may prevent endometriosis recurrence. This is why diet, lifestyle, and complementary methods that support whole-body health are essential considerations when healing from endo.

Conversely, once endometriosis lesions are established they don't just respond to body ecology, but actually start to contribute to the equation. It's how endo can increase the level of stress hormones in the body by creating chronic pain or other health challenges, impact the reproductive, urinary, or digestive system through tissue damage or associated inflammation, create disruptions in the nervous system through pain that never ends, and so much more. In this way, it's almost like endometriosis becomes a bodily system of its own (think of it as you now have twelve!)— one reason why endometriosis is considered a full-body disease, both impacting and being impacted by a whole-body ecology gone rogue. This is why expert surgical removal of lesions is currently considered the "gold standard" treatment for endo removal, and an important step to consider. All of this we'll touch on in-depth in the coming chapters.

Yet, suppose we can tip back the scales from sickness to health, from inflammatory to soothing inputs for all our bodily systems. In that case, we may stand a fighting chance against endo. If you stop the inflammation in its tracks, you may be able to stop endo-ing. If you've met or heard of women who managed their endo to the point where it no longer causes them problems, then you've seen this in action.

The Ecology of Endometriosis

Endometriosis both reacts to and contributes to the functioning of your eleven body systems, which can either support progression, stabilization, or regression. This is one way endo is a full-body issue.

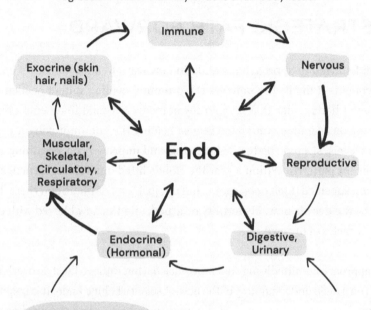

Soothing Inputs Support Stabilization

Beneficial movement

Sleep

Proper breathing patterns

Hydration

Lovely friendships

Proper nutrition

Happy/content mental and emotional state

Outside time

Self-compassion

Healthy microbiome

Inflammatory Inputs Support Progression

Poor breathing patterns

Poor sleep

Sedentary

Dehydrated

Anxious/ stressed

Poor nutrition

Excess screen time

Chemical exposure

Dysbiosis

Low-quality friendships

Gut or reproductive tract infections

> **If you stop the inflammation in its tracks,**
> **you may be able to stop endo-ing.**

A STRATEGIC PATH FORWARD

When I started to approach my endo in new ways to address endo's many components, I finally began to see the profound healing shifts I needed. At the time I had no idea that my journey of recovery would first benefit from focusing on seemingly unrelated issues: healing the gut, improving my nutrition levels, sleeping better, de-stressing, and improving my breathing and movement patterns. Within a year the clouds lifted, my vigor returned, and the pain subsided. I felt *good* again, and not just for a day here and there, but for nearly a decade now. My fertility returned, and I'm now blessed with two little miracles of my own.

This approach admittedly may not be a quick fix, but rather a lifestyle overhaul, based on a deep understanding of the newest science behind endo. It is inspired by my own path and by those of the many women I've had the privilege of working with over the years. So I ask, what if you could find the triggers that contribute to your own endo inflammatory cascade, address them to free up your immune system to function correctly, and feel your own endo ease? Or, after surgery, how can you best prevent endo from returning and the slew of symptoms from creeping back? These are the questions this book answers by looking at endo from a modern perspective: as an inflammatory disease rooted in immune dysfunction.

Chapter 2:

Doctors, Diagnosis, and Endo Confusion

Doctors are the gateway to our disease. They are the ones that can give a diagnosis, proper advice, referrals, and treatment ... or not. In the case of endometriosis, sadly it's often the latter. It's a well-known fact that there's an average wait time of 7–10 years for an endometriosis diagnosis. This becomes maddening when we remember that endo can be a progressive disease, advancing and scarring for as long as it goes untreated. One of my clients waited over 15 years for a diagnosis and was told after surgery, "It looked like a war zone in there." Not something you want said about your reproductive organs.

Yet, we *need* doctors to get a proper diagnosis and care. That's why, in this chapter, we will discuss how to better tap into the medical arena: doctors, diagnosis, where endo confusion stems from, and how to be your own best advocate.

"EXCUSE ME, ENDO WHAT?"

If you're surprised to find endo isn't simply a hormonal, gynecological, or "period problem," you're not alone. Endo is a complex disease that is poorly understood by most, including doctors and patients. As the *New York Times* eloquently stated in a 2021 article, "[Endometriosis] suffers from a branding problem: It falls into the abyss of 'women's diseases' (overlooked), diseases that don't kill you (unimportant), and menstrual problems (taboo)."[6]

Unfortunately, the foundation of the misunderstanding may start at the medical level. Some doctors' understanding of endo may stem from an antiquated endometriosis theory that they learned in medical school decades ago—and perhaps that some schools are still teaching today. Due to a variety of factors, there is a 17-year lag between when research is *released* and when it is *applied* in the field of medicine. In other words, nearly two decades will pass before the findings generated by research today are made available to your doctor. Perhaps this is why up to 63 percent of general practitioners feel uncomfortable diagnosing and treating endo, while as many as half are unfamiliar with its main symptoms.[7]

In addition to all this, for women, there is a frustrating level of pain that has become normalized in our society. If you've ever been turned away by a doctor who told you that your debilitating period pain is a normal part of a woman's cycle, you'll understand what I mean. Too often, women with excruciatingly painful periods are told their pain is "just part of being a woman." Many of us end up in the ER with pain so intense we think an organ must have ruptured, and still we are brushed off and told to go home. Almost every endo client I've seen has a horrifying endo story in which she was left in complete agony, ignored or misunderstood by her medical team, sometimes for years.

This medical void in understanding the reality of endometriosis, torpedoes our ability, as sufferers, to heal. It is what drives the thousands of stories you've heard about patients being brushed aside. Even from the most well-meaning doctors, you may have been told "there's really *nothing* else we can do." It leaves us on cycles of hormones, pain medications, and undergoing rounds and rounds of poorly done surgeries, only to find ourselves with symptoms remaining. We exhaust our options, forfeit our fertility, and may develop such a reduced quality of life that it can lead to suicidal thoughts or actions.

All of this sets the stage for societal confusion as we endo patients, suffering under a mountain of symptoms without much direction, start to seek self-treatment. Perhaps you've heard that having endo means you *simply* have far too much estrogen and that by lowering your systemic estrogen levels your endo will cease (even if it makes you feel awful, or you see no improvement at all).

Or maybe you've read about a new endo diet that will *simply* heal your endo if you cut out many different types of foods (even if you feel miserable). I had one client who tried a vinegar and maple syrup cleanse for 10 days after being told by a *chiropractor* that it would help "clean her endo out."

This societal confusion may even extend to friends, family, or alternative care providers, who may tell us that the pain we experience is due to trauma, or having too much anxiety. It may even manifest in truly appalling ways, such as when Dr. Drew Pinsky, a doctor and host of the popular show *Loveline*, called endometriosis a "garbage bag diagnosis," and claimed that endo was not a real disease, but rather an imagined issue stemming from sexual abuse.[8] Or, for a more far-out interpretation of how your pain is all in your head, Dr. Stella Immanuel claims that endo is caused by people having sex in their dreams with demons and witches.[9] It doesn't really get much more confused than that.

And while none of this is fair, knowing the level of misunderstanding around endo should help you feel a little less crazy when you're told that you *may* need to know more about endo than your doctor to get the care you need and deserve. No, you weren't destined to have stage 4 endometriosis ravage your body. It could have—and should have—been stopped years before.

A BETTER WAY FORWARD

The truth about endo is that, between endo specialists, nonprofits, surgeons, and complementary care providers, we know a lot about endo and how to address it. If caught early, and taken seriously through comprehensive care, endo many never become the tragedy it is today. This is an important change in perspective from the mainstream dialogue you may have been told, that there is little we can do besides managing symptoms.

The first step of this better plan is to get a diagnosis or even a suspected diagnosis. Many other issues can cause endo-like symptoms (some of which may be more easily treated), and you need to know what you're dealing with in order to best move forward.

While there's no absolute consensus on the best next steps for *everyone* after a diagnosis, there are two approaches among the experts I spoke with that stand out.[10] One recommendation is to immediately have a professional excision surgery after diagnosis to remove the endo and give your body a clean slate to heal.[11] This plan comes with merit for many who have long awaited a diagnosis or have easy access to an endo excision specialist. Because endo can progress if not treated, contributing to a slew of issues from full body pain to allergies, digestive issues to infertility, a swift diagnosis and surgery (followed by the complementary care recommended in this book) may be just what some bodies need.

The other recommendation is first to give yourself 6–12 months to see whether the body therapies known to help endometriosis—the focus of this book—work for you. If you can actively slash the inflammation and your endo responds, you may find your endo much more manageable. If your symptoms aren't budging after that period, then a consultation with an endometriosis surgical specialist is promptly recommended.[12] This is an approach many of us may consider who lack the resources to obtain an expert surgery at this time or prefer to consider a more natural approach before committing to surgery.

Understanding the differing approaches recommended by experts in the field allows all of us to more advantageously work within our budgets, goals, and with our medical team to formulate the best plan of action for our own bodies. In the following pages, we'll discuss all of this, including when to suspect endo, getting a diagnosis, speaking to doctors, and why integrative care is important.

ADVOCATING FOR AN
OPTIMAL APPROACH

While your own path with endo will be based on care available to us today, know that there *is* an ideal plan we should all advocate for future generations. Use your voice to support changes in endo care that look more like this, so our daughters have a better fighting chance against endo!

1. **Endometriosis should be screened for routinely:** Catching endo early can mean a total difference in preserving our quality of life and fertility, which is why we should all be screened regularly for endo just as we are for cervical cancer. While this will be easier as more diagnostic technologies are uncovered (such as menstrual blood, serum, or urine sampling, for example), doctors could presently use symptom questionnaires and physical exams to offer red flags for suspected cases.

2. **Suspected or diagnosed endometriosis cases should be immediately referred to endo specialists:** If you have cancer on your toe, you will be sent to an oncologist (cancer doctor) rather than a podiatrist (a foot doctor). Endo should be treated similarly, with immediate referrals to an endometriosis specialist who can help patients discover their own unique endometriosis "footprint" (stage, the scope of present damage, and the best plan to move forward with integrative care options). Some fantastic places currently offer comprehensive treatment like this, two examples being the Vital Health Endometriosis Center and the Center for Endometriosis Care. If caught early, and taken seriously through comprehensive care, endo many never become the tragedy it is today.

3. **Insurance should cover the process:** Most insurance will not cover the extended care many of us need, including a properly done excision surgery or consultations with experts. For this reason, we must *all* advocate for insurance companies to cover the proper types of care we need.

WHEN TO SUSPECT ENDOMETRIOSIS

The signs and symptoms that most people with endo experience vary widely. The most common symptoms are *dysmenorrhea* (pain associated with your period) and infertility, though not everyone with endo experiences these issues. In fact, some women may not even know they have endo because their symptoms seem so unrelated to their menstrual cycle. Understanding the diversity of endo symptoms may help speed up your diagnosis.

You may be able to relate to some of the most common signs and symptoms of endometriosis, including the following:

- **Pain**. While pain is not everyone's main symptom, for many it is. It may occur at menses, ovulation, randomly or constantly, with sex or physical activity, urination, or defecation—which is obviously different from solely being "period pain." One reason for this wide variety of pain symptoms is that endo lesions grow more sensory nerve fibers than normal tissue does. Sensory nerve fibers alert our brain to stimuli—they are how you *know* when you step on a sharp rock or have an itch on your arm. In a highly inflammatory environment, the high number of sensory nerves can send constant alert signals, leading to the various manifestations of endo pain that many of us have experienced: everything from stabbing sensations in the gut or pelvis to feeling as if someone is wringing your uterus out like a wet towel, to pulling, throbbing, burning, even itching.[13]
- **Bloating, IBS, and GI distress**. The severity of digestive woes we experience in the endo community is so common that there is a slang term for it: endo belly. Not to mention that many of us will receive either a misdiagnosis or a co-diagnosis with Irritable Bowel Syndrome (IBS). If you have endo, chances are that you also suffer with issues ranging from uncomfortable bloating to life-altering GI tract distress.
- **Hormonal imbalances**. There is often a link among thyroid, adrenal, and sex hormone imbalances in the endo sufferer, and many of us suffer from accompanying symptoms that can include anything

from personality-changing PMS to weight gain, excess facial hair, cold extremities, heavy periods, and more.

- **Fatigue**. Chronic fatigue is a reality for many sufferers. Very different from just feeling tired, those suffering from chronic fatigue may not be able to even take a shower or prepare food without energy-regulation troubles.
- **Immune issues**. Those with endo often suffer from allergies, getting sick often, rashes, colds, feeling rundown, or asthma—as well as autoimmune diseases. A whirlwind of immune chaos in addition to the endo.
- **Depression and anxiety**. There is a strong link between having endo and mental health challenges, such as anxiety, depression, or even suicidal thoughts. According to a recent poll, nearly half of those with endo who experienced symptoms had suicidal thoughts.[14]
- **Fertility challenges**. It's estimated that about 1 in 3 of us will have trouble conceiving (although please note, *this does not imply that 1 in 3 of us will never go on to have children*). If you have been trying to conceive for over a year without success, and other issues have been ruled out, you should consider seeking an endo diagnosis even if you have no other symptoms. Endo is sneaky like that.
- **Every other random symptom in the book**. I've worked with a variety of clients who have symptoms few others seem to have. Pain in the feet at menses (yep), full-body rashes in the week before menses, shoulder pain, joint pain, and endo flare-ups at the oddest times. So if you personally suffer from symptoms you haven't seen listed anywhere, you're not alone. Remember, endo is a full-body disease that affects us all differently.

If you have some of these symptoms and suspect endo, it's time to talk to your doctor. Even a basic physical examination by someone well versed in endo can help *lead* to a diagnosis. Although a physical examination of the pelvis alone is not enough to confirm anything, an experienced gynecologist can often identify issues in the pelvis that might prompt a suspicion of endometriosis. In some advanced cases, the uterus may become so "stuck" with endo-associated adhesions that it no longer moves/responds to physical manipulation the way a healthy uterus does. Pelvic masses and/or an enlarged uterus (often due to adenomyosis or uterine fibroids) may also be identified in an examination.

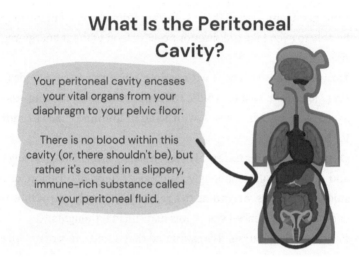

Ultrasound is another tool that can hint at endo (such as viewing free-flowing blood in the peritoneal cavity), or visualize certain types of progressed forms of endometriosis, like *endometriomas* (endometriosis cysts on the ovaries). Typically, by the time an ultrasound is able to discern an endo cyst, the endo is fairly advanced and the patient will likely benefit from further investigation and often excision surgery.

The use of magnetic resonance imaging (MRI) is becoming more popular for assessing the severity of endometriosis. MRI is not particularly helpful for identifying the more superficial types (this is where exploratory surgery can really shine), but it *can* be helpful in identifying the more severe types of endo, like endometriomas and deep infiltrating endo. An MRI can help your providers visualize abnormal pelvic masses and tissue that has been changed in some way (a clue there is something abnormal happening), particularly in the colon, bladder, and reproductive organs.

Together with an examination, discussion of symptoms and family history, and perhaps some imaging, you may get your *suspected* endo diagnosis.

GETTING AN OFFICIAL DIAGNOSIS

Sometimes being diagnosed with suspected endometriosis is as far we get for a while, since the only way to get an *official* diagnosis is through an exploratory laparoscopy. A laparoscopy requires anesthesia while a surgeon inserts a camera through your navel to see what's happening inside. Understandably, many of us opt to wait on this procedure.

Waiting is not necessarily a bad plan when faced with the limited endo specialist care we may have access to. If you take your "suspected" case seriously and work to address your symptoms *as if they're all related to endo* (as per Part 3 and 4 in this book), you may find your body responding beautifully as symptoms fade. However, if your symptoms persist past the 6–12-month mark without any change, it's time for a look inside.

When faced with surgery as the only diagnostic tool, you may ask, "Are my symptoms bad enough to warrant surgery?" If you've been experiencing chronic pain, unexplained infertility, or other intense symptoms long enough to even *consider* exploratory surgery, then yes, these symptoms warrant further investigation. Many other issues can cause pain and infertility, but if it's endo it's necessary to know what you're dealing with for treatment purposes. For example, if you're dealing with infertility due to endometriosis, you may not be able to get pregnant without addressing it. Early diagnosis is essential to preserving quality of life, so please be brave and seek answers.

Adenomyosis (endometriosis-like tissue growing within the musculature of the uterus) is more challenging to diagnose because it requires a positive biopsy and often there are no visual signs of it on the uterus. MRIs and ultrasounds can be helpful once adeno masses grow large enough to discern (like a fibroid or cyst), but for those of us suffering from small fragments throughout the uterus, a diagnosis may be elusive. For those of us without an official diagnosis (like me), suspected adeno based on symptoms may have to suffice until diagnostic technology improves. For others who are *truly* ready to consider a hysterectomy, at that point adeno may then be diagnosed when the entire uterus can be inspected.

While options for accurately diagnosing endo are currently limited, there are some exciting non-invasive diagnostic tools coming down the pipeline, such as sampling menstrual blood (how easy is that?) or even looking at genetic sequencing to clue providers in on endo without the need for invasive measures.[15]

ENDO IS AN EQUAL-OPPORTUNITY DISEASE

Endo affects us all equally without political, racial, or even gender divides (it has in rare instances affected men). Keeping ourselves informed may be especially important for women of color, transgender, and gender non-binary individuals who are statistically less likely to be taken seriously by medical professionals. Please understand that when I use the words *female* and *woman* throughout this book, I do so with the best of inclusive intentions.

UNDERSTANDING YOUR DIAGNOSIS: THE DIFFERENT STAGES OF ENDO

Endometriosis is currently diagnosed based on "stages" of disease:

- **Stage I or Minimal:** limited superficial lesions.
- **Stage 2 or Mild:** more abundant lesions, often with deeper "roots."
- **Stage 3 or Moderate:** an abundance of lesions both deep and superficial, one or more small cysts, limited adhesions.
- **Stage 4 or Severe: an** abundance of deep lesions, one or more large cysts, thick adhesions.
- **Should there be a Stage 5?** In the future there may be a Stage 5 for the even more advanced Stage 4 cases associated with *severe* adhesions.[16]

Please know that it's common for your diagnosis level not to coincide with the symptoms you're experiencing, especially your pain. I remember getting a Stage 2 diagnosis after my first surgery and feeling like a total fake because I swore my pelvic pain warranted a Stage 4 diagnosis. Alternatively, women with Stage 4 endo may not have any noticeable symptoms and discover their diagnosis only during a surgery or investigation for something else, such as infertility.

In addition to stages, there are currently four different types of endo—which is why it's considered a *heterogeneous* (remember, having different types) disease:

1. **Deep Infiltrating Endo (DIE).** This is the most invasive type of endo and penetrates 5mm or more under the peritoneal surface. These lesions are considered very active and are strongly associated with pelvic pain symptoms.[17] Deep infiltrating endo is considered an advanced and progressive form of the disease, meaning it's probably been around for a while. According to some surgeons, because DIE is associated with terrible pain, these sufferers may be the ones whose symptoms benefit most from a professional, wide-excision surgery.

2. **Ovarian Endometriotic Cysts (Endometriomas).** Endometriomas (aka "chocolate cysts") are ovarian cysts that tend to respond very poorly to medical treatment. They have the potential to destroy healthy ovarian tissue, which may contribute to premature or early ovarian failure, problems with ovulation, decreased ovarian function, and infertility. They too are considered an advanced form of disease, even without other diagnosable forms of endo.

3. **Superficial Endometriosis.** The least severe form of endometriosis (technically speaking), in which endometriotic lesions are found superficially in the peritoneal cavity. It's important to note that just because a lesion is superficial does not mean that it won't cause pain.

4. **"The Rest."** This is a holding place for the many other types (and subsets of those types) that are expected to surface upon further investigation. Remember, there are already 65 potentially different varieties of endo already isolated, so "the rest" may end up being a long list. Just as there are over 100 different types of cancer and autoimmune disorders, we may have many types of endo to be diagnosed in the future.

SPEAKING WITH DOCTORS

Talking about proper endometriosis care will often start with your general practitioner (GP) and/or OB-GYN, the gateways to your diagnosis and treatment plans. Some of us have kind, understanding, dedicated doctors. If you have one like this, make sure to tell them how much you appreciate them! I personally had an incredible GP who, upon hearing my very initial complaint of deep pelvic pain, told me she suspected endometriosis, scheduled an immediate ultrasound, and referred me to a gynecologist she knew on the island I live on who cared for endo patients. Years later she advocated for my insurance company to pay for surgery (my second) on the neighboring island of Oahu with a better surgeon than was available on Kaua`i. I credit this doctor for saving my fertility, and my sanity—especially since my own endo presented as constant deep pain *except* at menses, which is confusing if you know endo only as painful periods.

Many of us are not so lucky, having had frustratingly poor experiences with doctors. Like the doctor who told you to "just get a hysterectomy and adopt" or the one who said to "take pain medications and get on with your day." They're the ones who won't refer you to a gynecologist, push Lupron or Orlissa as the first line of defense, or even stop you in your tracks from seeking a diagnosis. *Sigh.*

To differentiate between these two types of care, let's call them "excellent care" versus "substandard care." Substandard care can come from a regular GP, a gynecologist, or even an endometriosis specialist if they don't take your case, concerns, or symptoms seriously. Ever had a doctor smirk at you for bringing up an alternative viewpoint or not agreeing with their treatment suggestion? That's substandard care, regardless of the degrees framed on the wall.

Alternatively, you may be lucky to find excellent care from your local GP, OB-GYN, or even a pediatrician—caring and empathic individuals who may not be endo experts but who take your case seriously, go to bat to get you referrals, and never dismiss your concerns. They're the ones that listen when you show up knowing more about the disease than they do, and support your case.

That's because what makes care excellent isn't necessarily how much your doctor knows about endo theories of pathogenesis or whether endo is heterogeneous or multifactorial; *the most important principle is how much they care about you.* You are the main character of this story, not your endo, and only when someone focuses on you and your symptoms (rather than the specifics of a textbook case of endo) will you find your voice heard and symptoms properly addressed. You may need to develop a bit of a thick skin when dealing with substandard medical professionals and learn that when you don't like how you're being treated, you can decide to find another doctor with more compassion.

The role of second opinions is also important to understand, as even a kind doctor can give poor medical advice. In fact, I recommend seeking second opinions regularly, *especially* when dealing with surgeries or recommendations for strong hormonal treatments. If a doctor wants to cut out a piece of you right away or put you on strong pharmaceuticals, it's always worth taking the extra time to understand whether there's another option. If you're confused in any way about even a simple recommendation, never hesitate to reach out to a different medical professional. Doing so will put the control back into *your* hands.

Unfortunately, racism within the medical community is yet another hurdle for many living with and seeking treatment for endo, and it can make communicating with doctors an even bigger challenge. This is an ugly side of medicine, and one that has gone unaddressed for far too long. We know that people of color are less likely to have their pain taken seriously, less likely to be prescribed painkillers, and less likely to get an accurate endometriosis diagnosis. Racial disparities in health care are well documented, so finding a vetted doctor whom you trust is important.

A BETTER STRATEGY: INTEGRATIVE CARE

While doctors are the gateway to diagnosis and conventional medical treatments such as pharmaceuticals and surgery, Western medicine has not been shown to sufficiently conquer endometriosis for the majority of patients. It's great for treating broken bones, infectious diseases, and heart attacks (what I'd call acute issues). However, conventional medicine is simply not set up to properly treat chronic diseases. Western medical doctors who excel at treating acute issues may find themselves unequipped to best treat the millions of people who, like you and me, are sinking under an overwhelming tide of symptoms. Nearly every chronic disease in the world will develop from a variety of factors and many of them stem from a whole-body ecology gone rogue. Endometriosis, cancer, autoimmunity, diabetes... they are all diseases with "no cure," and rates are skyrocketing.

This is where *integrative care* shines as a better approach for those of us dealing with a chronic disease like endo. Integrative care combines the best of Western medicine (such as surgery, and pharmaceuticals if needed), with complementary strategies that address a patient's total health needs, be they physical, mental, emotional, dietary, environmental, or spiritual. It refers to the *many* components that may be needed to heal a disease that developed thanks to *many* factors—epigenetics, environmental pollutants, bacteria, inflammation, diet, lifestyle, and more. Addressing these many issues will take a multi-faceted approach—why integrative care supports the use of all healing tools as needed, including:

- **Diet and Lifestyle**: nutrition, movement, daily chemical exposure, mental health. These are what I'd consider the foundations for healing from an inflammatory condition, since your choices can either induce or reduce inflammation in the body.
- **Conventional Medicine**: treatments for endo that you'll find at your doctor, surgeon, or medical provider. To be sure, some women have been able to clear their symptoms and live a pain-free life thanks to conventional interventions such as professional excision surgery alone.

- **Complementary and Alternative Medicine (CAM)**: therapies often considered to be part of a holistic framework, such as acupuncturists, herbalists, nutritionists, movement teachers, or stress coaches.

If you've tried some integrative therapies or diet and lifestyle shifts before, or even had a professional excision surgery, and nothing so far has helped, don't despair. First, it's important to remember how diverse endometriosis is and that you are not broken if you've tried what you think is "everything" without success. I implore you to keep seeking new solutions, I applaud you for reading this book, and I recommend that you continue to seek out new types of integrative medicine presented in these pages that you may not have tried yet.

Another aspect to consider is that the specific therapy you tried, though perhaps beneficial for another person, may not have been targeted to your specific needs. For example, if your ongoing pain is rooted in pelvic floor dysfunction but you only tried acupuncture, you can see why your pain would persist. And again, for some of us nothing will budge without surgery.

This is why a true integrative approach to endo can (and often should) include the best of both conventional methods of care *and* holistic modalities to yield a strategic path forward for the endo patient. Consider them tools in the endo-toolbox to help your own body to stop *endo-ing*.

However, to create *your* best integrative healing plan, we first need to take a few steps back to better understand the problem of endometriosis: where it comes from, how it is activated, and what triggers may be fueling your inflammatory fire. While understanding the complexities of the pathogenesis of endometriosis may seem unimportant when you just want to feel better, know that it will help you do just that! It will help you put your endo back to bed.

This is what we'll learn in the next section.

THE PROMISE OF THE SLIDING
SCALE OF REMISSION

We most often hear about "managing endo symptoms," but I'd like to introduce a different word to your endo arsenal: *remission*. While remission does not equate to a cure, it implies the suspension of your endo symptoms. Remission levels come in many forms. For example, full remission means you no longer experience any of the symptoms that you previously had, and thus can feel like you're (amazingly) cured. Partial remission can mean many things depending on the person, with the symptoms presenting on a sort-of sliding scale. It may mean you feel much better most days, but still occasionally experience symptoms.

Finding remission may include any combination of the inputs discussed in this book. Once in remission, you may still notice a recurrence of symptoms at times of high stress or with inflammatory lifestyle choices. But often once you've reached a comfortable area of remission, even if you have a flare-up, you can find your way back to being symptom-free by returning to the personalized "endo lifestyle" that brought you to remission the first time.

PART II:

The Perfect Storm: How Endometriosis Develops

For too long endometriosis has been seen as a mysterious woman's condition with no known cause or cure. Yet, there are thousands of studies available to show endo is not as mysterious as we're led to believe. While it's important to note that some of this research is in its infancy (done through research in Petri dishes or on animals, rather than humans), or still in theory form, there is still much we can glean from putting all of the research together. In this section, we will explore the *myriad* of ways endo may develop, how endo-like cells establish into a fully-fledged endo lesion, as well as what factors are promoting chronic inflammation as we speak. In the following five chapters, we will finally be able to understand *what* our disease is.

Chapter 3:

Making a Monster: The Creation of an Endo-Like Cell

Before we develop an endometriosis lesion, the first step of "getting endo" begins with the creation of an endometriosis-like (endo-like) cell. These appear to be related to the cells within the endometrial lining of your uterus (the ones that shed and regenerate each month with menses), yet are distinctly different: more like jacked Navy SEALs than cushions of fertility. These cells are often highly sensitive to estrogen and very resistant to progesterone, meaning there's lots of growth without much cooling. They can avoid normal cellular death and immune cleanup processes, and become pain factories. These cells are *great* at migrating, self-healing, and invading into the smallest nooks and crannies (which may be associated with the start of adenomyosis in the uterine wall).[18]

This begs two questions: how did normal endometrial cells turn into these monstrous creations, and how did they end up outside of the uterus?

ENDO TERMINOLOGY

Endometrial cell: a normally behaving cell of the endometrium, the inner lining of the uterus that sheds each month with menses.

Endo-like cell, or **endometriotic cell**: Similar to an endometrial cell (bleeds cyclically, regenerative, responds to hormones) but different, this cell behaves like endometriosis (aggressive, proliferative, extra estrogen-sensitive, progesterone resistant, etc.). Yet, this cell is not yet endometriosis.

Endometriosis: When an endo-like cell is activated into an endometriosis lesion, established with blood supply and nerves. When you have an endometriosis lesion you *officially* have diagnosable endometriosis. We will discuss this in the next chapter.

Monster Maker #1: Genetics

You are born with genes inside every cell in your body, each with a specific set of instructions that inform cells how to work. This is referred to as *genetics*. You inherit a combination of genes from your parents, grandparents, and all your ancestors before them. Unfortunately, it's estimated that a little over half of us (51 percent of us, to be exact) may be born with the genes that predispose us to develop endo.[19]

For example, a protein-coding gene called BCL6 may set our endometrial cells up for progesterone resistance.[20] Another gene (NPSR1) may contribute to some of the pain and inflammation we face.[21] As research continues, expect to see a long list of genes that will become associated with endo. For now, just know you may have an assortment of them.

Because of genetic inheritance, your odds of developing endometriosis increase significantly if you have a family history of the disease, especially on the maternal side.[22] This is true for me, having cousins, grandmothers, and aunts whom all dealt with endo-like symptoms (some had terrible menstrual pain, others had miscarriages, and one had zero symptoms but later discovered stage 4 endo when getting her "tubes tied"). It's probably true for many of you as well. You might want to ask your female relatives how tolerable their menstrual cycles were and see what you discover in your own family history.

Unfortunately, family lineages of endometriosis may lead some women to put off finding treatment options because they've been told by their mother, aunts, or grandmothers that painful periods are normal—they managed to live with them, after all—and it's nothing you can't discreetly bear once a month. By now, you know that debilitating and painful periods are *never* normal, though they are common (big difference).

Some genes associated with endo are linked with other diseases as well, such as the autoimmune diseases celiac disease, lupus, and Hashimoto's thyroiditis, among others.[23] This is why we sometimes refer to these as "sister diseases" since those of us with endo are often more likely to develop these in tandem with endo.

While genetics obviously plays a role in inheriting "endo genes," it doesn't automatically mean you will develop an endo-like cell. Instead, there is another factor deeply involved in changing the behavior of your endometrial cells: epigenetics, the study of how triggers from our own lives may change the way our genes behave and open the door to endo.

Epigenetics: Training an Endometrial Cell to Behave Like Endo

Pop quiz: If corn has 32,000 genes and a tree has 45,000, how many genes do humans have? Nope, not 50 million—only about 25,000! Fewer than corn. It's mind-boggling when we think about just how complex we are.

To understand how it's possible for humans to have fewer genes than corn (or trees, for that matter), I'd like to introduce the concept of epigenetics. Epigenetics is how genes can change their behavior (for better or worse) depending on what "information" they pick up. Now it makes sense how we can have fewer genes yet be so complex, because our genes have the ability to change their behavior so profoundly.

Epigenetics works like this: when your genes are exposed to strong triggers, they change their behavior. These triggers can be good or bad. For example, chemical triggers can be good (exposure to lots of nutrient-rich food) *or* bad (household toxins); behavioral triggers can include feelings of deep contentment *or* high stress levels; or physical triggers like healthy levels of exercise *or* sedentarism. In fact, gene behaviors can turn "on" or "off" based on any number of lifestyle experiences you have throughout your entire life, and indeed they can be incredibly beneficial, or not.

These genes are not mutating, however. Rather, the changes that occur are known as epigenetic alterations: changes in gene *behavior* (something that is reversible) rather than changes in the genetic code itself. Epigenetics makes a lot of sense when talking about survival since it allows our bodies to adapt to our constantly changing environments in order to have the best chance of survival. Epigenetics helps explain how humans can thrive in so many different environments, eating so many different diets, in different climates, being different sizes and with different skin colors—yet we're all still genetically human.

Yet, gene expression isn't choosy and will respond to *any* prolonged and intense triggers, good or bad. If we have too many inflammatory or chemical triggers signaling "danger" to our genes, our cells may adopt aggressive behaviors in a last-ditch effort to simply *survive* in a world that feels unsafe. That means if the genes within your normal endometrial cells are constantly facing down a barrage of negative triggers (i.e., stress, chemical exposure, bacteria, etc.—see image), epigenetic changes may tell these cells to behave even more like endometriosis.

When that happens, what was once a normally regenerative endometrial cell that naturally bleeds cyclically each month, may now also become estrogen-sensitive, progesterone resistant, aggressive, invasive, proliferative, and can avoid normal cell death. Yes, it's starting to resemble endometriosis even more.

You may be wondering what these triggers are. While there may be many, here I'll discuss two well-researched epigenetic triggers associated with the creation of an endo-like cell: endocrine-disrupting chemicals and chronic inflammation. [If you want to see a few epigenetic abnormalities an endo-like cell is famous for, see Appendix 1].

Monster Maker #2: Endocrine-Disrupting Chemicals

One reason that environmental toxins and pollutants are part of endo's multi-factorial disease is that they can epigenetically alter endometrial cells, changing their behavior to be more like endo. Endocrine-disrupting chemicals (EDCs) are one class of chemicals that are particularly damaging. By interfering directly with the endocrine (hormonal) system, EDCs have the power to produce adverse developmental, reproductive, neurological, and immune effects, and unfortunately they are just about everywhere.[24]

One EDC associated with endo is a class of chemicals called dioxins. They are nasty by-products of industrial and farming processes that linger in the environment for decades. They're known to be potent endocrine disruptors and linked to a variety of diseases, including endometriosis. Their epigenetic effects are potent, and there is concern that these can be passed down inter-generationally (meaning you could have inherited these epigenetic changes from your mother or even grandmother). Dioxins have been shown to interfere with cellular vitamin A metabolism, which is important for normal cell death—something you *really* want when it comes to endo.[25] They can also contribute to progesterone resistance and create abnormalities with the Homeobox A10 gene, which affects fertility.[26]

But dioxins aren't the only chemical caught red-handed helping to create an endo-like monster. Phthalates are another group. Used to make plastics durable and fragrances last longer, they're found in everything from synthetic floor tiles and carpets to lipstick and your favorite-smelling shampoo, body wash, baby powder, and perfume—yes, even if marketed as "all-natural" (because of an FDA loophole, if you see fragrance/parfum as an ingredient it almost certainly has phthalates in it). When normal endometrial cells are exposed to phthalates they not only show signs of inflammation and oxidative stress but also become more invasive and proliferative, much like the behavior of an endo-like cell.[27] A 2021 review pinpointed 13 different studies showing people with endometriosis to have a much higher level of exposure than people without endo (we have higher levels of phthalates in our blood, urine, and/

or peritoneal fluid), illustrating just how much phthalate exposure and endo may go hand in hand.[28]

Bisphenol A, commonly called BPA, is another well-known EDC associated with endo. BPA is used primarily to make plastic products, as well as a protective coating for things like food and drink cans, hot coffee cups, and thermal receipt paper. It's basically everywhere. Exposing normal endometrial cells to BPA has been shown to significantly decrease progesterone receptors (creating an estrogen-dominant cell), strengthening the argument that BPA may also be involved in the development of endo-like cells.[29]

There are more EDCs associated with endo as well. I will introduce you to more of them in Chapter 15, as well as a plan to help reduce chemical exposure. For now, know there are many.

Those With Endo Have More Toxins In Their Bodies Than Those Without

These toxins may be partly responsible for helping to create an endo-like cell, as well as contributing to immune dysfunction, helping to illustrate the chemical-endo connection.

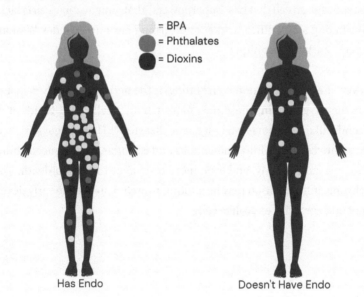

= BPA
= Phthalates
= Dioxins

Has Endo   Doesn't Have Endo

Monster Maker #3: Chronic Inflammation

If an endometrial cell is exposed to inflammation for too long, it can start to behave more like endo. The way this happens is through a side effect of chronic inflammation: the suffocation of your cells. This is called *hypoxia*. Without oxygen, your cells cannot function—as you'll know if you've ever had a leg fall asleep from sitting the wrong way.

Where did the oxygen go? An area suffering from tissue damage will immediately have less oxygen thanks to the blood supply being partially cut off from blood vessel damage. In addition, chronic inflammation will mean the area is teeming with millions of immune cells that also need oxygen. These little guys suck up oxygen at an exponential rate, meaning that an area that is already low in oxygen from poor blood supply now has an increased demand for oxygen, resulting in chronic oxygen starvation. Hypoxia ensues, creating an environment so hostile to human cells (that need oxygen to survive) that it can epigenetically alter their behavior.

To survive this, our normal endometrial cells (or any precursors to endo-like cells) have a last-ditch epigenetic survival tactic: turning into a *mesenchymal* cell, a type of stem cell that has "superpowers" that your average cell is lacking. It's like taking a lazy office worker and turning her into Wonder Woman—a pretty cool survival technique.

However, if either the endometrial lining or the peritoneal cavity is in a state of *chronic* oxygen debt, these new mesenchymal cells start to adopt even more endo-like behaviors—an epigenetic disaster.[30] These behaviors include increased invasiveness into small nooks and crannies, an enhanced ability to migrate around the body, and even more resistance to cellular death. This is why chronic inflammation may be another prerequisite for the early development of an aggressive endo-like cell.

Making an Endo-Like Cell

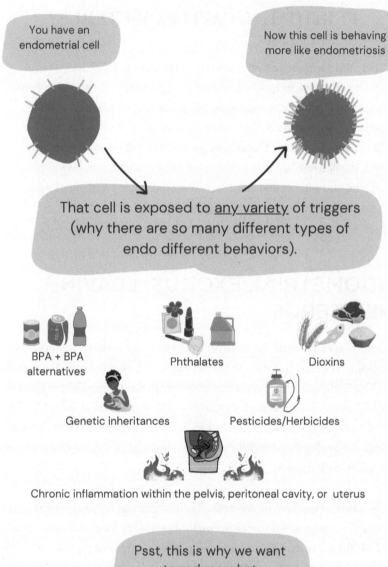

You have an endometrial cell

Now this cell is behaving more like endometriosis

That cell is exposed to <u>any variety</u> of triggers (why there are so many different types of endo different behaviors).

BPA + BPA alternatives

Phthalates

Dioxins

Genetic inheritances

Pesticides/Herbicides

Chronic inflammation within the pelvis, peritoneal cavity, or uterus

Psst, this is why we want to reduce what exposures we have control over!

WHY WOULD WE DEVELOP CHRONIC INFLAMMATION IN THE PERITONEAL CAVITY OR UTERUS?

There are numerous drivers linked to endo that we'll discuss in the following chapters, including bacterial overgrowths in the reproductive tract or gut, chemical exposure, excess blood, lack of antioxidants, sedentarism, and more. Once endo is established, it will also contribute to the equation. If the tissue damage and ensuing inflammation never end, it will damage tissue further (that fire-breathing dragon torching your insides without end), and blood vessels become so damaged they can no longer deliver enough oxygen-rich blood.

ENDOMETRIAL EXODUS: LEAVING THE UTERUS

An endo-like cell is now developed thanks to these genetic and epigenetic alterations. The next question that arises is how that cell moves throughout the body. Endo has been found anywhere from the peritoneal cavity to the bowel, bladder, diaphragm, lungs, kidney, skin, nose, and more! To help understand how these cells migrated so far away, numerous science-backed theories are available, with different theories perhaps working for different types/placement of endo.

One area that's been heavily researched is how you can be born with an endometrial cell already outside of the normally placed endometrium, in something called Müllerian rests.[31] This would happen soon after conception when two "simple" Müllerian ducts within the embryo develop into the fallopian tubes, uterus (including the endometrium), cervix, and top third of the vagina. Even healthy women without endo can have some endometrial cells misplaced in Müllerian rests, which may not necessarily be problematic. However, if you have the specific genetic and epigenetic alterations we discussed, these misplaced cells may start to behave more like endometriosis. This becomes even *more* problematic when this person begins menstruating and the cells have no escape route for the shed blood, contributing to inflammation. Being born with misplaced endometrial cells helps explain why some people have pain with first menses, certain types of adenomyosis, and even the rare endo found in men.

Other theories help explain how endo can make it *far* away from the uterus. These theories speculate that endo-like cells may disseminate through the lymph or circulatory systems (very similar to how cancer metastasizes), by metaplasia (the conversion of one type of tissue to another), or through physical means such as an unintended transplant through surgery (i.e., some women have developed endo on a C-section scar). And because endometrial cells are regenerative, they may have the "superpower" to reconstruct anywhere outside of the uterus.[32]

The most controversial theory explaining one way endo-like cells may migrate is known as the theory of retrograde menstruation, something you may have heard briefly mentioned at a doctor's visit or read about online. Retrograde menstruation is the normal back-flow of a small amount of menstrual blood from the fallopian tubes into the pelvis each cycle. Because nearly all women experience this, it's considered a normal part of menses. In the case of endo, however, the theory suggests if you have abnormal cells already existing within the uterus, they may be able to migrate into the peritoneal cavity this way.[33]

The reason it's so controversial is that it's been falsely labeled as "the cause" of endometriosis for decades, which has needlessly undermined our ability to secure proper treatments. The belief by some physicians that stopping menstruation can cure endometriosis may fuel their belief that stopping periods will stop endo (which it doesn't), or that endo sufferers need recurrent surgeries to constantly remove it—even though the original surgery may not have been effective in the first place. Others may incorrectly believe that performing a hysterectomy can cure endometriosis without removing the endometriosis itself. These myths perpetuate old-fashioned treatments and demonstrate why it's crucial to truly understand how different types of endometriosis may develop so that we can better develop individualized treatment plans. Again, we deserve better.

The Potential Starting Places of Endo

It may be possible for endo-like cells to originate within the endometrial lining of the uterus, and/or outside of the endometrial lining in Müllarian rests. From these starting points, they can migrate throughout the body.

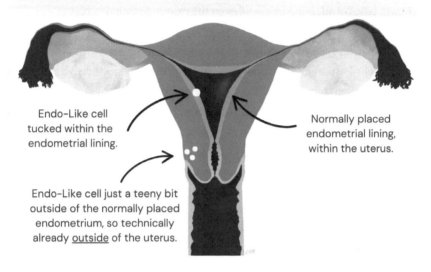

Endo-Like cell tucked within the endometrial lining.

Normally placed endometrial lining, within the uterus.

Endo-Like cell just a teeny bit outside of the normally placed endometrium, so technically already <u>outside</u> of the uterus.

THE GREAT DEBATE: ENDO ORIGINS

Were we born with an endo-like cell already created, or did the transition happen after birth? Was that endo-like cell placed in the uterus, or outside of the uterus? These are big questions within the endometriosis research community—why it's an ongoing scientific discussion! While many researchers actually believe any/all of these possibilities could hold true depending on the person (i.e., not all endo is created equal, and some people may indeed be born with an aggressive endo-like cell already placed outside of the uterus, while others may take a number of triggers to develop an endo-like cell), know that certain groups in the endo field have strong opinions on specifics. I leave it to science to further uncover the mysteries of endometriosis, and here in the book simply explain what research has so far uncovered.

A NEW PERSPECTIVE: DIFFERENT TYPES SPURRED BY DIFFERING CIRCUMSTANCES

The unique genetic inheritances we receive at birth, combined with epigenetics, are the main reason we develop any endo-like cells at all. The fact that there are so many different types of genes we could inherit, or epigenetic behavioral changes we could pick up, explains why there are different types of endometriosis (i.e., why it's *heterogeneous*), and how it can develop in different ways (i.e., why it's *multifactorial*). Altogether, it shows how various types of endo can behave quite differently:[34]

- While most endometriosis lesions will regress during pregnancy, sometimes deep lesions actually progress.
- Some types of endometriosis grow slowly and barely spread, while others grow and spread at a rapid rate.
- Certain types of deep endometriosis lesions are associated with cancer, while others are not.
- There is a wide variety of inflammation levels around what appear to be similar types of lesions, meaning that the immune reaction is widely diverse among different types.
- Progesterone resistance in endo lesions varies from non-existent to very pronounced. This may be why progesterone therapy, a widely recommended treatment for endo pain, varies widely in its efficacy from significant to none at all.
- While most endo requires estrogens to grow, some can develop without much estrogen, as seen in men or women more than 10 years after menopause (who aren't taking hormones).

Genetics and epigenetics also help us understand how endo affects our bodies differently:

- Why there's such a wide array of symptoms experienced by endo sufferers.

- Why different treatment options work well for some people and not for others.
- How each type of endo may benefit from identification and *unique* treatment after diagnosis, rather than implementing the same blanket treatment strategy for all types.
- Why some endo appears to be more aggressive and other endo is more slow-growing.
- How your normally placed endometrial lining (i.e., within the uterus) may not be so normal to begin with.[35]

Overall, we can thank genetics and epigenetics for creating a recognizable endometriosis-like cell.

TAKING BACK CONTROL

Genetics and epigenetics allow us to understand many things about endo, perhaps most importantly reminding us that *endometriosis is no one's fault.* You didn't "get endo" because you used toxic cleaning products, had unprotected sex, or because your mom ate a lot of canned tuna when she was pregnant; it's much more complex! Rather, genetics and epigenetics show us a *myriad* of factors that may contribute uniquely to each case of endo, factors that are out of our control. So repeat after me: "Endometriosis is not my fault." Good.

Next, the study of epigenetics is awesome because, as it turns out, epigenetic expression *is not written in stone.* Just as consistent negative inputs can flip the switch toward disease, so too can positive inputs flip it toward health. In fact, research shows that by shifting our body ecology to one of health, we can also turn "off" many bad genes associated with disease. This was demonstrated in a recent study on people living with an autoimmune disease called ulcerative colitis (an inflammatory bowel disease).[36] When the participants applied a diet called the Paleo Autoimmune Protocol, which focuses on nutrient infusion and removes inflammatory-food triggers, they found that after 6 weeks a total of 324 "bad" genes associated with the disease had epigenetically changed for the better while the inflammatory responses had decreased significantly. One patient went into remission.

While that's not to say we simply flip off the "switch" for endo (akin to having a total cure)—at least not yet—studying epigenetics is enormously encouraging. It allows us to see that how we approach our body ecology can either mitigate or exacerbate the effects of epigenetics, which may make a big difference in how our endo behaves. By removing triggers known to increase the likelihood of endo behavior, we may be able to give our body a better fighting chance. Science is right there, with brand-new endo research recommending that clinicians focus on preventing additional epigenetic incidents by reducing environmental harms and oxidative stress to better manage endo.[37]

But while genetics and epigenetics appear to account for many unique behaviors and anomalies that define endometriosis *cells* as we know them, unless the cells become full-blown endometriosis *lesions* that have blood supply, nutrients, and plenty of oxygen, these cells may not cause any problems. So what's the big factor that drives a wayward endo-like cell to become an endometriosis lesion? And why doesn't the body get rid of it? To answer these questions, we need look no further than the immune system.

Chapter 4:

Your Immune System Establishes Endo Lesions

Once endo-like cells appear within the body, it is the job of your immune system to clean them up. This is what a normally functioning immune system does; it finds abnormal and/or mutated cells and removes them. This may be why very active microscopic endometriosis lesions have been documented in healthy women, which seem to appear and disappear without progressing to cause pain or damage.[38]

Moreover, research has shown that while up to 10 percent of fetuses may be born with endo-like cells in the deep cul-de-sac tissue, less than 4 percent end up actually developing activated endometriosis in those areas.[39] This means something *happened* to activate those cells into active endo lesions.

So, why do some women have the precursor to endo that never turns into the problem of endo-lesions? For people with endometriosis, it appears that inflammatory triggers and immune dysfunction turn a premonition of endo into the real deal. Not only do we have an immune system that's not "cleaning up" endo-like cells as it should, but it's also responsible for activating endo-like cells into fully established endo lesions! Without these triggers, it's possible your endo-like cell might never have developed into the disease you're facing today.

MEET YOUR IMMUNE SYSTEM, IN HEALTH AND IN CONFUSION

To understand how the immune system is so implicated in endometriosis, we need to understand exactly what it does. Your immune system is one of the most intricate and important systems of your body. Best known as your body's protector, it essentially runs a 24/7 surveillance operation to ensure your survival in a world that is literally crawling with invaders (think of all the bacteria, dust, mold, viruses, toxins, etc., you may inhale, touch, swallow, or otherwise encounter in a day). Not only does it brilliantly utilize inflammation—the immune system's "fire-breathing dragon"—to keep you protected from all of this *stuff,* it also works diligently to clean up shop and keep your human organism functioning at the top level. It removes damaged, dead, or otherwise potentially problematic cells that naturally occur. It repairs the bodily structures suffering from natural wear and tear, mending damaged tissue. This is how the immune system doesn't just attack but also mends and heals.

As one of your eleven major body systems, the immune system also requires a wide variety of soothing inputs to best perform. It basically requires the *exact same* healthy inputs that your genes do to best behave: proper nutrition and hydration; outdoor time; healthy friendships; and balanced microbial communities, hormones, and energy levels. It also needs *low* levels of stress, chemical exposure, and sugar. It communicates with your other ten systems to make sure all are in sync. This balanced body ecology benefits your immune function and keeps inflammation at tolerable levels.

Unfortunately, many of our daily behaviors have radically shifted from what our bodies depended on just a few hundred years ago to keep inflammation levels in check (toxic chemical exposure, poor nutrition, sedentary lifestyles, etc.). For many of us, this means our nervous system is overstimulated as we *chronically* experience anxiety, sadness, stress, or anger, our hormonal system is off-kilter as we breathe in toxins and get poor sleep, and our gut microbiome is imbalanced from food choices, pharmaceuticals, and lack of outdoor play. And if these factors never get pulled back into balance, the immune system starts to become very confused. It begins to think the body is being attacked from all angles, and it will protect you the best way it knows how: inflame. No cleaning up, no repair, it just inflames until the "danger" ends. In this state, your immune system is on overdrive, slowly becoming exhausted and confused as it struggles to identify the real problem. When it can't take anymore then immune dysfunction occurs, which, in our case, creates an ecosystem ripe for *endo-ing*.

A DYSFUNCTIONAL IMMUNE SYSTEM ESTABLISHES ENDO

Immune dysfunction is very different from the immune system simply needing extra support, say, by taking zinc and vitamin C to shorten the duration of a cold. It actually indicates that it's not behaving properly. It's often doing things it shouldn't, while not doing things that it should. You may be surprised how many diseases you're familiar with that are also rooted in immune dysfunction.

For example, nearly all conditions associated with chronic inflammation, including acne, kidney stones, asthma, rosacea, and some forms of arthritis, have some level of immune dysfunction. Even chronic allergies present an aspect of immune dysfunction and are another part of the immune picture that many of us with endo deal with on a regular basis.[40]

I'm sure you've heard of autoimmune disorders, which are more serious diseases of immune dysfunction. These are chronic diseases that occur when the immune system becomes so confused that it begins to inflame and attack a normal part of your body—your healthy cells, tissues, or organs. There are more than 100 known autoimmune disorders. You may be familiar with some of the better-known types, such as celiac disease (where your own immune system attacks the villi of your small intestine), multiple sclerosis (where your immune system attacks the myelin sheath around your nerves), or Hashimoto's thyroiditis (where your immune system attacks your thyroid gland). There's really no better example of a confused immune system than one that attacks your own body. And while endometriosis is not considered an autoimmune disorder (as of now there are no known auto-antibodies specifically associated with endo) it is still considered an "autoimmune-associated" disorder due to its chronic inflammatory nature and link with other autoimmune diseases.

Cancer is another potent example of immune dysfunction, wherein your immune system can no longer distinguish an aggressive, destructive, and abnormal cell (the types of cells your immune system should be cleaning up) from the healthy one next door. Moreover, it's often the immune system that established the cancerous cells as full-blown cancer, connecting them to blood supply and (mistakenly) fostering their growth—similar to how it behaves with endo. In fact, endometriosis behaves so much like cancer that we sometimes see it described as a benign (non-lethal) cancer-like tissue.[41] [But don't worry, as painful as endo can be, it is not cancer and it will not kill you.]

So, where exactly does endometriosis fit into this immune-dysfunction picture? How is it a disease of chronic inflammation that, despite not being acne, cancer, or autoimmune, behaves similarly to each in some ways? It turns out that it's a unique disease, with specific facets of dysfunction that turn an endo-like cell into an endo lesion and continues with a progression of lesions once established. Immune dysfunction is so implicated in endometriosis that it appears no matter how the original endo cells came to be, the disease can't come to fruition without the participation of a dysfunctional immune response, including these four components:

Part 1: Establishing your endo lesion

Your immune system is the culprit that transforms a potentially harmless endo-like cell into a full-blown endo lesion by helping these microscopic endo-like cells to root down, establish blood, nutrient, and oxygen supplies, and grow.

Visualize it: you have an endo-like cell. That cell shouldn't be there—it's not normal—but right now it's not necessarily a problem either. But, because of some trigger, your immune system hears a call for help and rushes inflammatory immune factors to the scene of what it assumes is a wound in need of healing or bacteria in need of killing. In swoop the immune factors that are crucial for mending damaged tissue that may be bleeding, may need a ton of inflammation to kill off pathogens, and may need sewing back up. Macrophages, platelets, estrogen, cytokines, and more are all there to save the day! Or they should be...

Instead, when these inflammatory immune factors arrive, they mistakenly believe that the endo-like cell looks like it needs saving rather than destroying (maybe because it slightly resembles an *endometrial* cell, or maybe because the immune system is just plain confused). Quickly the immune system activates and/or integrates that cell into your tissue, and establishes a blood and nerve supply to supply the tissue with oxygen, blood, and nutrients to ensure their growth. This is called *neoangiogenesis*, the creation of new blood vessels.

To add insult to injury, estrogen itself is used as a crucial immune factor to help with healing, so estrogen will also be shuttled to any site of inflammation.[42] This becomes very problematic since endometriosis uses estrogen to activate and grow.

The Immune System Establishes Endo Lesions

First: Immune cells "see" renegade endo-like cell in need of oxygen.

Then: Confused immune factors "sew" the endo-cell to your tissue by establishing blood and oxygen supply. Now it's an established endo lesion.

"What is that?"
"Dunno, Let's save it?"

Great Job!

Help!

Immune Cells

Endo-Like Cell

Now an Endometriosis Lesion

Now, thanks to a dysfunctional immune response, you officially have an active, established endometriosis lesion.

LOVE SCIENCE?

For the complex details behind the immune dysfunction of endo, please see Appendix 2.

Part 2: The Janitor Asleep on the Job

The part of your immune system capable of seeking and destroying abnormal cells should be on high alert every day. This is exactly what it is trained for—to *obliterate* anything it doesn't recognize as normal before it can damage your body, be it damaged tissue, old or abnormal cells, pathogenic bacteria, viruses, pre-cancerous cells, or even excess blood where it shouldn't be found. Let's call this part of the immune system the "immune janitors." These immune cells continually sweep up debris to keep your body functioning at its best.

In the peritoneal cavity, immune janitors are at work at all times, flowing freely through the peritoneal fluid (the fluid that lines the organs within the pelvis that acts as a sort of lubricant so that your organs don't stick together). Truly, it's a microenvironment within itself that is saturated with a host of specific immune cells ready to clean up and remove any problematic cells—such as normal retrograde flow or a little bit of tissue damage. However, in the case of endometriosis, there appears to be a significant level of dysfunction preventing the endo-like cells and inflammatory debris from being removed. In other words, the janitor is asleep on the job.

So while there appears to be an *increase* in certain immune factors that enhance the growth, adhesion, migration, and invasion capacities of endo cells (per Part 1), there is a simultaneous *decrease* in the surveillance immune factors within the peritoneal cavity that would give endo cells the boot. The immune system's inability to clean up endo cells seems to play a pivotal role in their persistence and progression.

The Immune System Lets Them Stay

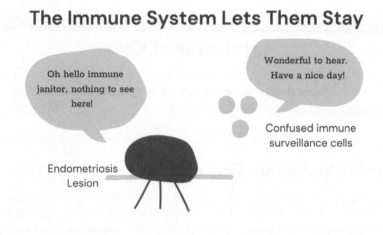

Part 3: A Systemically Dysfunctional Immune System

Immune dysfunction isn't observed only at the site of endo lesions, it is also observed throughout the entire body—another reason why endometriosis is considered a full-body disease. While it's not totally clear whether the systemic immune dysfunction in the endo body begins before or after the endometriosis lesions take hold, it's obvious that endo-related immune dysfunction affects the *entire* body, with widespread abnormalities in the levels and behavior of circulating immune factors.

Systemic inflammation and immune dysfunction also account for myriad other not-so-obviously-related endo symptoms that drive many of us crazy. For example, those with endo are more prone to developing allergies, skin problems, hypothyroidism, celiac disease, chronic fatigue syndrome, fibromyalgia, chronic joint pain, and frequent headaches—all diseases and symptoms associated with chronic inflammation and immune system dysfunction. New research even hypothesizes that autoimmunity may be a contributing factor in the pathogenesis of endo for some of us.[43]

This widespread immune dysfunction can create a sort of whack-a-mole situation where endo patients feel like they're struggling to manage all their symptoms at once. It contributes to what feels like a body on fire—and perhaps leaves confused doctors telling you it's all in your head.

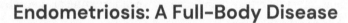

Endometriosis: A Full-Body Disease

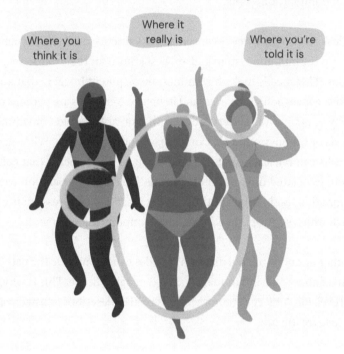

Part 4: Endometriosis Lesions Create a Unique Immune Environment

Once endo-like cells are established as endometriosis lesions, you officially have endometriosis as the disease you know. Now, these lesions produce their own estrogen and inflammatory immune factors, exacerbating the progression, pain, inflammation, and immune dysfunction.[44] They also produce lactic acid, which acts as a kind of "invisibility cloak" so janitorial immune factors get confused, contributing to the immune system's inability to clean up the cells or lesions.[45]

This means that endometriosis lesions are no longer just responding to immune factors. They are also producing them *and* confusing them—thus becoming an integral part of the immune equation (and now a rabid contributor to your body ecology). And because all this is happening within the peritoneal fluid, increased levels of oxidative stress may begin to affect your surrounding organs, creating either pain (such as when urinating or defecating), or intra-abdominal adhesions.

Endo lesions also show heavy concentrations of active mast cells, which are key players in the immune system and are best known for their role in response to allergies.[46] Mast cells make histamines, those potent buggers that stimulate sneezing, congestion, puffy eyes, and itchiness. Mast cells are perhaps one reason why so many endo sufferers deal with rampant allergies, or why allergies (to foods or the environment) can increase endo symptoms. When activated, mast cells can release histamines and tryptase, components that contribute to endo-associated fibrosis and inflammation. Their association with pain, inflammation, and even infertility is why mast-cell suppression is one lens through which science is looking at endo symptom management.[47]

Few other immune-related diseases (besides cancer) involve the pathological growth of abnormal, inflammatory, and damaging tissue. This is why professional excision surgery to remove lesions is often described as a necessary step in disease treatment.

WHEN INFLAMMATION BECOMES CHRONIC

The big question I kept coming back to was why is there chronic inflammation in the peritoneal cavity in the first place, and why won't it stop? You *really* don't want your immune system attacking this delicate area that houses your vital and reproductive organs. It turns out that chronic inflammation within the peritoneal cavity may have existed for some of us even *before* the establishment of our endo lesions, and some of it may be continuing to fuel your endo today.

Here are five culprits that can cause chronic inflammation. They have been studied in direct relation to endo:

Pathogenic bacteria. Pathogenic bacteria from the intestinal tract or genital tract can migrate into the peritoneal cavity due to either retrograde menstruation or intestinal permeability. If these bacteria keep coming (for example, if the infections of the gut or reproductive organs are not adequately addressed), the inflammatory immune response becomes chronic. Over time this can lead to tissue damage, which—you guessed it—creates an inflammatory environment that may set the stage for future endometriosis to thrive.[48]

Iron overload. Iron overload is caused by too much blood in the peritoneal cavity. If you have a very heavy, thick, clotted, or longer-than-normal monthly flow, it may saturate your peritoneal cavity once a month thanks to retrograde menstruation. Although the majority of women experience retrograde menstruation without a hitch because their immune system clears out the debris, this immune response seems to be subpar in endo sufferers.[49] Iron overload can be terribly inflammatory, and may even affect you *pre-endo* if your body is dealing with an exceptionally heavy flow one full week per month.[50] And once endo lesions are established, they will also bleed each month, contributing to the issue.

Estrogen. The presence of estrogen is a big factor in chronic inflammation associated with endo. Estrogen fuels endo growth, especially when it has little to no progesterone to cool it down. Even normal levels of estrogen in the body can feed endometriosis growth since endo is so estrogen sensitive.

Endocrine-Disrupting Chemicals. When inside the body, EDCs can create cellular damage, leading to inflammation. Those with endometriosis have been shown to have higher levels of EDCs in their peritoneal fluid (the slippery immune-rich liquid that lines your peritoneal cavity).[51]

Established Endo Lesions. Growing endometriosis lesions damage healthy tissue in their wake, and *any* tissue damage screams for more inflammation to "sanitize" the scene. Even more, established lesions produce some of their own inflammatory immune factors.

There are additional factors that may contribute to inflammation in the peritoneal cavity.

Sedentary lifestyles directly atrophy the musculature that encases the peritoneal cavity: the obliques, glutes, pelvic floor, and so on. Over time, atrophied muscles lose vasculature (the much-needed blood and oxygen supply), which may lead to oxygen reduction in the peritoneal cavity.

High levels of stress inform your immune system to prioritize inflammation in case the danger you're stressed about results in you being attacked (and inflammation is already "on-site" to sanitize the wound). Unfortunately, this process can also be triggered by non-dangerous though stressful moments such as work, news, or too much doomscrolling on social media. When stress becomes chronic, so does inflammation.

Poor breathing and movement patterns may cause slight pressure damage to your reproductive organs, increasing inflammation.

While these issues haven't been studied in direct relation to endo, their impact has been studied in-depth in relation to our overall health. I believe they are worth mentioning because most of us deal with sedentary behaviors, poor breathing, and chronic stress as part of our daily lives. My endo clients who mitigated these factors as part of their overall treatment have expressed an improvement in their symptoms. I'll discuss how to address these factors in the coming chapters.

CHRONIC INFLAMMATION CHRONICALLY DAMAGES

Too many unaddressed triggers lead to inflammation so prolonged that it starts to create its own damage. Imagine the fire-breathing dragon scorching and scorching, damaging not just the trigger (like bacteria), but also *you*. This is called *oxidative stress*—damage produced by inflammation.

When You Eat Plenty of Antioxidants

STEP 1
Tissue damage occurs for whatever reason. Inflammation is called to the scene

STEP 2
Radical immune ninjas are sent to destroy any invaders that are causing trouble

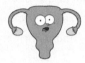

STEP 3
Done! Now handcuffs are deployed to subdue ninjas

STEP 4
All good! Invader destroyed, ninjas handcuffed, body happy

Not Enough Antioxidants? Uh oh

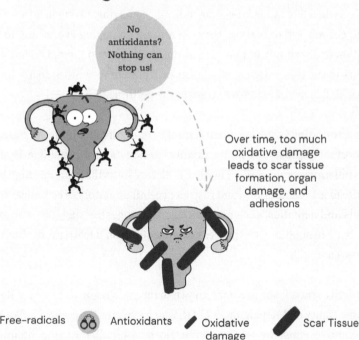

Your Immune System Establishes Endo Lesions

Oxidative stress happens thanks to free radicals (also known as reactive oxygen species), one of your immune system's weapons of choice. Free radicals are, well, pretty radical in that they can d-e-s-t-r-o-y cellular membranes at an incredible rate—a great weapon to have in your immune army. Think of them as wild ninjas with swords, slashing everything around them to pieces. The way free radicals are stopped is by being paired with an antioxidant; it's like the ninja needed some handcuffs, and antioxidants act as such. Antioxidants are not usually a problem to find within a healthy body under normal conditions.

However, in the context of significant and chronic inflammation—leading to a *lot* of free radicals—these wild ninjas are often left without antioxidant handcuffs. In this situation, free radicals don't spare a human cell over a pathogenic cell; they will damage your cells and your tissues just as easily as they destroy a virus or pathogen. You need *a lot* of antioxidants to subdue the billions of ninjas if you have chronic inflammation. If you're low on antioxidants, the destruction will continue.

This is when free radicals become radically damaging. Living in an area doused with chronic inflammation, they zip around damaging everything in sight... and there are simply not enough antioxidants to stop them. Oxidative stress refers to the tissue damage that ensues. Those of us with endo are known to have high levels of oxidative stress in the peritoneal cavity.[52]

It's astounding just how much damage free radicals can do. It's incredibly important to consume a high amount of antioxidants every single day to quell this inflammatory cascade. This is why dietary shifts that promote high levels of antioxidant consumption and restrict pro-inflammatory/free radical-forming foods and activities, such as smoking, drinking, stressing, etc., can support the body in subduing the process of *endo-ing* (you'll learn more about this in Parts 3 and 4).[53]

Oxidative stress leads to what's known in the endo realm as a cycle of Repeated Tissue Injury and Repair, or *ReTIAR,* which explains the cyclical inflammatory immune response we see in endometriosis. After all, the same inflammation that's arriving at the scene to "save the day" ends up causing damage itself since it never gets the message to STOP. This leads to more damage, more hypoxia, and more oxidative stress. Chronic damage without healing will eventually lead to scar tissue formation and intra-abdominal adhesions, both of which are the result of a prolonged and abnormal immune response. They represent the culmination of years of immune-based inflammation.

TAKING THE INFLAMMATION AND IMMUNE EQUATION SERIOUSLY

The biggest reason to care about the inflammation and immune-dysfunction aspect of endometriosis is that you have it in your power to do something about it. Many inflammatory triggers related to endometriosis *can actually be addressed* and, for many of us, a dysfunctional immune response can be retrained. If you've had friends or family members who put their issues of immune dysfunction into remission (whether it be cancer, autoimmunity, or, heck, acne), you can understand that this is possible. You don't have to live in inflammatory despair forever, adding more conditions or symptoms to your life every year. By adopting a new endo lifestyle, stabilize your endo and/or symptoms, and start to reclaim your life.

So how do we do this? To calm our worst symptoms, it is helpful to understand more about what is causing them. So let's take a look at some of endo's most significant inflammatory triggers: bacteria and hormones.

The Story of Endo Pathogenesis

2 At some point, the body amounts an immune attack (maybe it recognizes that the endo-like cells are in the wrong place, or maybe there's bacteria, excess blood, tissue damage, or some other trigger).

2b If the immune system is overwhelmed thanks to chronic inflammation and immune dysfunction, it "mistakenly" establishes that endo-like cell into an endo lesion, with established blood and nerve supply. You now have endometriosis.

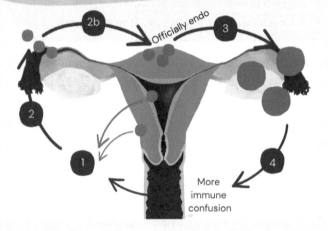

1 An endo-like cell appears in a place outside the uterus. But no worries, it's just an "endo-like cell", not really a problem yet

3 Without addressing the inflammatory triggers, endo grows and progresses into advanced forms (such as deep infiltrating or ovarian endometrioma). Scar tissue and organ/tissue damage ensue.

4 All the while, the improper immune response stops the clearance of these abnormal cells, and mistakenly continues with chronic inflammation. This becomes cyclical in nature.

Chapter 5:

Endo's Secret Little BIG Trigger: Bacteria

Bacteria may be the most potent trigger of endometriosis you've never heard of. In some ways, bacteria may be the "smoking gun" behind the continuous inflammation that drives endo. In fact, there is an intricate relationship between bacterial imbalances (known as *dysbiosis*) and endometriosis establishment, progression, immune dysfunction, and endo symptoms. The good news is that dysbiosis can be addressed, which may help you reduce your symptoms or even slow (or stop) the endo-ing.

To understand the relationship between bacteria and endo, you first have to understand a little bit about the human microbiome. Your microbiome consists of around 10,000 microbial species on or in the body (think the gut and beyond, including the skin, mouth, intestines, eyes, sinuses, vagina, uterus, *everywhere*), which make up a total population of some trillions. Although the microbiome makes up a small percentage of our bodies by weight (1 to 3 percent), it's estimated to outnumber our human cells 10 to 1, meaning we have substantially more microbial genes than human genetic code in our bodies! These little microbes are quite literally our evolutionary partners and are so crucial to both our survival and our ability to thrive that some scientists believe the microbiome should be considered a pseudo-organ. In the future, it may indeed be added to our list of body systems since, without it, you would die just as if someone removed your liver.

You can also think of your microbiome as a cellular periscope because our human genes rely on it for gathering important information. Everything you eat, drink, touch, and inhale will interact with some part of the microbiome in your mouth, nose, skin, vagina, or gut. By taking in clues as to what's happening outside your body, it influences how your body reacts on the inside. A healthy and vibrant microbiome is absolutely essential for proper immune function, procreation, and mental health.

This is especially true of the relationship between your microbes and your overall health. Our bodies (and microbes) are suffering under the weight of modern, industrial living. The hyper-sanitization of food, the addition of preservatives, lack of diversity and fiber in the diet, antibiotics, birth control, toxic chemicals, pain killers, and more—all of these act like a lawnmower over our delicate microbial populations, slowly whittling down certain beneficial species and allowing others to overgrow like inflammatory weeds. This imbalance within the species that make up the microbiome is called *dysbiosis,* and it's linked to just about every symptom of poor health—from insomnia and joint pain to acne and arthritis—as well as diseases of inflammation and immune dysfunction such as endometriosis.

The Sad History of the Modern Microbiome

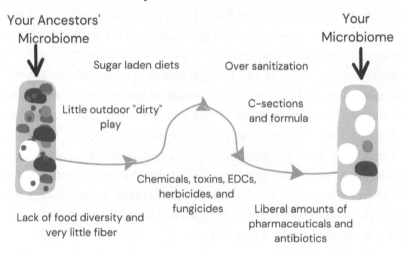

Your Ancestors' Microbiome

Sugar laden diets

Little outdoor "dirty" play

Lack of food diversity and very little fiber

Chemicals, toxins, EDCs, herbicides, and fungicides

Over sanitization

C-sections and formula

Liberal amounts of pharmaceuticals and antibiotics

Your Microbiome

ENDO-DYSBIOSIS – GOOD GUYS VS. BAD GUYS

Those of us with endo may be dealing with dysbiosis across various micro-biome sites. Starting with the gut, the average endo sufferer may have fewer *gram-positive* bacteria (think of these as the "good guys") and more *gram-negative* bacteria, such as *E.coli* or *Strep* (considered the "bad guys" when there are too many).[54] While gram-negative bacteria aren't totally bad, per-se, we want their populations kept to a minimum, since they produce toxic and highly inflammatory compounds called lipopolysaccharides (LPS). The immune system despises LPS, and as such it will provoke an enormous inflammatory response in the body whenever it encounters them outside of the digestive tract.

This is why, if you have more inflammatory microbial populations than beneficial ones, it can quickly become problematic. And, unfortunately for some of us with endo, we may have so many "bad guy" gram-negative populations that they *dominate* our gut microbial communities![55] Because of its inflammatory nature, dysbiosis like this may even be implicated in the development of endo itself.[56]

But it doesn't stop at the gut. The "bad guys" have been shown to proliferate throughout the peritoneal cavity as well as the reproductive and genital tract. For example, endo sufferers have been observed to have the following: [57]

- Inflammatory microbe populations in the uterus and peritoneal fluid;
- A significantly altered cervical microbiome;
- More *Strep* in their cervical mucus;
- Higher concentrations of *E. coli* in their peritoneal fluid;
- Four to six times more *E. coli* in their menstrual blood; and
- Higher levels of *Streptococcus* and *E. coli* in the endometrium.

With this high level of gram-negative bacteria seeming everywhere from our gut to our menstrual fluid, it may not come as a surprise to know that we endo sufferers altogether end up having higher concentrations of LPS in our peritoneal fluid.[58] This is deeply problematic, and the immune system sees an emergency as it expedites an enormous inflammatory response.

THE GREAT MIGRATION

How did gram-negative bacteria and LPS migrate to your endo lesion? The truth is that bacteria found in certain parts of the body may not be as isolated from *the rest* of the body as you may think. For example, beneficial bacteria within the intestinal tract will seed other parts of the body, as you may have observed if you've ever taken probiotics orally and watched a yeast infection or athlete's foot clear up. Conversely, pathogenic bacteria from the intestinal tract have been observed in the lymph nodes, liver, spleen, kidney, and even in the bloodstream.[59] This process of bacterial movement is called *bacterial translocation,* and it's important to understand if we are to stop the great migration of bacteria to endo lesion ground zero (being, wherever your own endo lesions are), where it has been shown to directly fuel the growth of endometriosis lesions through the creation of an inflammatory response.[60]

Perhaps the foundational site implicated in the great migration is the intestinal tract, home to the majority of your microbiome. The cellular lining of the intestine is just about as fragile as can be: incredibly, it's only one cell thick. That means without abundant protection, the insides of your gut are *one cell away* from leaking into your bloodstream. To prevent bacteria (and LPS) from escaping, your gut has a built-in defensive system that includes a lot of protective mucous and hefty immunosurveillance. However, if you have any issues within your intestinal ecology—*i.e.,* gut infections, inflammation, food allergies, dysbiosis, etc.—the defensive measures can quickly be overcome. This is called gut hyper-permeability, a.k.a. *leaky gut,* and when it develops pathogens from the intestinal tract can more easily migrate into the rest of the body, prompting an immune attack. Unfortunately, one preliminary study shows that potentially *all of us* with endo may have leaky gut to some degree.[61]

Healthy Gut

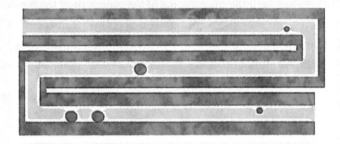

The thick mucous lining keeps bacteria, LPS, toxins, food particles, and everything else inside your digestive tract.

Leaky Gut

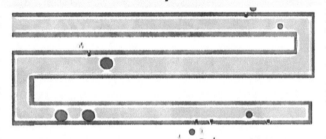

Damaged lining allows particles to break through your thin cellular wall. Now pathogens, bacteria, LPS, and partially digested proteins can leak into your bloodstream, prompting an inflammatory reaction (with each meal).

This may also be how we develop a slew of odd food allergies, as the immune system starts to think that tomato protein (for example) leaking into the bloodstream is the enemy.

Immune Cells

But the gut microbiome isn't the only storage facility that can translocate bacteria. It turns out that nearly any site in the body can seed bacteria from one site to another, be it the microbiome of the mouth or of the reproductive tract.[62] This helps us make sense of why you may be three times more likely to develop endometriosis if you have Pelvic Inflammatory Disease (PID), an infection of the peritoneal fluid, or why our risk of developing endo is significantly increased by having genital infections.[63]

Address Bacterial Overgrowths, Stop The Great Migration

Gut, oral, vaginal, uterine, or ANY dysbiosis + translocation = bacterial onslaught and subsequent inflammation at your endo lesions.

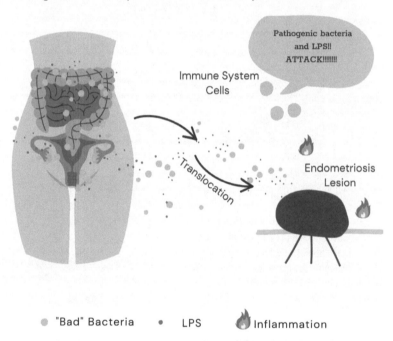

All of this information should help paint the picture of the vital importance of addressing infections and overgrowth, both in the gut and reproductive tract (or, heck, in the mouth, sinuses, or wherever *you* have a chronic infection), as well as healing any residual leaky gut. To stop the cyclic inflammation, we *have* to stop the bacteria. All of this we'll talk about in-depth in the coming chapters.

WHICH CAME FIRST: DYSBIOSIS OR IMMUNE DYSFUNCTION?

When Hippocrates said "All diseases begin in the gut" some 2000 years ago, he wasn't far off. The gut is actually the home of the immune system, where many immune cells are grown and *trained* in how to behave through a bacteria-immune conversation.[64] When bacteria become imbalanced (dysbiosis) the conversation can quickly become skewed, directly influencing the behavior (or, misbehavior) of certain immune components. This is why leaky gut and dysbiosis are associated with autoimmune disorders, chronic allergies, skin problems, hypothyroid, celiac, chronic fatigue, fibromyalgia, joint pain, and frequent head-aches—many symptoms shared by endometriosis sufferers. When the immune system is called upon day and night to address an issue that shouldn't exist, it never gets to rest, clean up, and repair other damaged tissues and cells elsewhere.

Specifically for those of us with endometriosis, gut dysbiosis may direct-ly train our immune cells to misbehave in specific ways. This includes immune cells unable to "see" or clean up endometriotic debris as they should, the immune system misbehaving by *inducing* inflammation in the pelvic cavity, increasing prostaglandin levels (which contributes to pain), and supporting the rooting down of endo lesions.[65] (See Appendix 3 for the details). It begs the question of which came first, endometriosis lesions or the dysbiosis associated with it?

DYSBIOSIS, ENDO, AND INFERTILITY

Reproductive tract dysbiosis may be a big factor when it comes to infertility, something that up to a third of women with endo may deal with at some point (of note, "infertility" does not mean you can never have children, but rather refers to someone who has tried to conceive for over a year with no success). In fact, one study demonstrated that 42.3 percent of women with endometriosis and infertility issues also had chronic *endometritis*, an acute and prolonged infection of the endometrium lining.[66] Endometritis is associated with recurrent miscarriages, as well as with the same strains of bacteria associated with endometriosis. Because nearly half of infertile endo patients may be dealing with this infection, I believe it's important to investigate. In this case, a simple antibiotic treatment could dramatically improve fertility.[67]

Even if you don't have a diagnosable infection, you may have a subclinical infection (basically some *serious* dysbiosis), as 81.5 percent of women with endo were shown to have uterine pathogenic bacterial colonization to some degree.[68] These high amounts of pathogenic bacteria will produce LPS, which can directly cause endometrial or tubal damage, prevent implantation, reduce sperm motility, and even kill sperm. In an IVF study analyzing successful outcomes, women with less LPS in the reproductive tract were much more likely to have a successful embryo transfer than those with more LPS.[69] The connection is so powerful that I always remind folk to be extra careful with pregnancy precautions during a gut-healing protocol. As the bacteria become more balanced, this seems to be the time when surprises most often happen—as has happened with my clients and even with me for my happy surprise second child. Healing the microbiome is a top priority for infertility cases.

ENDO BELLY, CHRONIC YEAST INFECTIONS, AND OTHER SYMPTOMS OF DYSBIOSIS

Dysbiosis of any kind can cause digestive disorders, either minimal or detrimental, something most of us know all too well. Endometriosis and digestive complaints are so common there's even a slang word in the community for it: Endo Belly. This is a general term for the enormous bloating associated with endometriosis, perhaps accompanied by diarrhea, gas, constipation, or a mix of everything. For some, Endo Belly is painful. For others, it can be embarrassing. And for many, it comes with a diagnosis of IBS (irritable bowel syndrome) or worse.

The problem with the name "Endo Belly" is that—for some of us—it gives more blame to endometriosis than it should. For example, while 93 percent of women with endo report having gastrointestinal issues, perhaps only 3 to 37 percent have endometriosis of the bowel, highlighting the larger role played by the bacterial component in some of our worst gastrointestinal symptoms.[70] It shouldn't be surprising to hear that large pathogenic overgrowths may cause or exacerbate many of the gastro issues we suffer from (chronic bloating, diarrhea, constipation, abdominal pain, gas, you name it). Dysbiosis stemming from the gut and digestive tract aggravate endo and can make us feel just plain lousy.

One type of dysbiosis associated with endo that is known to cause unpleasant digestive symptoms is called Small Intestinal Bacterial Overgrowth, or SIBO. SIBO happens when bacteria (either beneficial or not) overgrow in the small intestine. Your large intestine should house the majority of the bacteria in your gut (and where fermentation of fibers should occur). However, large amounts of bacteria residing instead in your delicate *small* intestine can cause serious issues. Food fermentation by large numbers of bacteria should *not* be happening here. But when an overgrowth of bacteria migrates mistakenly to this sensitive spot, you can get *extreme* bloating, reflux, terrible-smelling gas, chronic diarrhea and/or constipation, and you can generally feel sick.

If you have terrible digestive symptoms (perhaps with an IBS diagnosis to boot), you may not be surprised if you find that you have SIBO. One small study actually uncovered that 80 percent of women who had both endo *and* significant digestive distress were positive for SIBO.[71] Not only that, but SIBO is also highly associated with IBS, perhaps accounting for up to 84 percent of IBS cases.[72] This is incredibly important to note for the many of us who suffer from an IBS co-diagnosis, which is pretty common.[73]

IS IT DYSBIOSIS, OR ENDO?

The truth is, your digestive issues may stem from your endo directly (which is why some who surgically remove their lesions see an immediate reduction in gastro symptoms) or they may stem from dysbiosis. Or maybe a combination of the two. Yet, if dysbiosis is contributing in any way, understand that it's treatable. SIBO, for example, is a clinically diagnosable gut infection that needs to be eradicated. Once eliminated, you may notice a dramatic reduction of your endo and gastro symptoms. Or, if you have an overgrowth of *Strep* or *E. coli*, you can eliminate those as well while reducing the amount of LPS in your system.

Another symptom of dysbiosis can be excess estrogen. This is because your estrobolome (the part of your microbiome that helps process estrogen) can be disrupted by bacterial dysbiosis. This misinforms your gut to reabsorb the estrogen that your liver had so nicely bound up and thrown in the intestinal "trash" and sends it back into circulation.[74] This can make dysbiosis a potent contributor to estrogen excess in some cases.

And of course, chronic gut dysbiosis is widely associated with inflammation and immune dysfunction on a grand scale—which is why those with endo often suffer from additional symptoms or conditions associated with excess inflammation as previously mentioned, including autoimmunity, allergies, chronic fatigue, joint pain, and frequent headaches.[75]

Dysbiosis of the reproductive tract can make things painful, irritated, itchy, smelly, and uncomfortable. It can make sex painful, or is perhaps the reason behind those recurrent UTIs or yeast infections. On the other hand, you may have no obvious genital symptoms but find yourself struggling with infertility, pelvic pain, or terribly painful periods as a result of bacterial reflux into the peritoneal cavity, where it stokes a wildfire of inflammation every month.

MEND THE MICROBES, HEAL THE ENDO

Addressing dysbiosis at the gut and reproductive tract level may help you directly treat some of your worst endo symptoms, if not your endo lesions themselves. Just as we see LPS and pathogenic bacteria fostering endometriosis, so too do we see the beginnings of research uncovering the relationship between the reversal of dysbiosis and regression of endometriosis.

In a fascinating 2019 study, researchers treating endo-induced mice with antibiotics observed their lesions shrink to one-fifth the size and with a less proliferative capability, while immune factors related to endo were all reduced.[76] But, when they were then re-inoculated with the same "bad" bacteria through their food, the endometriosis lesions again grew and progressed, demonstrating just how linked microbial overgrowths in the gut may be to the growth and progression of endo.

In another study, endo-induced mice were also induced with dysbiosis.[77] Half of these mice were left alone and the other half were supplemented with a gut-healing nutrient called butyrate—an important SCFA known to repair the intestinal barrier. What they found was that the untreated mice developed larger endo lesions, while the mice supplemented with butyrate developed fewer and much smaller lesions, again demonstrating the endo-gut cross-talk.

I AM NOT A MOUSE! A NOTE ON ENDO STUDIES

Because there is limited funding for endo research, studies are more often conducted in vitro (in a petri dish), or on non-human subjects such as mice. This type of research is the "tip of the iceberg" since, without large human cohort studies, we are unable to generate *reliable* results that span the broader population. Still, the research we have today allows us to see trends and develop plausible theories that can be further investigated. For example, if a theory works on mice, those results can be further investigated in humans to reveal more information. It's imperfect and slow and explains why there are still so many theories about pathogenesis, treatment, or anything in between. Consequently, what we know today will continue to evolve as new information is discovered. This book is a snapshot of the research available today and will be updated as new information emerges.

We also see research showing that substances with helpful antimicrobial properties such as berberine may be able to positively impact endo. Berberine is a natural antimicrobial compound with an affinity for LPS which has been shown to reduce the inflammatory components associated with both LPS *and* endo.[78] It's even been shown to increase endo cell death and reduce the proliferation and invasiveness of adenomyosis tissue (when endometrial tissue grows into the muscular wall of the uterus) by up to 60 percent.[79]

Thanks to this new research, a new picture is emerging on the *direct* relationship between bacteria and endo: the specific types of immune dysfunction, the progression and establishment of endo lesions, and some of the life-altering digestive symptoms many of us deal with. It may be that, for some of us, bacterial contamination started the rampant pelvic inflammation in the first place, and it is continuing to spur our pain and disease progression today. For some, bacteria may pave the way for the familiar factors of chronic inflammation, oxidative stress, tissue damage, and hypoxia.

This is why getting to the root of your own bacterial issue should be a top priority. Doing so doesn't have to be rocket science; there is plenty of research showing how nourishing diet and lifestyle changes can change the microbiome in as little as days to weeks. Swapping out processed, refined foods for fiber- and nutrient-rich whole foods, removing chemicals from our house and skin and beauty routines, minimizing stress and anxiety, eschewing antibiotics unless absolutely necessary, playing outside, starting a garden and digging in the dirt—all of these can help, and I'll address them in the next sections. Of course, you may also need some professional help if your specific type of dysbiosis is severe, and working with a well-trained professional who can test, diagnose, and treat you to get rid of any overgrowths or infections will be essential for some. With that inflammation-provoking bacteria gone, some of your endo symptoms may also be alleviated, such as digestive symptoms, pain, anxiety, depression, or even infertility.

Chapter 6:

Hormones: Are They Really the Enemy?

While endometriosis is first and foremost an inflammatory condition, it's estrogen we hear about most when it comes to pathogenesis, progression, and treatment. That's because endo *is* an estrogen-dependent disease, meaning it depends on estrogen to grow. Think of estrogen as endo food: endo eats estrogen, endo lesion grows, growth damages the surrounding healthy tissue, damage invites more inflammation and activates lesions, and active endo lesions produce more inflammatory factors. The cycle continues. This is why controlling estrogen levels has been the main treatment strategy for years.

Still, much of what we think we know about the relationship between endo and estrogen is misconstrued. First of all, we *need* proper estrogen levels to feel well, so estrogen is not necessarily the enemy. And while estrogen lesions themselves feed on estrogen, having endo does not simply mean you, as a person, have too much estrogen. You might, or you might not. In addition, progesterone and stress hormones are often the missing links in the endo-hormone discussion.

WHAT ARE HORMONES?

Hormones are essentially chemical messengers. There are around 70 in the human body that help regulate everything from digestion to sleep, happiness to stress, reproduction to immune function. Based on the inputs they receive from the outside world (via your emotions, chemical skin absorption, sleep, sunlight exposure, etc.) and the inside world (communication between your eleven body systems) they support the healthy, happy functioning of your body ecology.

Hormones connect to cellular receptors where they attach and are then absorbed into the cell to be used. Imagine that hormones are information "delivery trucks" on the road, while cellular receptors are the "mailboxes" hormones are delivered to.

And while we often want to zoom in to fix one single hormone level at a time (like estrogen), all 70 hormones work together in a symbiotic way. It's a vast and complex system of communication that relies on many players to either create hormonal balance or foster a disease state (*endo-ing*, for example).

This may be why there appear to be numerous hormones associated with endo, either in prevention and mitigation, or establishment and progression. Vitamin D, for example, is in fact a hormone that's made in the kidneys and is important for immune function. Interestingly, researchers found those with the lowest levels of vitamin D had the largest endometriomas (endometriosis-filled cysts), and that the lower your vitamin D levels, the higher your risk of developing endometriosis.[80] Also, insulin is a hormone created by the pancreas to control blood sugar levels, and excess insulin may foster some of the immune dysfunction associated with endo.[81]

Yet, the four hormones that steal the center stage for endo time and time again are the stress hormones cortisol and adrenaline, and the sex hormones progesterone and estrogen.

ESTROGEN AND PROGESTERONE

Estrogen is a fantastic hormone that promotes cellular building and growth—it gives cells permission to grow. This is a useful and necessary function for many processes in the body, such as muscle and tissue repair and the rebuilding of the uterine lining each cycle after menses. It's *absolutely necessary for health* and contributes to strong bones, nourished skin, balanced moods, and a healthy libido and menstrual cycle. Estrogen is why women going through menopause (either natural or chemically induced) may develop challenging symptoms—hot flashes, mood swings, loss of libido, vaginal and skin dryness, and premature aging—as their estrogen drops dramatically, and why those with low estrogen may develop osteoporosis. Proper levels of estrogen make us feel good, whole, and healthy.

And we can't truly understand estrogen without also understanding progesterone, a female sex hormone produced mainly by the ovaries after ovulation (so yes, healthy ovulation is tantamount to healthy progesterone levels). Progesterone is vital for a healthy luteal phase (the two weeks between ovulation and menses), fertility, pregnancy, and menstruation. Not only that, but progesterone fights inflammation and aids in proper immune system behavior. You can see why it would be an important part of the endometriosis discussion. Think of estrogen as the "grower" and progesterone as the "soother." It is why you need these two to be in balance just like you need balance on a teeter-totter. We need both for healthy bodies, moods, and fertility. Unfortunately, hormone levels both localized (at the site of the endo lesions) and systemically may be skewed in the endo body.

Hormonal Imbalance at Endo Ground Zero

If you've heard estrogen is endo's arch nemesis, it's because, yes, endo depends on estrogen to grow. Think of estrogen as endo food that signals rapidly for lesions to grow, grow, grow, damaging healthy tissue in its wake (which, of course, invites plenty of inflammation). And, unfortunately, endo is known to be able to throw back a hefty amount of estrogen. What research has found is that endo cells are epigenetically altered to have increased levels of estrogen receptors, from a few more to *a lot* more (up to 140 times more!), meaning endo can gorge.[82]

But there is also an imbalance in progesterone receptors, with endo cells observed to have low to undetectable levels.[83] This leads to something called progesterone *resistance*, meaning even if there is plenty of progesterone available, your body may not be able to use it since there are little to no "docking sites." Without the cooling power of progesterone, the effects of estrogen will be exacerbated even more.[84] Essentially this means double trouble: lots of endo-lesion growth, barely any cooling.

Estrogen Sensitive & Progesterone Resistant

Note that the level of hormonal sensitivity in lesions may be quite different between sufferers, and even perhaps between lesions within the same sufferer! This often makes the hormonal treatment equation unique to each case (for example, why oral contraceptives or progesterone work great for one person, but not another).

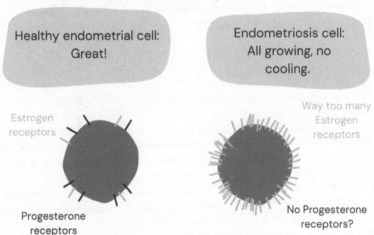

Healthy endometrial cell: Great!

Endometriosis cell: All growing, no cooling.

Estrogen receptors

Way too many Estrogen receptors

Progesterone receptors

No Progesterone receptors?

The difference in receptor levels is one reason why endo may affect us all so differently, from some hormonal treatments working excellently for one sufferer and poorly for another, as well as helping explain how different types of endo behave. Indeed some sufferers with intense hormonal sensitivity may see endo rapidly spread or progress while others with low sensitivity may find their endo slow-growing. Even more, you can have different levels of receptors in different lesions within the *same* body (maybe yours, for example), making the hormonal discussion even fuzzier and especially reminding us why hormonal treatments aren't able to address this disease all on their own.[85]

Beyond hormonal receptivity, there is another element that comes into play in the localized endo environment: endo makes its own estrogen, which is obviously problematic when it feeds on it. But here comes something wild—while endo tissue may make a teeny bit more estrogen on its own, it may make up to *48 times more estrogen* when provoked by inflammation![86] This is how inflammation may be more implicated than we realize in creating the enormous estrogen "avalanche" that endo is famous for.

The Estrogen–Inflammation Equation

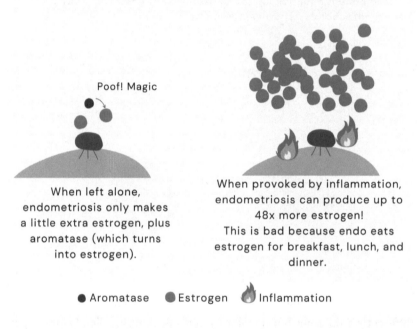

Poof! Magic

When left alone, endometriosis only makes a little extra estrogen, plus aromatase (which turns into estrogen).

When provoked by inflammation, endometriosis can produce up to 48x more estrogen!
This is bad because endo eats estrogen for breakfast, lunch, and dinner.

● Aromatase   ● Estrogen   🔥 Inflammation

If left unchecked, this issue can become cyclical: endo eats estrogen, endo grows, growth damages tissue, damage invites inflammation, inflammation provokes endo to make more estrogen, endo eats more estrogen, and on and on. This is how the localized hormone equation becomes deeply implicated in all stages of endometriosis development, pain, and growth. It's one of the reasons why, if left undiagnosed and untreated for too long (i.e., the 7+ years it typically takes to get a diagnosis), endo gets dramatically worse, building on itself each menstrual cycle and often resulting in worsening pain and scarring of the pelvic organs.

Systemic Hormones, a Different Story

The other factor in the estrogen-progesterone story for many of us is an imbalance in the number of hormones circulating through the whole body, known as a *systemic hormonal imbalance*. Namely, many of us deal with something known as estrogen dominance. However, this term does not necessarily mean we have too much estrogen coursing through our bodies. While the localized area of your endo may be highly estrogenic (as you just learned), there's no guarantee you are overflowing with estrogen. The opposite could easily be true, and perhaps why some sufferers feel even worse when they diligently work to lower their estrogen.

Rather, estrogen dominance means having excess estrogen *relative to* progesterone—the teeter-totter is off balance. This can look very different depending on your body. Here are some potential scenarios in the endo body:

- Normal estrogen and progesterone levels, yet you have progesterone resistance
- Normal estrogen levels but low progesterone levels and/or progesterone resistance
- Low or even very low estrogen levels and *really* low progesterone levels and/or progesterone resistance
- High estrogen levels and normal progesterone levels and/or progesterone resistance
- *Really* high estrogen levels and high, normal, and/or low progesterone levels or progesterone resistance

The Many Faces of Estrogen Dominance

Estrogen dominance doesn't necessarily mean you have too much estrogen. Rather, it refers to an imbalance when estrogen dominates over progesterone. With endo, it could look like any of the following.

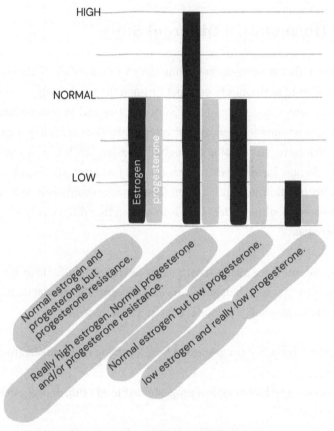

Note That:

- You can have endo and have high, normal, or even low amounts of circulating estrogen.
- You could have normal levels of progesterone, yet battle with progesterone resistance which creates symptoms of deficiency.
- This is why it's imperative to test before diligently working to balance your own unique "hormonal fingerprint."

Frustratingly for diagnosis, symptoms of estrogen dominance can be similar across the board, whether your own imbalance is due to high or low estrogen levels, or low to very low progesterone levels. Symptoms include what a lot of us with endo deal on the regular, including heavy/thick/clotted or painful periods (the type of periods we *don't* want), terrible PMS symptoms, premenstrual spotting, lack of abundant fertile quality cervical fluid at ovulation (also known as "egg-white" type discharge that happens mid-cycle), moodiness, painful or swollen breasts, acne, and/or a short luteal phase (the time between ovulation and menses that should be 12–14 days).

While the level of imbalance can look different for each of us, estrogen dominating over your progesterone will communicate to your body to grow cells and inflame tissue. Without enough progesterone, you won't be able to balance out the estrogen response, which is absolutely essential to cool estrogen growth and modulate the immune response. This is why, *if* you have estrogen dominance, you will probably do well to naturally increase your systemic progesterone levels (as I discuss in Part 4). Doing so may start to mitigate the potentially life-altering symptoms associated with an estrogen-progesterone imbalance that many of us with endo suffer from.

Stress Hormones: Cortisol and Adrenaline

The other hormonal elephants in the endo room are your stress hormones, namely cortisol and adrenaline. Psychological stress is the umbrella term for all the negative emotions you can experience (think anger, jealousy, anxiety, depression, nervousness, etc.), and cortisol and adrenaline flood the body when it feels these emotions come on. But cortisol and adrenaline can also be produced during times of chemical or physiological stress, stimulated by anything from blood sugar dysregulation and caffeine to poor sleep patterns. These chemical or physical stressors cause your body to increase systemic stress hormones, even if your mental state feels fine.

While our bodies are made to deal with stressors in short bouts, they are not hardwired to deal with stress that never ends. And in today's fast-paced, tech-heavy, and sugar- and caffeine-laden worlds, our stress can become chronic. This will begin to affect immune system behavior, which relies on complex communication links between the hormonal and nervous systems to know when to prioritize an immune attack (inflame) or tissue repair.

When your body is ramped up with fight-or-flight hormones, your nervous system kicks into *sympathetic mode* where inflammation is prioritized. This would make ancestral sense since a body in a fight-or-flight mode would *actually* be in a life-or-death scenario (not just being canceled on social media), so the immune system would prioritize inflammation in case you need to heal a wound fast. Conversely, when you're peaceful and relaxed, the switch is flipped to *parasympathetic mode* where healing, rejuvenation, and repair are prioritized.

Unfortunately, high levels of both cortisol and adrenaline are associated with endometriosis establishment *and* progression. This is thanks to the hormone–immune conversation, where a constant surge in adrenaline tells the immune system to produce many of the *exact* inflammatory immune players endometriosis relies on to thrive.[87] Not to mention that chronic stress promotes "stress-induced immune dysregulation," which has been associated with a state of chronic low-grade inflammation.[88] This may be why mice subjected to chronic stress tests developed endo lesions twice the size of those without chronic stress.[89] Conversely, blocking adrenaline production has been noticed to *stop* the rooting down and progression of endo.[90] This is how stress becomes an actual endometriosis lesion provoker and grower, much more than just affecting symptoms.

And while so many in today's world are dealing with chronic stress, those of us living with a health condition like endo may have even more. In fact, studies have shown that over two-thirds of women with endo have mild to high levels of stress, while 57 percent of women with endometriosis reported so much chronic anxiety they viewed it as a *personality trait* compared to 8.3 percent of women without endo.[91] This is so different from experiencing a stressful event that then passes and we're calm again. Nearly two-thirds of us believe it's part of who we are at our core—we're just "stressed people" who are chronically anxious, fluttery, worried, nervous, or overwhelmed. It may be due to your endo that you feel this way (chronic pain and emotional wear can do that), or it may be because society as we know it has done that to us. Probably a bit of both. Unfortunately, a chronic stress mindset like this may be directly fueling endo-ing in the body.

Symptom-wise, stress continues to be an endo-provoker. Over time, a chronic stress response will affect your master regulator of stress hormones (called the Hypothalamic-Pituitary-Adrenal Axis, or HPA), creating dysfunction. Dysfunction can look different depending on how long your body has been dealing with stress. Initially, you may be stuck in an alarm phase, where your body is no longer picking up cues that your "threat" is gone and instead keeps you in a fight-or-flight response. You may now constantly feel anxious, worried, agitated, or "wired but tired," yet are unable to relax.

When the alarm stage goes on for too long, cortisol levels will eventually start to drop. While this may not sound problematic at first, know that cortisol isn't *just* used for stress but also for proper wakefulness, rest, and moods. If your cortisol level is blunted, you may find yourself in a state of deep exhaustion—chronic fatigue if you will—something many of us with endo are known to have. You may not be able to wake up easily, nor perform your daily tasks without crumbling. You may have brain fog, be irritable, and be unable to focus. I was there too, with chronic fatigue being one of my worst symptoms, something so different from being just "tired" that many days it would feel like a Herculean effort to simply get up and take a shower.

HPA dysfunction is associated with endo in numerous other ways. Low cortisol is associated with the type of incapacitating pain women with endo experience,[92] while high cortisol levels were significantly higher in endo patients dealing with infertility.[93] In fact, being stressed during ovulation may reduce your chances of conception by nearly 50 percent![94] You may have noticed your own symptoms of stress directly affect your own cycle, either through reduced production of healthy cervical fluid at ovulation, delayed ovulation or irregular periods, increased PMS symptoms, or more painful or heavy periods. Are you beginning to see the stress–endo connection more clearly?

TAKING BACK CONTROL

I hope that looking at the relationship between endometriosis and hormones through this lens helps you cultivate new respect for estrogen, progesterone, cortisol, adrenaline, and the wide variety of hormones in general. Truly, estrogen is not the enemy: your body wants and needs healthy *balanced* circulating estrogen levels to thrive! In the context of endo, the challenge becomes finding a healthy balance within the body.

Instead, we can be more strategic about the two hormonal fronts that may be affecting the endo: hormones directly at the lesion site, and systemic levels of hormones. Addressing both may truly help us feel better symptomatically, and may even slow endo disease progression. While your own systemic hormonal imbalance will be unique to you, there is plenty we can all do to benefit our body ecology to help our hormone signaling. I will discuss this in Chapter 14.

LOOKING AT CHRONIC INFLAMMATION AS THE SUM OF MANY PARTS

To summarize, there are still many factors that may be driving endo-related inflammation, either fostering endo locally or contributing to immune dysfunction systemically. Here are some of what we've already touched on, or will in the sections to come:

Iron Overload: Excess blood in the peritoneal cavity can lead to iron overload, which is very inflammatory in this should-be-blood-free zone. Heavy, clotted, and/or thick periods may contribute through retrograde menstruation, as will endo lesions once established.

Chemicals: Endocrine-disrupting chemicals (EDCs), fire retardants, herbicides, pesticides, the list goes on. Each of these may play a prominent role in promoting inflammation *and* immune dysfunction, both within the peritoneal cavity and systemically.

Oxidative Stress: Too many free radicals + not enough antioxidants = cellular damage.

Nutrient Deficiencies: Your body needs nutrients to feed your immune system during times of inflammation. Without enough specific nutrients, it's possible for your body to be unable to heal from inflammation, contributing to the inflammation cycle.

High Levels of Blood Sugar or Insulin: High levels of glucose are associated with increased free-radical damage; too much insulin is associated with the type of immune dysfunction that allows endo lesions to stay and grow. This, altogether, creates more damage, which thus invites more inflammation.

Inflammatory Fats: Our modern diets are often stuffed with omega-6 fats, a type of fat that feeds the inflammatory process.

Sedentary Lifestyle: As muscles atrophy (which they naturally do when not being used), the body must constantly repair the inflammatory damage of muscle loss.

Sleep Deprivation: Even one night of botched sleep increases levels of inflammation in the body.

Stress: High levels of stress hormones (adrenaline and cortisol) tell your body there is danger near. In response, it heightens levels of inflammation in case you're attacked.

Endometriosis Lesions: Once established, lesions will produce their own inflammatory immune factors and excess blood. And, as they grow, they will continue to damage surrounding tissue, which increases inflammation even more.

Chapter 7:
A Strategic Path Forward

Learning that endometriosis is a disease of chronic inflammation with immune dysfunction may seem initially daunting. But I can assure you that it doesn't necessarily have to be. There is so much within our control when it comes to reducing inflammation and modulating our immune response to reduce your endo symptoms! When inflammation is the root of the problem, we can make some incredible inroads to healing by zapping the inflammatory triggers.

This brings us to the complex yet rewarding job of formulating your personal healing plan. Because there are two areas of inflammation in the endo body, we will focus on a two-pronged approach to correct the inflammatory triggers that may be affecting you: address inflammation at the localized site of your endo, as well as systemic, body-wide inflammation. Indeed, most people today have many *constant* inflammatory triggers that eventually become too much for the body to bear, triggers that have even become normalized issues like too little sleep, too much sugar and ultra-processed foods, not enough movement, and way too much stress.

These behaviors have a profound impact on your inflammatory burden, as well as your immune function. This is why you may experience an endo flare with certain food choices or after a terribly stressful month, or why diet and lifestyle changes alone have dramatically stopped endo symptoms for some lucky ones. Once you adopt new lifestyle behaviors to remove the triggers, you will allow your immune system to cool its jets and perhaps slow or stop the process of endo-ing.

When Inflammation Is the Problem, Address the Inflammation

We have too much inflammation, both localized and body-wide, altogether contributing to advancing our endo and causing the immune system dysfunction associated with it

Solution: A Two-Pronged Approach

Address the localized inflammation at the site of your endo lesions

- Remove gut and/or reproductive tract infections
- Ensure your periods aren't thick, clotted, and heavy
- Eat boatloads upon boatloads of antioxidants
- Bring blood flow back to the peritoneal cavity and reduce intra-abdominal pressure
- Remove endo-provoking chemicals
- Consult with an endo surgeon about removing endo lesions

Address the additional issues of systemic inflammation triggering the immune system dysfunction

- Address chronic stress
- Food triggers/allergens
- Chemical exposure
- Movement issues
- Sleep issues
- Incorrect breathing patterns
- Have more fun. Laugh
- Eat lots of veggies
- Be outdoors
- Reverse nutrient deficiencies
- Balance blood sugar
- Everything else in the following chapters

THE WHOLE-BODY APPROACH TO REDUCING INFLAMMATION

In the pages that follow, you will learn about some of the best diet and lifestyle techniques shown in research to support the endo body. As a Nutritional Therapist, my job is to teach these methods to help shift a body that suffers from inflammation, hormonal imbalances, gut issues, stress, and immune dysfunction (basically one that may be radically endo-ing), to one that is deeply nourished—body, mind, and soul. This approach has helped many sufferers find a new normal, one without chronic misery. When we change certain inputs for the better, we *can* re-regulate the immune system, lower inflammation, balance hormones, and support overall health. A massive amount of research supports this.

In fact, I consider nutrition an important, if not essential, step to begin healing anew. The food you eat has the ability to *create* inflammation, or *soothe* the immune system. It can repair muscles and tissues, or it can cause the body to get bogged down under too many inflammatory triggers. It can create chronic, unrelenting stress in your body (i.e., are you often "hangry," shaky, or irritable when you're hungry?), or it can help balance your moods and cycles. It can either *create* immune dysfunction or help heal from immune dysfunction. Certain healing diets have even been shown to literally change epigenetic expression from a diseased state back to a normalized state.[95] Yes, this can all happen through our food choices.

While there isn't an "endo diet" we could easily prescribe to everyone, after pouring through the research, four distinct dietary foundations emerged that not only reduce symptoms, but may also potentially reduce the size, progression, and intensity of endometriosis lesions. That's an endo-healing diet we all can agree on. The foundation of this dietary approach includes:

1. Reversing under-nutrition + increasing antioxidants
2. Balancing macronutrients (i.e., fats, carbs, and proteins)
3. Removing triggers
4. Balancing the gut microbiome

And while what you put into your body will make a big difference when it comes to healing, it's not the only thing that will influence your endo. Equally important are how you move your body, how your mental health fares, and what chemicals you're in contact with. These are what I consider the "lifestyle" aspects of health or disease.

Each of these facets contributes to the functioning (or dysfunctioning) of your bodily systems, directly affecting your immune and hormonal systems, and also your endo. It's why I like to remind clients that we often have 99 inflammatory problems, and established endometriosis lesions are *just one* of them. Utilizing diet and lifestyle strategies to balance your immune system's inflammatory response and create a healthy whole-body ecology is your ticket to reducing your endo symptoms. This will be the main focus of the next two sections of this book.

Although I'm not a medical professional, the following sections will also touch on other treatments known to address endo: oral contraceptives, pain medication, surgery, and certain Complementary and Alternative Medicine (CAM) treatments shown to help support healing. Together, I hope this information will begin unraveling some of the best options that may benefit the average endo sufferer.

THE IMPORTANCE OF SURGERY

Please note that while holistic care is an important part of healing from endo (and the focus of this book), it simply does not take the place of surgery when you need one. Indeed, there is a wide swath of endo experts that believe surgery is so important that *everyone* should have their endo excised in order to truly heal. This is why surgical removal of lesions by an endometriosis expert is considered the "gold standard" in treating the disease because it (quite literally) removes the diseased tissue. So while you implement holistic care options in your life, please don't be sidetracked into thinking that diet and lifestyle factors alone can "treat" your own case of endo. If you're not feeling improvement please be honest with yourself, consult with an endo expert, and never ignore lingering or returning symptoms as they can be signs of endo progression. See Further Reading for many incredible books and films that dive deep into the topic of a properly done surgery.

Stopping Cyclical Inflammation

Inflammation that never ends leads to a repeated cycle of tissue injury and repair (ReTiar). This is a cycle that promotes endo-ing. Luckily, there are many factors we can address through integrative care to minimize this inflammatory response, the focus of the next chapters..

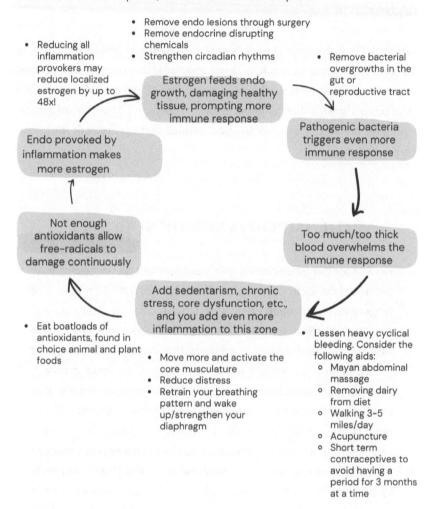

- Reducing all inflammation provokers may reduce localized estrogen by up to 48x!

- Remove endo lesions through surgery
- Remove endocrine disrupting chemicals
- Strengthen circadian rhythms

Estrogen feeds endo growth, damaging healthy tissue, prompting more immune response

- Remove bacterial overgrowths in the gut or reproductive tract

Pathogenic bacteria triggers even more immune response

Endo provoked by inflammation makes more estrogen

Not enough antioxidants allow free-radicals to damage continuously

Too much/too thick blood overwhelms the immune response

Add sedentarism, chronic stress, core dysfunction, etc., and you add even more inflammation to this zone

- Eat boatloads of antioxidants, found in choice animal and plant foods

- Move more and activate the core musculature
- Reduce distress
- Retrain your breathing pattern and wake up/strengthen your diaphragm

- Lessen heavy cyclical bleeding. Consider the following aids:
  o Mayan abdominal massage
  o Removing dairy from diet
  o Walking 3-5 miles/day
  o Acupuncture
  o Short term contraceptives to avoid having a period for 3 months at a time

TIME TO HEAL

Discovering that endo depends on a rogue inflammatory response that has gone a bit haywire thanks to immune dysfunction, gave me a new direction, as I hope it does for you. It showed me that there may be another way out of the cycle of endo pain and despair. When we stop the inflammatory triggers, it may help the body stop *endo-ing*. When we replace negative triggers with soothing inputs, we can calm our symptoms, slow or reverse progression, or even find a place on the remission sliding scale. If we get an expert surgery, we can change our health trajectory in the course of hours rather than suffering for decades. Many endo sufferers have successfully walked this path before you, and I encourage you to give this type of healing an opportunity.

And still, I want to be very clear. Depending on your unique case of endometriosis, you may need more professional support beyond diet, lifestyle, or even surgery, to fully rectify the amount of illness you may be dealing with. I've had women reach out to me over the years with *many* issues that would need more professional guidance— such as autoimmune diseases, SIBO infections, continuous monthly vaginal bleeding, and the list goes on. Complex cases like these often take skilled professionals to address. So although this book touches on numerous issues associated with endo and the *basics* of how to address them, it is simply no substitute for working with sophisticated medical professionals when needed.

If you're ready to start healing anew, let's move on to the next chapters to learn how to heal endo.

Part III:

Healing with Nutrition

Nutrition may be considered one foundational pillar to healing from endo. Without adequate nutrients or antioxidants, we won't be able to quell an inflammatory response. If our blood sugar is imbalanced, it could lead to endo progression and tissue damage. If we continue to eat foods that provoke inflammation, we may be contributing to immune dysfunction. Yes, all through the foods we eat. In the following chapters, we will discuss how proper food choices aren't just important for healing from endo, but essential.

Chapter 8:

A Nutrient-Dense Diet

Consider nutrient intake as the most important starting point for any endo-healing diet. That's because every one of your eleven body systems requires ample amounts of nutrients to do their jobs. Nutrients allow your body to think quickly, have stress resilience, fight inflammation, make babies, balance hormones and support immune function. In fact, your immune system has one of the highest nutrient demands in the body, and low nutrient intake *alone* can foster a certain level of immune dysfunction![96] If you're not eating enough nutrients, your body simply won't be able to perform the many essential tasks it needs to do for optimal health. This is why nutrients aren't just important for healing from endo, they are essential.

The problem is that most of us don't fully understand what nutrition really is. I certainly didn't for years. Like many of us, I was raised in a diet culture where it was "good" to restrict "bad" foods, although what was considered good and bad seemed to be based on opinion and new diet trends more than anything else. Instead, the study of nutrition is really about understanding both the balance and overall quantity of nutrients your body needs to function: vitamins, minerals, polyphenols, amino acids, fatty acids, and more. Nutrients are the fundamental ingredients in the chemical reactions that your body needs to survive and thrive. In fact, your body performs trillions of chemical reactions *per second*, with each reaction depending on an assortment of specific nutrients. No nutrient fuel, no chemical reaction, and your body will begin to feel lousy.

NUTRIENTS VS. CALORIES

To better understand how nutrient fuel differs from fuel from calories, let's pretend we're baking cookies. You can imagine the oven is heated on calories, while your ingredients are the nutrients. Even if your oven is very hot with plenty of calories, if you don't have enough ingredients (nutrients) your cookies will be of poor quality, even though the oven is hot as can be. This is where the terms "Stuffed yet Starved" and "Overfed and Undernourished" come from, acknowledging that while calories today are ubiquitous, nutrients are not, and deficiencies are contributing to a public health epidemic of disease.

NUTRIENT DEFICIENT, THE ENDO NORMAL

To better understand which nutrients we should be consuming regularly, the USDA has a nutritional framework called the Recommended Daily Intake, or RDI. The RDI is based on the *lowest* amount of a nutrient needed to prevent acute deficiency. For example, the RDI for vitamin C is set at 75 mg/day for an adult woman to prevent scurvy (an acute vitamin C deficiency). The problem is that the RDI *doesn't* tell us how many nutrients we need for optimal health—i.e., how much vitamin C you would need to not just prevent scurvy but also to optimize immune function, fertility, stress resilience, or even healing from endo. Research has clues, those with endo benefit from a whopping 1000mg/day, thirteen times the recommended intake![97] As you can see, it may be easier than we realize to be running a deficit.

Unfortunately, nutrient deficiencies are widespread in today's world—yes even in wealthy industrialized countries such as the United States. A recent US National Survey found that nearly *all* Americans aren't getting adequate levels of many nutrients; for example, 94 percent are deficient in vitamin D, 88 percent in vitamin E, 100 percent in potassium, and 52 percent in magnesium.[98] Thanks to the ubiquitous rise in highly refined and processed foods, we're quickly becoming a nation that is both stuffed with calories, yet starved for nutrients. And, unfortunately, if you analyze published literature linking those with endometriosis and their nutrient intake, something will quickly become very clear to you: *those with endometriosis appear to be more undernourished than their non-endo counterparts.* It's one part of the multifactorial problem of endo, and it is important because under-nutrition may be partly to blame for your endo pain, progression, severity, infertility, hormone imbalance, brain fog, immune system dysfunction, and more.

Under-nutrition becomes even more problematic when dealing with a chronic inflammatory condition like endometriosis, which often makes our nutrient requirements *higher* than our non-endo counterparts (meaning we need to consume more nutrients than a healthy, disease-free person does). This may be due to:

- **Increased immune needs:** if you have an enormous chronic, inflammatory attack happening inside, your immune system will burn through nutrients like wildfire. Thus, you will need more vitamins and minerals than someone without chronic inflammation.
- **Tissue damage that ensues from oxidative stress:** constantly mending tissues will require more nutrients. Someone with chronic inflammation may need 1.5 to 2 times *more* protein than a healthy individual.[99]
- **Excess free radicals:** to quell free radicals, we may need a lot more antioxidants. High levels of free radicals are perhaps why endometriosis sufferers were found to have fewer antioxidants in their systems, even though they were consuming the same amount of antioxidants as their non-endo peers. This suggests our nutrient need is much higher than our disease-free counterparts due to our chronic inflammatory battle.[100]

Even though our endo bodies may have higher nutrient needs, we may unknowingly experience nutrient loss through diet and lifestyle choices that rob us of critical nutrients. Stress, caffeine, hormonal birth control, and alcohol each deplete a variety of nutrients, including calcium, B vitamins, vitamin C, sodium, potassium, vitamins A and E, and magnesium.[101] So if you are living a high-stress life while drinking alcohol and caffeine and taking oral contraceptives (as many of us are), you can start to understand how precious nutrients may also be flushing all too easily out of your system.

The inability to properly absorb nutrients may also play a pivotal role in endometriosis-related deficiencies and nutrient loss. Knowing the majority of us with endo present with digestive issues of some degree—such as chronic diarrhea, inability to fully digest proteins or fats, dysbiosis, increased gut permeability, and intestinal inflammation—we can assume that most people with endo will have some level of difficulty absorbing nutrients, even if they're eating the most nutrient-dense foods on the planet. These digestive issues *literally* mean nutrients are flushed down the toilet, another reminder of why healing your gut should be priority number one.

Taken together, this explains how you may not have an *acute* deficiency (like scurvy), but rather may develop a set of symptoms due to *subclinical* deficiencies that can also cause serious issues. This is well illustrated by the example of vitamin D. While acute deficiency leads to rickets (the softening of bones in children), a subclinical deficiency is associated with symptoms such as depressed immunity, back pain, fatigue, depression, and fertility issues. If that sounds like a lot of your endo issues, you may not be surprised that endo sufferers are more than *twice* as likely to be deficient in vitamin D, which may even play a role in the severity of your endometriosis diagnosis.[102]

Of course, vitamin D is just one missing nutrient of many associated with endometriosis. A 2015 paper on diet and endometriosis confirms that numerous dietary nutrients *directly* influence endometriosis expression, as well as hormonal balance, normal cell death, cell signaling, and more.[103] So interwoven are nutrients with endometriosis, the paper concludes that nutrient-deficient diets "may be involved in [endo] genesis and progression" and that diet alone is "a promising tool in the prevention and treatment of endometriosis." Yes, you heard right: prevention *and* treatment.

ENDO DIETARY CONFUSION 101

If you've heard that you're supposed to avoid eating a long list of foods if you have endo, please know that most mainstream endo-diet recommendations come from an extraordinarily limited number of *observational studies*. These types of studies analyze dietary or lifestyle patterns mainly through generalized questionnaires rather than controlled experiments, leaving us with some confounding information. On one hand, we see conflicting information. Some studies suggest that eating more fiber and more fruit increases endometriosis risk while eating more dairy decreases risk (something many of us would cringe at).[104] Whereas others say exactly the opposite.[105] There are studies observing that red meat consumption is associated with endometriosis and others not at all.[106] One study claimed that increased fruit consumption upped endo risk while another claimed it decreased endo risk.[107] Confusing, eh?

This is why I believe it's greatly misleading to use limited studies like these to create specific diet recommendations for a complex disease like endo. Not only are they unable to inform us on the correct approach, but highlighting what to restrict without advising what foods to replace them with is also a surefire way to create a nutritionally empty diet (like one based on gluten-free pasta and low-fat almond milk over cereal). Instead, I recommend clients with any food restriction mindsets swap their focus to nutrient infusion!

THE ENDO-9

To reverse nutrient deficiencies, we need to shift our focus away from an old "endo-diet" belief in restricting foods to a new perspective that will start to heal our bodies: *eating as many nutrient-dense foods as possible.*

Nutrient density refers to the number of nutrients found per calorie of food. For example, 500 calories of cookies will have a very different impact on your genetic expression and immune function than 500 calories of salmon, since there are simply more vitamins and minerals per bite in salmon.

When you use nutrient density to guide your food choices, it means you can be eating far more nutrients while consuming the same number of calories. This is the mindset needed to reverse under-nutrition: *replace* the foods that have little to low nutrient density (toast, pasta, chips, baked goods, desserts, cereals, rice, etc.) with the most nutrient-dense foods on the planet: **cold-water fatty fish, seafood, organ meats, seaweed, healthy fats, egg yolks, bone broths, a few fruits, and tons of vegetables.**

You may be alarmed to realize that you don't eat many of these foods, either in quantity or at all. Please stick with me as I explain exactly why these foods are pivotal to healing through the lens of nine nutrients, which I call "The Endo-9". These nine nutrients are particularly essential for immune system re-regulation, antioxidant status, anti-inflammatory support, and healing from endo.

The Endo-9 are:

- Magnesium
- Zinc
- Iron
- Vitamin D3
- Vitamin A
- Vitamins C & E
- Omega 3s (EPA + DHA)
- Phytonutrients

ERIN'S STORY

Before I met Katie my fatigue was overwhelming to the point where just taking a shower would exhaust me and send me back to bed. The pain, always a 10/10, left me trembling in fear for the next flare-up. My career, my independence, my joy, my finances, and my health had left me, and what remained was a shell of a human with no hope of ever living a normal life. Katie changed that with the Heal Endo approach, and to this day I tell everyone she gave my life back to me. Her approach to my situation was so *individualized*, which was something I had not encountered from anyone along my healing journey yet.

In my case, the biggest obstacle to tackle first was food. I was severely malnourished, so I switched gears to start eating as many nutrient-dense foods as possible. I was so excited to focus on adding foods in, instead of taking them away. Because we went slowly at my own pace, creating lifestyle changes rather than implementing "diets," I was never intimidated or overwhelmed by her suggestions, which is huge considering I lived in a perpetual state of overwhelm at this time. As I built up strength, I increased my daily goals to include more cooking, exercise, and mindfulness. I added targeted supplements. I focused on eliminating anxiety and learning how to mitigate stressors that would zap my health.

I was unwavering in my dedication to the Heal Endo approach. Although it took a few months, my health transformed and I was able to participate more in life. Within a few more months, I was almost back to my normal self. A few more months after that, and no one would have any idea that previously I had been so ill I couldn't get out of bed. Katie's approach quite literally worked a miracle for me. If you haven't tried it, I recommend you give it a go!" - Erin, USA

Magnesium

Magnesium is a mineral used by the body to help muscles relax or contract, cope with stress, and send messages through the nervous system. Deficiency is important for endo sufferers to understand because magnesium is a *vital* supporting factor in anti-inflammation and antioxidant activity—which is perhaps why low magnesium intake has been associated be an increased risk factor for developing endo.[108]

How could this be? Turns out, a deficiency in magnesium alone can release inflammatory cytokines, acute-phase proteins, and excessive free radicals—numerous components endometriosis requires to establish and progress.[109] Deficiency is associated with increased levels of oxidative stress and a weakened antioxidant defense, more factors endometriosis requires to establish and progress.[110] If you don't have enough magnesium, consider yourself likely to be endo-ing.

Painful periods and severe PMS are additional symptoms of magnesium deficiency, both of which many of us with endo can relate to!

Women with painful periods have been shown to be much lower in magnesium than those without period pain.[111] In fact, supplementing with magnesium at even just 250 mg/day was shown to significantly reduce or relieve painful menses as well as other PMS symptoms, including headaches, depression, muscle and back pain, anxiety, water retention, and cravings.[112] One study found supplementing with magnesium significantly reduced pain in 21 out of 25 participants after only 6 months by reducing prostaglandins, an immune factor implicated in the inflammation and pain associated with endo.[113] One large 2017 review article declared the "picture that emerges indicates that magnesium supplementation is effective in the prevention of [period pain], [PMS], and menstrual migraine."[114]

Testing for magnesium deficiency is challenging since about 99 percent of it is stored in the muscles, bones, teeth, organs, and other tissues, and only 1 percent is found in the blood. Still, there are basic symptoms you can follow. Early signs of deficiency may include fatigue and lethargy, anxiety, or weakness, while more advanced stages of deficiency may involve migraines, constipation, PMS, painful periods, and muscle spasms. Fun fact: muscle/foot/leg cramps at rest are more associated with magnesium deficiency, and leg cramps with exercise associated with potassium deficiency. But, if you have endometriosis, PMS, painful periods, muscle cramps, and inflammation it's probably safe to assume you're deficient to some degree.

Food Fix: Foods rich in magnesium include nuts, seeds, beans, vegetables, cacao, and herbs. But because soils have become so depleted of magnesium (perhaps why we consume less than half the amount our ancestors did 100 years ago!), it may also be wise to supplement.[115] If you talk to your doctor and decide to supplement, consider 500 mg of magnesium glycinate a day. It's absorbed much better and doesn't affect the bowel like the more commonly used magnesium citrate. Consider supplementing simultaneously with vitamin B6 which supports magnesium uptake within cells.

Zinc

Zinc is a powerful antioxidant and anti-inflammatory mineral that acts to quell inflammation, scavenge free radicals, support the immune system, heal wounds, and support fertility. Pretty cool.

Unfortunately, simply having endometriosis may be a significant reason to suspect you are deficient in zinc. Women with endo have been found to be *highly* deficient in comparison to their non-endo peers.[116] One 2014 study even suggests that zinc is found to be so low in women with endo it could actually be used as a marker to detect women at high risk of endometriosis (as well as be used to immediately help support infertility cases).[117] That's because zinc is necessary for procreation, with deficiency alone found to decrease egg size, cause problems within egg cells, and prohibit an egg's ability to properly divide after fertilization.[118]

Because zinc is a critical antioxidant, reversing deficiencies can significantly reduce inflammatory markers and oxidative stress.[119] Perhaps this is why zinc treatment given in the days preceding menses has been shown to reduce menstrual pain.[120] So if you're deficient in zinc, you may be dealing with some infertility issues, menstrual pain, immune dysfunction, and inflammation to boot. All the things we need to stop endo-ing.

Symptoms of zinc deficiency may include cuts that are slow to heal, hair loss, acne, an underperforming immune system, and/or chronically coming down with *something*, white spots on fingernails, or (oddly enough) a reduced sense of taste or smell. If you want further testing, you can measure zinc levels via a blood test.

Food Fix: Zinc is by far best absorbed from animal foods. Best options include red meat (beef, lamb, bison, etc.), organs (liver or kidney), seafood, or shellfish. Eating these foods on a regular basis will be important for those of us with chronic inflammation. Plant-based options like seeds, nuts, and certain grains and legumes are considered secondary sources because they are not as easily absorbed. This is why the RDI for zinc is set 50 percent higher for vegetarians (12 mg instead of 8 mg/day) and why long-time vegetarians and vegans have consistently been found to be significantly lower in zinc status than omnivores.[121]

While meeting (or exceeding) the RDI is important, supplementation may be an essential step to reverse already existing deficiencies. If you have strong symptoms of deficiency (see above), talk with your doctors about supplementation. Functional medicine doctors often recommend 30 mg zinc taken daily for three months (you don't want to supplement for too long at high doses as it can knock other minerals out of balance, such as copper). I recommend seeking out quality brands that have been third-party tested, such as Pure Encapsulations.

Iron

Iron is best known for energy production. It's an essential ingredient to make hemoglobin, a protein within blood cells that carries oxygen to where it's needed in the body. No iron, no oxygen to muscles or organs, *including* your ovaries, eggs, uterus, and pelvic cavity. Perhaps that's why iron is necessary for both healthy ovulation and a proper immune response.[122] You can see why iron is extremely important to us endo sufferers dealing with fatigue, infertility, and immune dysfunction.

Iron deficiency becomes extra problematic when talking about oxidative stress-related inflammation (the type of damage created by free radicals, and a key characteristic of endometriosis). It's well documented that iron deficiency increases oxidative stress by reducing the number of antioxidants in the system.[123] In fact, researchers found that by supplementing anemic participants with iron for six weeks, there was a significant decrease in oxidative stress. All of this means that iron is much more important to your antioxidant and anti-inflammatory activities than you may have realized, and it's one reason why iron supplementation is recommended for those with anemia to heal the antioxidant defense system.[124]

Those with endometriosis may be more likely to be iron deficient (anemic) than those without endo. This could be due to numerous factors, including heavy menstrual bleeding, digestive disorders that prevent proper iron uptake, or chronic inflammation that also reduces iron levels. It's why, if you have endometriosis, you may need even more iron than someone without endo to maintain proper iron sufficiency.[125]

Iron deficiency symptoms may include fatigue, bruising, headaches, shortness of breath, dizziness, or pale skin (think symptoms of oxygenated blood not getting where it needs to be). As someone who's had anemia, I can attest that being deficient in iron can make you feel like your body is made out of lead. Of course, you can also be subclinically deficient in iron and have no outward symptoms—which is why testing is key.

Luckily, iron levels are easy to test for. So, if you are reading this and have endometriosis, *please go get tested*. If you're deficient, you may start feeling a little better within mere days of supplementing. You'll want to ask for a CBC to look at your serum blood levels, and additionally a ferritin test that measures your *stored* iron. Some doctors may be hesitant to order a ferritin lab test because of insurance pushback, but they might be more comfortable ordering it if you describe your anemia symptoms. (Of note, most Western medicine doctors view ferritin levels above 11 as okay, but for optimal health, energy levels, and fertility you will want your ferritin to be at least 50 ng/mL.)

Food Fix: For menstruating women who are omnivores, the RDI for iron is 18 mg iron/day, although as someone with endometriosis you may need more.

The best iron-rich food sources are animal products because they contain a highly absorbable form of iron called heme iron. Best options include a 3.5-oz portion of chicken liver (9.9 mg), canned oysters (6.65 mg), beef liver (6.3 mg), or ground beef (2.68 mg), although nearly all animal foods will have iron to some degree.

Plant options contain the less absorbable form, non-heme iron, so vegetarians and vegans must consume nearly double the amount of iron (1.8x more) to meet the basic vegetarian quota set at 32.4 mg/day. Best sources include dark leafy greens, broccoli, beans, and grains. Because 32.4 mg/day is a challenging amount to ingest daily, vegetarians are consistently found to have lower iron stores than non-vegetarians.[126] Meeting the basic RDI of plant-based iron would include eating about 5 cups of *cooked* spinach (equivalent to 55 cups raw) or 17 cups of cooked broccoli every day, which is why a vegetarian or vegan may consider continuous iron supplementation.

TO GET MORE IRON, TRY THESE TIPS:

- **Combine heme iron, non-heme iron, and vitamin C in the same meal.** Research shows that eating animal- and plant-based iron at the same meal increased the absorption of plant-based iron by about 250 percent, compared to a meal without animal-based iron.[127] Additionally, consuming iron with a rich source of vitamin C may increase iron absorption by up to 414 percent.[128] Think grass-fed beef patties over a bed of lightly sautéed spinach and bell peppers.
- **Cook with a cast-iron pan.** This alone can increase the amount of iron in foods between 2 and 21 times, depending on the acidity of the food being cooked. For example, an egg cooked in a cast-iron pan has 2 mg more iron than an egg cooked in another pan, while tomato sauce would have a whopping 5 mg more iron per 3-oz serving.129 These pans are an amazingly effective and simple way of increasing iron content.

- **Avoid dairy products, teas, or coffee with your iron-containing meals,** as well as avoid acid blockers like Tums. These prohibit iron uptake, so even if you're eating iron-rich foods your body won't be able to properly absorb it.
- **Eat liver.** Liver is an iron superhero, among other nutrients, although the taste is something to be acquired for most of us. Baby steps include liver paté, ground liver hidden in burgers or chili (seriously, this works), or even desiccated liver pills for the truly squeamish.
- **Supplement.** If you test first and know you're deficient, it's important to work with a professional to reverse deficiency, since too much iron can be just as problematic as too little. When supplementing, consider a gentle iron that doesn't cause constipation, such as Ferrochel Iron Chelate by Designs for Health.

Vitamin A

Vitamin A (retinoids) is an invaluable fat-soluble vitamin used for immune function, reproduction, eye/skin/mucous membrane health, as well as antioxidant functions. Our immune system is somewhat of a binge drinker of vitamin A because of its anti-inflammatory superpower and critical role in enhancing immune function.[130] This vitamin has consistently demonstrated a therapeutic effect in addressing a variety of diseases. It's also *essential* for reproduction and embryo development, as well as essential for detoxifying BPA from the body (and remember, BPA is implicated in the creation of endo-like cells).[131] Even sub-acute deficiency may cause trouble conceiving, poor night vision, acne (skin health), dry skin or eyes, or put you on the "sick train" of constant illnesses.

When it comes to endo, vitamin A becomes extra important. If you remember back to the epigenetics of endo, endometrial cells go through a process where they become mesenchymal cells, proverbially turning normal cells into "jacked navy seals." These cells are now better able to migrate, infiltrate, and invade the nooks and crannies of the body, resulting in new lesions. Yet, vitamin A may be able to suppress this transition.[132] This may be why it's been demonstrated that increasing vitamin A availability decreases the size of endo lesions.[133]

Unfortunately, vitamin A is often a neglected nutrient in our modern diet, with 51 percent of Americans not consuming adequate amounts.[134] In addition, we may need *even more vitamin A than the non-endo population* (because vitamin A is quickly used up when faced with chronic inflammation and infection, both of which we contend with), making it even more imperative to ensure we're getting enough.[135]

Food Fix: To boost your vitamin A levels, consume it directly in the retinoid form. The *best* options for this include liver, grass-fed butter, egg yolks, and cod liver oil. Consuming 3 egg yolks *or* 4–7 tbsp butter (depending on whether it's grass-fed) *or* 1 tsp of cod liver oil per day (look for brands that are third-party tested for purity, such as Rosita's) will provide the RDI for one day. Eating liver will provide your RDI for the *week* in one single 3-oz serving! Another option to consider is 100 percent grass-fed beef, as it's been shown to have 7 times more vitamin A than grain-fed beef.[136]

When it comes to plant foods, know that plant-based beta-carotene is not vitamin A. While carotenoids are incredible antioxidants and polyphenols found most abundantly in orange-colored fruits and veggies, your body may not turn much into vitamin A. Due to deficiencies and simple body chemistry, some of us will convert no more than 5 percent of beta-carotene into retinoids.[137] This is why the 700 mcg/day recommendation for omnivores shoots up to 16,800 mcg/day for vegans. Ideally, we should all be consuming plenty of both retinol and beta-carotene, since each has an important (though somewhat separate) role.

Vitamin D

Vitamin D3 (cholecalciferol) is our fat-soluble "sunshine vitamin," although technically it's a hormone. It is essential for proper mineral metabolism, immune function, fertility, and more. It is also important for regulating normal cell growth and chronic inflammatory responses, increasing anti-inflammatory cytokine (a type of immune factor) production, and decreasing pro-inflammatory cytokines. Not surprisingly, multiple studies have found an association linking vitamin D deficiency with endometriosis.

Those of us with endo appear to be remarkably deficient in vitamin D3. In one study, researchers found 86 percent of those with endo to be deficient, and those with the lowest blood levels of vitamin D consistently had the largest endometriomas (endometriosis-filled cysts).[138] This is in line with another study that links lower vitamin D levels with a higher risk of developing endometriosis.[139] Another study concluded that vitamin D "modulates inflammation and proliferation in endometriotic cells, and a lower [D] status is associated with endometriosis," which is why vitamin D supplementation may be another therapeutic strategy for managing endometriosis.[140]

For fertility, vitamin D is also necessary for a healthy pregnancy. It's widely understood that women with higher vitamin D levels are more likely to conceive.[141] Notably, pregnancy success rates have been correlated with vitamin D levels because each additional unit of vitamin D3 in the follicular fluid may increase the likelihood of conception by 6 percent.[142]

The best source of vitamin D is the sun. Sounds simple, yet the challenges that arise with getting *enough* sun are many, including latitude, diet, over-applying sunscreen, and not being in the sun long enough—especially for dark-skinned people. A Caucasian person may need only 20 minutes of the midday sun on her mostly nude body (think bikini with no sunscreen) each day to get all the D she needs, while a very dark-skinned person may need 2 entire hours. Twenty minutes to 2 hours per day is more time than many of us with indoor jobs have, and sunbathing for vitamin D is not especially appealing in colder climates. Again, this makes testing and targeted supplementation imperative for many, which is quite easy and affordable.

Testing for deficiency is easily done with a quick blood draw. From a functional medicine perspective, your goal is to have your vitamin D levels at 50 ng/mL or above.

Food Fix: While the sun is the best source of vitamin D, you can also find it in animal products (from animals living outdoors absorbing the sun's rays), as well as in mushrooms. The RDI is 600 IU/day for women. You can get this from 1.5 tsp cod liver oil or a 4-oz serving of wild salmon, while other good sources include wild-caught cold-water fatty fish such as herring, sardines, and mackerel. Secondary sources include egg yolks (37 IU/yolk) and mushrooms (although these have the less-absorbable D2 rather than D3, which is the optimal version of vitamin D to consume). To note, if you're deficient you may need quite a bit more than this short term to bring levels up to sufficiency.

If you test and find you're deficient, speak with your doctor about supplementing with vitamin D3 up to 4,000 IU/day until you reach sufficiency (50 ng/mL or up). And as a reminder, if you need to supplement, please monitor your levels and stop when you are sufficient! As a practitioner living in an age of vitamin D deficiency, I've seen some folk taking a huge amount of vitamin D every day for years without any testing—they just assumed they needed it. Too much D will knock your other nutrients (such as A and K) out of balance, even leading to hypothyroid-like symptoms in some cases, so please work with your practitioner to get your levels up to proper sufficiency, and then monitor yearly as needed.

Vitamins C and E

Vitamin C can help both prevent tissue damage, and heal it once it occurs. It is an important antioxidant that fights free radicals and is essential for collagen synthesis. Vitamin E is an antioxidant, anti-inflammatory, and immune-supportive nutrient that helps thicken the endometrial lining, keeps your tissues healthy, scavenges free radicals, supports fertility, and, alongside vitamin C, has been shown to help manage endometriosis symptoms. Together these vitamins act as important "chain-breaker" antioxidants to end the free-radical cascade damaging your tissues (imagine those slashing ninjas) and leading to inflammation. This is also why we may need more than the average Jane.

One study that supplemented endo patients for two months with 1000 mg vitamin C and 1200 IU vitamin E (16 and 54 times the RDI, respectively) saw significant decreases in inflammatory markers within the peritoneal fluid.[143] Moreover, the study highlighted their pain-banishing superpowers: 43 percent of participants saw a reduction in chronic everyday pain; 37 percent reported a reduction in menstrual pain, and 24 percent noted a reduction in painful sex. The authors conclude that vitamins E and C "are a highly efficient alternative therapy to relieve chronic pelvic pain in women with endometriosis."

Another study examined how increased food consumption of these antioxidants could counter oxidative stress in women with endometriosis, with compelling results.[144] The researchers recruited women both with and without endo to eat a high-antioxidant diet, including 1050 IU beta-carotene, 500 mg vitamin C, and 20 mg vitamin E per day. The participants ate 8 servings (estimated around 4 cups total) of assorted fruits and vegetables per day for the beta-carotene and vitamin C, plus 4 tablespoons of pumpkin seeds and 3 tablespoons of peanuts to meet the vitamin E requirement. No supplements were consumed.

Interestingly, the study first uncovered that the women with endometriosis were consuming significantly fewer antioxidants before the study began compared to the women without endo, again highlighting the association between diet and endo. After switching to the high-antioxidant diet, the women with endometriosis made some dramatic gains. Their serum levels of these antioxidants rose after just the first month, and levels of powerful antioxidants made within the body (endogenous antioxidants SOD and glutathione) rose after only three months. Consequently, with the addition of so many helpful antioxidants from simple dietary changes, *the total level of oxidative stress these women were facing was clinically reduced.*

Vitamin C alone may directly counteract many endo-related symptoms we've accumulated. Increased consumption may raise progesterone levels in women struggling with deficiency (as many of us are).[145] Lower levels of vitamin C were also observed among women with recurrent miscarriages, perhaps due to the association between increased levels of free radicals in the pelvis and miscarriage.[146] It also appears to be quite an effective therapy for pain relief in chronically ill patients by acting as a mild anti-inflammatory, and chronic pain itself is a *symptom* of acute vitamin C deficiency.[147] One study even examined the effect of vitamin C on endo and found that the endometriosis volume was significantly reduced compared to those without vitamin C therapy.[148]

Although acute deficiencies in vitamin C or vitamin E are rare, subclinical deficiencies are not. Partly, this is because we may not be eating enough on a daily basis (89 percent of Americans don't get enough vitamin E), and also we may need to eat much more than the RDI if we have an inflammatory disorder like endometriosis.[149] If you imagine your inflammation is a wildfire and vitamin C and E are the water in your fire hose, you may need substantially more to keep the hose pumping water out full blast.

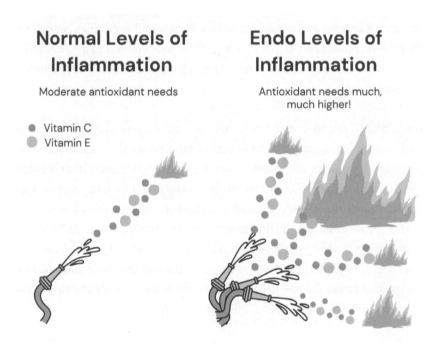

Normal Levels of Inflammation

Moderate antioxidant needs

- Vitamin C
- Vitamin E

Endo Levels of Inflammation

Antioxidant needs much, much higher!

Food Fix: Getting enough vitamin E takes diligence because it's found in high amounts only in certain foods. The best whole food sources include abalone (11 mg/cup), avocados (4.4 mg/avo), sunflower seeds (3 mg/tbsp), pure olive oil or red palm oil (each has around 2 mg/tbsp), almonds (2.1 mg/tbsp), and in lesser amounts in certain fruits and vegetables like broccoli, spinach, beet greens, or mango. Make sure to avoid vitamin E-rich foods that may be inflammatory, including wheat germ, canola, safflower, or sunflower oils (industrial seed oils which you'll learn about soon).

For vitamin C, the RDI for adult women is set at 75 mg/day, which is easily met by munching on ½ cup red bell pepper or one fresh orange—enough to prevent scurvy but not to fight inflammation and thrive. Sub-acute deficiency may slow the rate of collagen formation, leading to a number of issues such as slow healing, swelling and edema, and even joint pain since joints are made of collagen-rich connective tissue. Because vitamin C is also needed for healthy blood vessels, deficiencies are associated with increased bleeding, such as nosebleeds, bleeding gums, and even heavy bleeding with menses.[150]

While there is no defined amount of vitamins C and E that women with endo "should" be consuming, studies have shown that taking between 500 and 2000 mg/day of vitamin C is beneficial for pain, inflammation, heavy menstrual flow, and fertility.[151] Increasing vitamin E intake to between 20 and 800 mg/day has shown substantial benefit in reducing pelvic inflammation.[152] Even if you just focus on consuming the lower thresholds of 500 mg/day of vitamin C and 20 mg/day of vitamin E, your body will be better equipped to handle your endo-based inflammation. You can easily do this with some extra effort.

TIPS TO EAT MORE VITAMINS C & E

- **Eat 6–9 cups of fresh veggies per day:** I often see clients who believe they're eating plenty of veggies, although in actuality they're eating no more than 2–3 *servings*/day (about 2 cups). This may seem like a lot, but in the grand scheme of things, it's a drop in the pond. In order to reach that 500–1000 mg vitamin C mark, we consistently need a lot of fresh produce (it should make up the bulk of your plate), and most of us should focus on 2–3 cups per *meal*. This may seem like a lot initially, but you can slowly work your way up to it, and then you'll wonder why you hadn't been doing it all along. I will reiterate this recommendation throughout this book, because eating more vegetables has other significant benefits, and it is the cornerstone of the Heal Endo nutritional recommendations.

- **Buy local produce:** Vitamin C takes a nosedive after harvest, with some veggies losing up to 77 percent of it within a week.[153] Thus, the easiest way to improve intake is to shop at local farmers' markets, where produce is often picked the day of. In fact, you'll get much more vitamin C buying new or different types of vegetables at the local markets than you would buying foods touted as vitamin C rich (like oranges, peppers, or spinach) that have been imported from across the world. So be brave and try some new foods!

- **Don't overcook your veggies:** High or prolonged heat destroys vitamin C content, so people eating plenty of produce can still develop a deficiency if they consistently overcook it. The best way to retain vitamin C is to eat fresh produce raw or lightly cooked. Think lightly steamed or quickly sautéed. It should have some "crisp" left in it, rather than being a pile of mush.

- **Focus on your vitamin E foods:** If you can tolerate almonds and sunflower seeds, aim to eat a few tablespoons per day. Almond butter is an easy way to boost your vitamin E. Cook or drizzle your food with high-quality olive oil or sustainably harvested palm oil, focus on a large variety of vitamin E-rich plant foods like avocados and leafy greens, and even aim to eat that abalone (a kind of mollusk) if you can.

Omega 3s (EPA + DHA)

The omega 3s EPA and DHA are delicate polyunsaturated fats found most abundantly in cold-water fatty fish and seafood. They are renowned for their anti-inflammatory effects that support fertility, brain health, immune function, and healthy aging. They're an essential nutrient, meaning you need to eat them or you won't have any in your body; deficiency can lead to a cascade of issues ranging from dry skin and joint pain to clinical depression and ... endometriosis.

Numerous studies linking endo and omega-3-rich diets show pretty incredible results. One study found that increasing tissue levels of omega 3s suppressed active sites for inflammation in endometriosis.[154] It was also found that supplementing with DHA and EPA significantly decreased inflammatory markers in the peritoneal fluid and actually reduced the endometriosis implant size.[155] In another study, animals with more omega 3s had endometriosis lesions less than *half* the size and quantity of control groups.[156] Altogether, researchers conclude that omega 3s may be useful in reducing the inflammatory response of endometriosis.[157] When it comes to stopping the process of endo-ing, it becomes critical to have abundant of levels of these nutrients.

EPA and DHA have also been shown to help calm what is called an *arachidonic acid cascade*, which may cause intense endo pain as well as provoke a number of endo features, including cell proliferation, avoidance of normal cell death, inflammation, and rooting down of endo lesions.[158] Yikes. Instead of consuming less arachidonic acid (where some misplaced recommendations to reduce red meat consumption come from), you actually need to *increase* the amount of DHA and EPA you consume in order to slow down or prevent such an overreaction.[159]

Symptoms of EPA/DHA deficiencies include dry skin, slow cognitive ability, depression, fatigue, or joint pain, and unfortunately, nearly *all of us* may be deficient to some degree. A recent worldwide analysis looked at serum levels of EPA and DHA and found that nearly all North Americans are in the *very low* category.[160] In fact, not a single American participant tested in the optimal range![161] This means you may need a lot more than you think to not just meet your needs but reverse an existing deficiency.

Food Fix: The best sources of EPA and DHA by far are cold-water fatty fish and seafood, including salmon, herring, mackerel, sardines, anchovies, fish roe, and oysters. Affordable options include canned salmon, sardines, anchovies, and tinned oysters (which are actually very tasty on crackers). Other seafood and shellfish options also have beneficial amounts, although you'll want to avoid any larger fish that bioaccumulate toxins and heavy metals, such as shark, swordfish, tuna (except for skipjack), king mackerel, or marlin. You can also find EPA and DHA (albeit in lower amounts) in most products from animals that live as nature intended: think wild, hunted, fished, foraged, or 100 percent pastured or grass-fed.

Unfortunately for exclusively plant-based eaters, it's near impossible to get enough EPA and DHA without animal products. Although ALA is the plant-based form of omega 3 (found in omega-rich flaxseeds and walnuts), your body must *convert* it into EPA or DHA in order to use it, and humans appear to convert no more than 6 percent of ALA to EPA and 3.8 percent of ALA to DHA.[162] So in order to keep your levels optimal, it's important to ingest EPA and DHA directly from animals who've already done the conversion for us (the one exception is an algae-based supplement, which should be an absolute must if you're vegan).

To reverse an omega-3 deficiency, eat more cold-water fatty fish, seafood, shellfish, and grass-fed or pastured animal products, and consider quality supplementation. If you can, aim for up to one meal per day based around these foods (or at least every other day). When it comes to animal products, purchase 100 percent grass-fed if you can afford it since it has the best balance of fatty acids.

If seafood makes you queasy and you'd like to solely supplement, I under-stand—but hear me out. If you exclusively supplement, you'll be missing out on the myriad nutrients included in seafood that you likely need more of, such as selenium, zinc, vitamin D, and iodine. At the very least I ask you to try to begin waking up those atrophied taste buds, even if it's just one or two bites a week to grow accustomed to new flavors. I have a toddler and if it works for him (it does!), it will work for you. When you do supplement, know that low-quality fish oil supplementation is notorious for being rancid, and many are contaminated with dioxins and heavy metals. I recommend high-quality supplementation or none at all. One brand to consider is Nordic Naturals, which is third-party tested.

MIRIAM'S STORY

Since puberty, I suffered major bloating and IBS symptoms, intense pain episodes, wild mood swings, and more. My body was my enemy and I resented it and the rollercoaster I had to endure each month. I started following the Heal Endo approach not long after excision surgery which finally diagnosed me with stage 4 endo at the age of 37. It was such a relief to have a diagnosis and something to work with, and a plan to follow that was dedicated to helping women with this common yet elusive condition. I was desperate for change and just needed some direction and support.

I changed my diet significantly, and rather than avoiding certain foods, the focus was on cramming as many nutrients into my body as physically possible. I also employed a strict short-term elimination diet to help understand what my body reacted to. Surprisingly, I realized things I had previously eaten a LOT of (peanut butter, eggs, legumes) blew up my belly and left me feeling hungover. I now have a tailored diet for my unique body and horrify people by eating things like sardines and veg for breakfast! I went from grazing on snacks all day to not snacking at all (almost!). These changes have significantly reduced the discomfort and bloating in my gut, lifted my mood and brain fog, and probably most significantly feels like I've extinguished the fire in my belly, through my pelvis, and all the joints in my body by addressing my inflammation which in turn reduced my pain levels.

Under Katie's guidance, I've also focused on moving my body and pelvis regularly with yoga, walking, stretching, using stand up-desk, and letting go of strenuous cardio exercises. The focus is again on nourishment, blood flow, and trying (not always successfully) to calm my stress levels. Three years later I had another surgery for my endo and aside from endometriomas on my ovary there was minimal new growth. I'm determined and confident that I will never have surgery again. - Miriam, Australia

Phytonutrients

Phytonutrients should receive a standing ovation for having a profoundly beneficial impact on human health, and healing from endo. Phytonutrients (or phytochemicals) are a family of thousands of amazing plant compounds that research is just beginning to uncover. It's estimated that 5,000 phytonutrients have already been identified, yet a large amount still remains unknown.

Phytonutrients are powerful antioxidants and immune regulators, and are what give plants their unique color. You can imagine just how many phytonutrients there are when you think about the amazing variety of plant colors in the world. They're so important that over the next few decades we may even have an RDI for many of these, just as we do for vitamins and minerals today.

If you're not familiar with the name *phytonutrient,* you're probably more familiar with some of the subsets. *Flavanols* may ring a bell, a famous phytonutrient found in onions, garlic, cacao, green tea, kale, broccoli, and blueberries. Or you may have heard that some foods like dark chocolate, berries, and red wine are good for you because of phytonutrients like *resveratrol. Anthocyanidins* are phytonutrients found in high concentrations in black currants, blackberries, and blueberries, as well as in the skin of eggplant, red cabbage, and cranberries. In fact, many so-called "superfoods" like cacao, acai, mushrooms, and goji berries are actually "super" because of the concentrated amount of phytonutrients in them.

You could think of many phytonutrients as powerful plant medicines—indeed, many ancient cultures used these types of foods in elixirs or tinctures in folk medicine. If you think that's hocus-pocus, think again. Modern-day research supports just how beneficial they are to human health, and a number of these compounds have been studied in relation to healing from endometriosis.

Resveratrol is one that packs an endo-punch. It is found in foods such as grapes, wine, blueberries, cranberries, pistachios, and cocoa. There are numerous studies showing resveratrol to decrease the quantity, size, and/or volume of endometriosis lesions—one study found it to reduce the number of endo lesions by 60 percent![163] It was also shown to significantly increase levels of important antioxidants your body makes for you (SOD and glutathione) and thereby reduce pelvic oxidative stress.[164]

Curcumin, an active phytonutrient in turmeric, was used in ancient Asian folk medicine to address endo-like symptoms. Our ancestors may have been on to something since curcumin has been found to suppress the spread of endometriotic cells by reducing the form of estrogen that provokes endometriosis.[165] Another study demonstrated that curcumin could reduce endometriosis-related inflammation.[166]

Pycnogenol is a phytonutrient also known for reducing endometriosis symptoms. It comes from the bark of the French maritime pine tree (commonly called pine bark). One study that examined its effects on women with severe endometriosis pain showed that after just four weeks it reduced *all* participants' pain from severe to moderate without any other changes in diet or lifestyle, while an additional 5 participants became pregnant.[167] Another study reported that 100 mg of pycnogenol a day may significantly support pain reduction in women with endometriosis when taken in tandem with oral contraceptives. A whopping 57 percent of participants taking oral contraceptives and pycnogenol together reported a *complete* resolution of pain, while none of the women on oral contraceptives alone reported full pain resolution.[168]

Green tea polyphenols called *catechins* (epigallocatechin gallate, or EGCG) may also play a role in endometriosis suppression. In one study, EGCG significantly inhibited the development of endometriosis through anti-angiogenic effects (angiogenesis is the growth of blood vessels that connect your endo lesions to your body, like roots), resulting in the regression of endo lesions.[169] These results were similarly observed in another study, supporting the idea that "EGCG might be a promising therapeutic agent in the treatment of endometriosis, preventing the establishment of new endometriotic lesions."[170]

Want more? Okay. These studies found more endo-busting phytonutrients. *Silymarin* is the powerful phytonutrient in milk thistle that was shown to prevent endometriosis development through anti-angiogenesis and increase endo-cell death.[171] *Glycosylated flavonoids*, a phytonutrient in yellow sweet clover, lettuces, and more, was found to significantly decrease endometriotic areas and reduce inflammatory pelvic cytokine levels.[172] *Quercetin*, a flavonol found in fruits and veggies like onions, apple skins, lettuce, and cauliflower, slows the proliferation of endometriosis by increasing endo-cell death and upping antioxidant activity.[173]

Let's review what information we've collected:

1. Phytonutrients are found in every plant. They are potent anti-inflammatories and immune regulators.
2. A small number of phytonutrients are shown to directly aid in the healing of endometriosis and inflammation.
3. An *enormous* number (likely thousands) have yet to be investigated, but it is likely that many of them will also be really important to our health.

This is why we should focus on eating a wide variety of colorful, fresh plants every day to capture as many phytonutrients as possible. Some help our cells better communicate, some act as anti-inflammatories, some aid in preventing cellular mutations (critical), and many are super antioxidants. Although science will continue to pinpoint the specifics within one food at a time, we know they're in every plant, and our bodies need them.

Food Fix: The best thing about phytonutrients is that you don't need to fork out lots of money for pricey superfoods. There is an abundance growing all around you. A plant-centric diet (note: different from an *exclusively* plant-based diet) can truly benefit the endo body. To add more phytonutrients to your diet today, here are a few tips:

- **Eat a lot of fresh, local produce**: 6–9 cups of colorful vegetables per day, and a few pieces of fruit too if you want. If you can't find fresh veggies, frozen works as a great substitute.
- **Herbs and spices:** Your food should be full of them! They're an easy way to add phytonutrients *and* flavor at the same time. To learn, I recommend checking out some ethnic food cookbooks, since most in-

ternational cuisine is chock full of green herbs, ginger, garlic, turmeric, cinnamon, pepper, and/or other spices. Consider starting a small herb garden (even if you have a black thumb, perennial herbs are seriously so easy to grow). Think thyme, rosemary, oregano, and mint to start.

- **Eat the rainbow:** Different colors of plants offer you different health-promoting compounds, and nature offers us hundreds of different varieties of bananas, avocados, tomatoes, lettuce, eggplants, berries, broccoli, you name it. The global food system only wheels and deals with produce that can ship well, store well, and look pretty weeks later, so all this diversity isn't seen at your local Big Box market. Another great reason to run (don't walk) to your farmers' market this weekend.

- **Eat intense flavors and wild foods:** Bitter, astringent, spicy, sour— the more potent the flavor (and the more wild the plant), the higher the phytonutrient content. This is why fresh herbs, peppers, cacao, wine, deep purple berries, and wild-collected plant foods are less sweet and more intensely flavored and are regarded as some of the best sources of phytonutrients.

- **Drink tea:** One of the easiest ways to get phytonutrients. Look for herbal and organic varieties.

- **Eat it fresh or lightly cooked**: Like vitamin C, some phytonutrients arc heat sensitive. If you cook your produce, aim to keep some crunch.

- **Do this all before you go supplement crazy:** Nowhere do I find studies that say "women who eat poorly but take lots of phytonutrient supplements feel great." Rather, I see studies that observe that people who eat lots of phytonutrient-rich foods have a better chance at avoiding inflammation and immune dysfunction.[174] Food first, always, then consider supplementation.

Eat More Veggies

No matter who you are and how you eat, make sure your plate is loaded with a rainbow assortment of veggies. Here are some great examples of what those swaps look like:

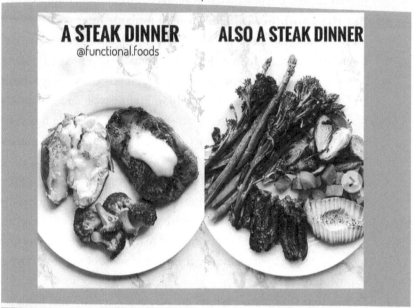

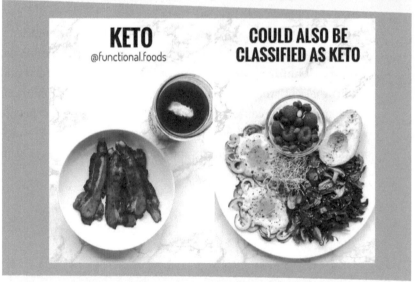

PHOTO CREDIT: DR. TYLER JEAN, @FUNCTIONALFOODS

WHAT ABOUT SUPPLEMENTS?

High-quality supplements may be extremely beneficial for many of us. Reversing iron, magnesium, zinc, and EPA/DHA deficiencies, for example, may take a higher level of nutrient intake than you would be able to consume through food sources alone. You might be dealing with such extreme levels of inflammation that you may need to consider consuming supplementary levels of antioxidants such as vitamin C, vitamin E, or phytonutrients daily as you work on the root cause. Yet, I stall with supplement recommendations because I so often see sufferers load up on hundreds of dollars of supplements first, and then wonder why they don't feel better.

Needless to say, we are not the Jetsons and cannot survive on vitamins as a side to nutrient-less meals. Thus, my recommendation is that you focus on food first and foremost. Spend the extra cash on quality nutrient-rich foods from local butchers and farmers' markets. After you dial in your nutrition, then consider supplementation—but only with high-quality brands, since so much of the supplement industry is poor quality (and even contaminated with toxic ingredients). To dial in your dosages, please consider working with a nutrition professional, or for an up-to-date list of supplement brands and dosage recommendations, check out www.healendo.com/supplements.

PUTTING IT ALL TOGETHER

Obtaining enough of the Endo-9 each day will mean a big shift in eating for most of us. It will mean our plates need to be piled high with a rainbow of assorted veggies, with our protein coming from seafood, organ meats, red meat (preferably 100 percent grass-fed), cold-water fatty fish, and meat on the bone (I'll discuss why in the following chapter). If you're a vegan or vegetarian it will be important to work with a practitioner to make sure you're meeting the mark on numerous key nutrients, supplement wisely, or perhaps consider adding in choice animal products for the sake of healing anew. By using the Endo-9 to guide food choices, you should start to feel gains as you begin to heal.

If you're curious about other nutrients not included in the Endo-9, know that yes there are plenty of others known to help endo (and create healthy bodies). B vitamins, sodium, potassium, iodine, copper, choline...the list goes on. These nutrients are crucial to the functioning of the body and many are associated with immune function, fertility, healthy epigenetic signaling, and even endometriosis. I could have taken this chapter and written an entire book!

Yet, if you focus on eating food following the Endo-9, you should be consuming a diverse, nutrient-dense diet that will provide the rest of the nutrients as well. For example, selenium is critically important for those of us with endo since deficiency is very associated with inflammation of the uterine lining. Yet, if you focus on eating nuts, seafood, and meat (which contain many of the other Endo-9 as well as selenium) you will meet your daily needs. If you focus on getting ample omega 3s from seafood, you'll also be getting a liberal influx of iodine and potassium. If you get your iron from liver, you'll easily be meeting your copper, B-vitamin, and choline needs. I am urging you to take action to heal your endo with simple steps, and not get kitchen paralysis or information overload.

To better understand how to get these micronutrients onto your plate, let's look at the macronutrients that contain them: carbohydrates, proteins, and fats.

Endo-9 Cheat Sheet

Here are some examples of primary sources for our Endo-9 for nutrient-dense success. Add secondary sources as needed, but please focus on these recommendations as the best options to address deficiencies.

From Plants

Plants should make up the bulk of your plate.

  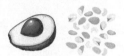

Magnesium

Nuts, seeds, beans, vegetables, cacao, and herbs.

Vitamin C + Phytonutrients

Fresh produce! The more freshly picked the better. Literally "eat the rainbow."

Vitamin E

Palm oil, nuts, seeds, nut butter, avocados.

From Animal

These should make up a smaller percentage of your plate. Think quality and nutrient density over quantity.

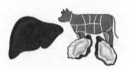 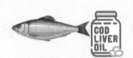

Iron

Liver, red meat, and oysters.

Vitamin D

Sunshine! Cod liver oil or fatty, wild-caught fish.

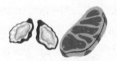 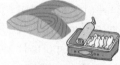 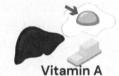

Zinc

Red meat, oysters and shellfish, organ meat, and seafood.

EPA & DHA

Cold-water fatty fish, such as salmon, herring, mackerel, sardines, anchovies.

Vitamin A

Liver, egg yolks, butter from grass-fed cows, cod liver oil.

Chapter 9:

Macronutrients: Carbohydrates, Fats, and Proteins in Balance

Macronutrients are the bigger nutrient groups we're more familiar with: carbohydrates, fat, and protein. Each is important for the functioning of the body, not to mention they're our source of all the Endo-9 *micro*nutrients you just learned about. And since carbohydrates, fat, and protein make up food as we know it, this chapter is about how to balance them properly to maintain healthy levels of *blood sugar,* another crucial factor needed to heal from endo.

BLOOD SUGAR IMBALANCE 101

Carbohydrates are pretty simple macronutrients, consisting of sugars, starches, and fiber. You can find them in all plant foods (with differing levels depending on the plant), as well as the more processed, refined varieties of foods we typically think of as "carbs"—pasta, bread, pastries, pizza, etc. In the gut, sugars and starches are broken down to *glucose* (our body's main form of fuel) and then absorbed into the blood to be transported around the body. This glucose in the bloodstream is called "blood sugar." Your body works hard to always have a small but steady stream of glucose circulating at all times, ready to feed your cells.

Your blood glucose needs to be kept at a very consistent yet minimal level throughout the day, with just enough to feed your cells but not too much to cause problems. To keep it at this very perfect level, we rely on a complex "braking system" to slow the absorption of sugars into the bloodstream so it drips in at a trickle rather than a rushing river. Fiber, fat, and protein make up this braking system. When we eat carbohydrate-rich foods in their fiber-rich natural form (i.e., fruits, veggies, grains, beans, etc.), and pair them in a meal with proteins and fats, the entire package slows the absorption of glucose to a slow drip.

When glucose does finally drip into circulation, it pairs with a hormone called *insulin*. Insulin escorts glucose to the cell door, where it politely knocks and hands over the glucose. It does this to every single cell in your body (there are trillions), from your eyeball to your cervix. Think of it like this: moderate levels of insulin + glucose = well-fed cell.

Unfortunately, most of us today eat a low-fiber diet based on refined flours, sugar, grains, and starches: store-bought bread, pasta, cereals, baked goods like cakes and cookies, frozen meals, pizza, breakfast cereal, soda, or other sweet drinks (yes, even organic or marketed as "healthy"). These "ultra-processed foods" are formerly whole foods, broken down via numerous processing techniques, stripped of nutrients and fiber, then rebuilt into something highly palatable. Sadly, they are also the foundation of a Standard American Diet (SAD) and contribute to the bulk of our diet for most of us, contributing nearly 60 percent of our calories and 90 percent of our added sugar intake![175] Think about that for a minute: the foods that we center our meals around are the very foods we should not be eating very much of. Stripped of fiber and nutrients, lacking quality protein and fat, and full of sugar and starch, these foods spike our blood glucose levels with every meal, snack, or sugary beverage.

When carbohydrate consumption like this dominates over quality protein, fat, and fiber, your blood sugar will start to *rollercoaster*—where your glucose, insulin, hunger levels, and energy levels spike and plummet all day long. When our blood sugar is low we can feel shaky or faint, "hangry" (hungry + angry), or we can become hypoglycemic. Blood sugar rollercoasters like this affect the vast majority of Americans.

Tracking Blood Sugar Levels

A blood sugar chart shows the difference between healthy and unhealthy levels of blood sugar and insulin. A spike and plummet of blood sugar is known as the "blood sugar rollercoaster."

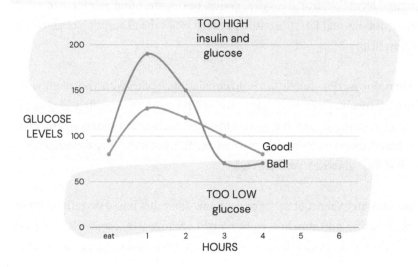

CRACKERS VS. COOKIES

When talking about blood sugar levels, pure starch and pure sugar are basically the same things in that they quickly break down into glucose within the body. So even though a purely starch food like a cheesy cracker may be savory in flavor, your body will react the same as if you had eaten a cookie. This means, in their most basic forms, starches and sugars are the same when it comes to blood sugar levels.

Even if you try to avoid sweets you may be surprised to learn just how much food producers add sugars to even our *savory* foods, such as pasta sauce, salsas, sausages, bacon, ham, bread, soups, sauces, ketchup, condiments, and many more. If you stroll through the supermarket and read labels, you may be surprised to find added sugars to nearly every product on the shelves. You may also be surprised to realize just how addicted to these foods you are or how you may not be able to go one single meal without sugar, even the hidden variety. I still vividly remember the first time I tried cutting out all sugars and had overpowering nausea from trying to eat eggs without first smothering them in sweet ketchup. Sugar addiction is real.

I even see sugar addiction spill over into the diets of clients who say they tossed all processed food and *only* eat whole, unprocessed foods. When I investigate, I see diets based on whole grains (pasta, bread, oats, rice, quinoa), sweet potatoes, beans, honey, homemade granola, smoothies, and lots of fruit. There's a sprinkling of low-starch veggies, little protein, and a little bit of fat but not much. In reality, these poor folk are stuffed to the brim with starch. Yes, there's some fiber, but not nearly enough to counteract the enormous quantity of starches and sugars they're consuming. On the island of Kaua'i, where I live, we call this "hippy sugar," and you may be drowning in it.

Here is an example of what that typical blood sugar dysregulation may look like in a day:

Mary wakes up in the morning and eats cereal with low-fat almond milk. Barely an hour goes by and she's already peckish, so she eats a quick snack bar stashed in her purse. An hour later she's hungry again, and kind of tired already. Oh dear, she grabs some chips and coffee and waits until lunch—but because she snacked all morning she's not ravenous, so she eats only half her lunch. Now afternoon rolls along and she's hangry, shaky, and exhausted— time for that pastry and maybe another coffee. Gosh, she feels bloated. And tired. Finally, it's dinner time, and Mary is desperate for something sweet afterward. Okay, maybe a late-night snack before bed, too. Mary wishes she wasn't so hungry and tired all day!

Sound familiar? For many of us hunger comes on fast, we're shaky and irritable, or perhaps we feel faint. We need constant sugar or caffeine jolts throughout the day to keep going. And because the majority of us deal with blood sugar dysregulation on a regular basis, it's become a cultural norm (kind of like painful periods—not normal, just common), which is why most of us may be on a blood sugar rollercoaster for years, if not decades. Unfortunately, blood sugar dysregulation may be *directly* influencing our endo.

HOW BLOOD SUGAR DYSREGULATION CAUSES TROUBLE IN THE ENDO BODY

A blood sugar rollercoaster means three things: sometimes you will have (a) excess glucose levels (b) excess insulin levels, or (c) too little glucose. Unfortunately, each may influence the way our endo behaves.

Excess glucose floating in the body is dangerous because sugar is highly reactive to proteins, which your body is made up of. This results in *glycation*, the process in which sugar reacts to proteins to create chemical bonds of "stickiness" (ever get a lollipop stuck in your hair?). Not only is glycation damaging in its own right, it also creates something even more damaging: Advanced Glycation End-Products, known as AGEs.

AGEs in the body cause damage by connecting to a type of cell receptor aptly called RAGE. When AGE connects to RAGE, it triggers a rapid generation of free radicals, which creates a tidal wave of inflammation and tissue damage.[176] This is how AGEs damage blood vessels, tissues, and organs: by causing so much damage to protein fibers that they become stiff, brittle, and malformed, eventually making it hard for blood and nutrients to get to where they need to be (one reason why diabetic patients can have their limbs amputated). But before something this extreme happens, you may feel like your joints hurt or you feel stiff, weak, or much older than you should.

Unfortunately, those of us with endometriosis may have significantly more RAGE receptors within our peritoneal and follicular fluid, as well as localized in certain endo cells.[177] RAGE reactions may also increase immune factors that promote the growth of endo "roots" that anchor endo to the tissue. This means we may react even more significantly to AGEs (and thus blood sugar imbalances) since we have more RAGE receptors at ground zero for our own inflammatory disease. And, in the case of blood sugar dysregulation, high amounts of circulating glucose can become the main contributor of AGEs within your body, creating a cascade of AGEs with each soda (or cold-pressed carrot juice), ready to blitz your peritoneal cavity with free-radical damage.[178]

Too much insulin is another story, one that may encourage the janitorial aspect of immune dysfunction associated with endo. Endometriosis cells are shown to have their energy metabolism a bit messed up because they produce more lactic acid than a normal, healthy cell.[179] Too much lactic acid changes the pH around the endo lesion so that immune surveillance factors can't function properly (kind of like creating an invisibility cloak around the lesion) thereby reducing endo-cell death.[180] Not only that but lactate is a key driver of cell invasion, "rooting down," and immune suppression—changes implicated in the establishment and survival of endo lesions.[181] Unfortunately, high levels of circulating insulin increase the rate at which your endo cells produce lactic acid, meaning *blood sugar dysregulation may directly contribute to more immune dysfunction, endo progression, and establishment.* If you've heard that "sugar feeds cancer," this is actually the same mechanism at play—and why it also appears that "sugar feeds endo."

BLOOD SUGAR AND HORMONAL CHAOS

But wait, the blood sugar roller coaster isn't yet over, because after the surge comes the crash. After your cells have slammed the door on insulin, your liver works frantically to convert the excess glucose into fat and store it away before it causes any more damage. But your hungry cells need a little glucose circulating at all times, so with a sudden shortage of glucose, you arrive at the well-known "blood sugar crash," a very stressful time for your body. You're shaky, hangry, grumpy, nervous, short of breath, and/or faint—signs your body is in desperate need of a glucose fix, even though you just ate two hours earlier. To keep you alive until you eat, your body releases stress hormones reserved for emergencies—cortisol and adrenaline.

If you remember back to Chapter 6, both cortisol and adrenaline are associated with endometriosis progression, chronic low-grade inflammation, and immune dysfunction. So, if your dietary choices are provoking you to release these hormones often (as it may happen numerous times *per day* for many of us), blood sugar dips will contribute to *endo-ing* as we know it, as well as lead to imbalances within your sex hormones, such as reduced progesterone or DHEA. And, as glucose is stored as fat instead of used for energy, those fat cells become an active part of your endocrine system (meaning they make hormones), including estrogen and testosterone. These fat cells also have ample insulin receptors on them, so while your other cells are stuck turning away insulin and glucose, making you both tired and hungry, your fat deposits offer up ample docking sites. This creates a vicious cycle between increasing weight gain and increasing estrogen levels (remember, your fat stores *make* some estrogen) and decreasing progesterone. Great, exactly what we endo-folk don't need.

"Sugar Feeds Endo"

Imbalanced blood sugar levels may directly affect the way your endo behaves.

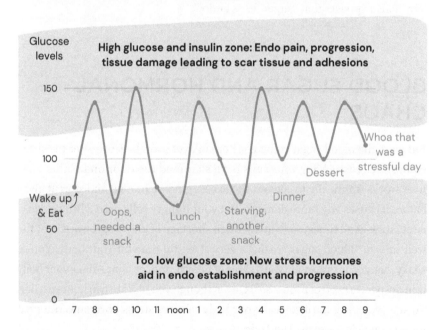

As a cherry on top, your insulin-resistant cells are secretly regretting that decision to turn insulin and glucose energy away. You may feel exhausted, hungry, and depleted, even though you're eating plenty of caloric energy.

With the possibility that imbalances in insulin *and* glucose levels may directly support the process of endo-ing, it seems that blood sugar dysregulation may be much, much more implicated with endometriosis than we realize.

TIME TO BALANCE

It should be apparent by now how blood sugar dysregulation is one of the biggest endo-enemies, and how some of the mainstream "endo diet" recommendations to limit proteins and fats that are exceptional tools to balance blood sugar may instead be fueling the endo fire. I've even seen some of my endo clientele suffering more from blood sugar issues than from endo. Fatigue, anxiety, unhealthy weight gain they're unable to lose, tremendous bloating, depression, pain (joints, period, back), and nervousness—all symptoms of endo, yes, but also symptoms of blood sugar dysregulation. This may be why some folk are shocked when their pain disappears or they get pregnant from balancing blood sugar alone. This is not at all to say that balancing blood sugar is everyone's silver bullet, but after watching clients who have witnessed miraculous turnarounds from addressing this issue alone, I now believe it's a true endo non-negotiable.

CLAIRE'S STORY

I had tried to conceive for two years without any success when I started the Heal Endo approach. I had Stage 4 endo and adenomyosis, and I was tired, frustrated, and fearful I'd never have children. After listening to my story and looking through my diet and lifestyle patterns, Katie helped me realize I was dealing with nutritional deficiencies and blood sugar dysregulation. I was thrilled to have two issues we could immediately address.

After implementing a plan to remedy these issues (including a lot of walking to combat insulin resistance, stress-reduction work, better sleeping habits, and blood sugar regulation dietary strategies), my overall health improved greatly. But, after three months, I was confused about why I was suddenly suffering from exhaustion again. Turns out I was finally pregnant—and now have a beautiful little boy!

While healing can take a long time for many, my story is a great reminder that sometimes we just need to find that missing "something." For me, by addressing my blood sugar dysregulation and eating a nutrient-dense diet, I was finally able to conceive. -Claire, UK

The great thing about balancing blood sugar is that it's achievable for just about everyone regardless of budget, and something we all should be doing long before more serious issues set in. The way you begin to accomplish this is by increasing the "braking system" of proteins, fats, and fiber while decreasing any overconsumption of sugars and starches. To imagine what this process looks like in real life, here's an actual conversation I had with a client about how to address her blood sugar rollercoaster:

Me: I see you're munching on a lot of snack foods throughout the day and have your meals based around high-starch foods, like this big bowl of oatmeal with raisins in the morning, a sandwich and crackers for lunch, and pasta for dinner. Instead, we want you to base your meals around protein, fiber, and fat, and slowly wean from the snacking.

Client: I can't, my doctor told me it sounds like I have hypoglycemia. If I don't snack, I feel angry and faint. I can't go more than two hours.

Me: Exactly, I want to stop you from having hypoglycemia.

Client: Wait, you can stop it? My doctor told me to eat simple sugars frequently so my blood sugar didn't dip.

Me: Hypoglycemia is more of a symptom of poor macronutrient balance. It's like getting a headache from being dehydrated and being told to take painkillers for it rather than drink water. In this case, consuming bigger meals with healthy amounts of fiber, protein, and fats are your "water" for this "headache."

Client: Oh my goodness, my head just exploded.

Maybe your head exploded too—it's that simple? Yes, in theory. Eggs or sausage plus a large side of veggies (topped with butter or olive oil) for breakfast. Huge salad of leafy greens with smoked salmon, avocado, pine nuts, and roasted beets for lunch. Kalua pork and cabbage for dinner with a small roasted sweet potato and coleslaw. Or perhaps tempeh curry made with veggies and coconut milk over a 1/2 cup serving of rice. Meals like this not only balance your macronutrients, they're crammed with our Endo-9.

To better understand which macronutrients to prioritize, let's check out each category together.

PRIORITIZE YOUR CARBS

Carbohydrates are not the enemy. They are the preferred form of fuel your cells and microbiome rely on! To create balance (the keyword), you simply want to choose the right carbohydrate-rich foods. This means avoiding the sugar- and starch-laden varieties and instead opting for the fiber-, nutrient-, and antioxidant-rich varieties such as *fresh veggies, fruits, tubers, squashes, beans, and maybe some grains.*

If all of this is new information to you, please don't overthink it at this stage; just make it a priority to buy fewer foods in boxes, bottles, or bags. Replace these with fresh or frozen vegetables, beans, fruit, and home-cooked grains.

Making simple swaps like these to reduce the overall quantity of sugars and starches in your diet will reduce your blood sugar and insulin load—altogether reducing the chronic inflammation bucket you're dealing with.

Cut Ultra-Processed Foods

Whether you fill up on donuts and soda or organic pasta and gluten free bread, make it your goal to replace ultra-processed carbohydrates with the nature made varieties (i.e. plants).

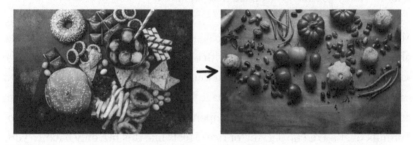

Prioritizing your carbs will also support your gut microbial health. Pathogenic and opportunistic organisms alike love sugars and starches, so a diet based around these foods will lead to flourishing populations of many of the bacterial species you don't want. The more pathogenic species, the less robust and less diverse your microbiome, and the more inflammatory issues you may develop.

In fact, eating a diet based on fiber-rich and lower-starch whole foods can alter the microbiome for the better in as little as 2 to 4 days.[182] You may have heard of "carb flu," flu-like symptoms, including headache and nausea, as well as bowel issues, which are the result of someone substantially lowering their carb intake. Part of the reason for this is the die-off of "bad" bacteria in the gut as the body works overtime to clear these buggers out—it's basically a detoxification reaction. That's how strong the high starch/dysbiosis connection is.

As a more advanced next step, you may start to prioritize *which* unprocessed carbs to eat more of than others. Without getting too caught up in diet fads (i.e., keto, Atkins, low-carb, carnivore, or anything else that wildly axes all carbohydrates), try following this gentle tier system:

First Priority: Low- to moderate-starch veggies. Consider *dark leafy greens, cruciferous cabbages, cauliflower, broccoli, fresh lettuce, herbs, jewel-colored roots, and bright orange squashes.* These should make up the bulk of your carbohydrates, varieties that will offer you more fiber with less starch, while contributing substantially more vitamins C and E, magnesium, antioxidants, and phytonutrients for your endo body. Aim to have these types of foods take up half your plate. Doing so will help you meet my often repeated recommendation of 6–9 cups of veggies per day.

Low-Moderate Starch Veggie Ideas

These should make up the foundation of your plate, adding a plethora of nutrients, antioxidants, and fiber, with low starch.

Artichoke	Eggplant	Salad greens
Asparagus	Hearts of palm	(arugula,
Baby corn	Iceberg lettuce	chicory, endive,
Bamboo shoots	Jicama	escarole,
Bean sprouts	Kohlrabi	radicchio, romaine,
Beans	Cooking greens (beet,	spinach, watercress,
Beets	collard, kale, chard)	lettuces)
Broccoli	Leeks	Scallions
Broccolini	Mushrooms	Snap peas
Brussels Sprouts	Okra	Snow peas
Bok Choy	Onions	Sprouts
Cauliflower	Bell peppers	Summer squash
Carrots	Poblano pepper	Spaghetti squash
Cabbage	Spicy peppers	Zucchini
Celery	Portobello mushrooms	Turnips
Chayote Squash	Radishes	Tomatoes
Cucumbers	Red cabbage	Tomatillos
Daikon	Rhubarb	Water chestnuts
	Rutabaga	

Second Priority: Fruit, beans/pulses, and higher-starch veggies such as corn, peas, potatoes, parsnips, taro, and yucca should be considered a side addition. When you eat these higher starch options in moderate to lower amounts (depending on where you feel the best), you will meet your needs for energy and satiety without overloading your body with too much sugar/starch (remember that starch, like sugar, gets broken down into glucose in the body). For example, if you ate 6 to 9 cups of fruit, potatoes, or rice every day, your insulin and glucose levels would be through the roof. Aim for these varieties to take up a quarter of your plate (or less).

Last priority: Grains. The most commonly consumed grains include wheat, rice, corn, and oats, and the grain-based products they're used in, like bread, pasta, baked goods, etc. While I'm not a "grain hater," I don't believe they deserve priority since they contain, on average, fewer nutrients and fiber, and much more starch than their vegetable counterparts. For example, if you put three cups of rice next to three cups of broccoli, you would find the grain pile had *much fewer* nutrients and *much more* starch. And while we're told to eat grains for fiber, there are much better options available. For example, 1 cup of brown rice only offers about 4 g of fiber, while 1 cup of raspberries offers 8 g, 1 cup of lentils offers 16 g, and 1 cup of avocado offers 10 g. And because, in our world today, most people are filling up on grains first and foremost before *any* other food group, I do believe it's necessary to single these foods out on the priority scale.

This is not to say no grains are allowed, but rather a suggestion to prioritize nutrient-dense and fiber-rich carbohydrates first, then add in grains as you feel necessary. Indeed, if you're in the "sensitive tummy" world of endo, you may feel very well with a few servings of low-fiber, easy-to-digest grains in a day. Conversely, you may feel a cultural attachment to grains, or uncomfortable giving them up for other reasons. If this is you, I simply recommend getting used to smaller portions to control the starch levels (such as 1/4 to 1/2 cup instead of one whole cup). Swapping out corn and rice for grains with more nutrients, (such as quinoa, teff, or buckwheat) can also help increase nutrient content, as well as soaking before cooking (please see the following text box on anti-nutrients). Cooking and cooling grains before eating can also increase levels of something called *resistant starch*, which is less likely to spike blood sugar and more likely to benefit your gut microbial communities.

If you prioritize carbohydrates in this way, you should fall in the moderate range of 100–150 g of carbohydrates per day, with up to 30 or even 40 g of fiber. This is the sweet spot for many of us. If you are a more serious athlete, you may find you need more carbohydrates. If you deal with significant blood sugar dysregulation, pre-diabetes, or diabetes, you may do well with less.

As a reminder, if you're on insulin-lowering medication always talk to your doctor before reducing carbohydrate levels.

ENDO TIP: DISSOLVE AWAY ANTI-NUTRIENTS

Phytates (or *phytic acid*) are found in all foods that were once the seed of a plant, including grains, beans, nuts, soy, and seeds. Phytates are also known as "anti-nutrients" because they bind to minerals within the food, preventing your body from absorbing them. They can also bind to minerals in the *other* foods you're eating at the same time, altogether robbing you of nutrients. Luckily, with some forethought, you can significantly dissolve phytate levels by pre-soaking, sprouting, or fermentation.[183] Aim to soak your grains and beans 24–48 hours before you cook them. If your body does well with nuts and seeds, soak them first in the same way, then dehydrate or roast on a low temperature to crisp them back up. While this may sound like an annoying extra step to think about, it becomes second nature after a while. I recommend setting a timer on your phone to alert you in the evenings as a reminder to soak any beans or grains for the next day. After a while, you will no longer need the reminder.

QUALITY PROTEIN

Protein-rich foods are an important part of the glucose braking system, and they are often also some of the best carriers of many of our Endo-9, including iron, zinc, omega 3s, and vitamin A. Moreover, when it comes to protein considerations for the endo body, there are two important factors: overall quantity consumed, as well as the quantity of specific amino acids.

Overall quantity: Consuming enough protein is extra important for someone with chronic inflammation, as we may need 1.5 to 2 times *more* protein than a healthy individual—between 0.54 and 0.68 g of protein per pound of your body weight per day.[184] That's because the longer the inflammatory response, the more tissue damage is done that needs repairing. It's almost like you're a bodybuilder whom every day needs extra protein to grow muscles and tissues, but instead of growing new muscle, you need that much protein just to help your body repair what's been damaged. This makes our endo-body protein requirements higher than we realize *just to prevent our muscle mass from being broken down by the body* (and that doesn't even take into account building muscle on top of that, folks). If you've felt muscle weakness, or seen muscle wasting, this may be one reason why.

To find your increased protein needs, multiply your weight by 0.54 and 0.68. For example, someone weighing 150 pounds would need to eat between 80 g and 102 g of protein per day. One pound of animal protein contains an average of 117 g of protein, so this person should eat one-quarter to one-third of a pound of protein per meal (or 113–150 g), a serving about the size of your palm (not your hand) in order to get sufficient protein. Vegetarians could consider 4 eggs *or* 1 cup of Greek yogurt with 1 oz almonds plus 1 tbsp chia seed, per meal, for the same amount of protein.

Important amino acids: Just as important as the amount of overall protein is actually the specific *type* of protein. Protein is the umbrella term for amino acids. There are 20 amino acids that act as the building blocks for every cell in your body, making up muscle, organs, skin, and tissue. In the case of chronic inflammation, three specific amino acids become very important to reduce levels of harm: glutamine, glycine, and cysteine.

Glutamine is the most abundant amino acid in the body and it becomes essential during periods of inflammatory stress, meaning you *need* to consume it in your diet if you have an inflammatory issue. In fact, during times of disease, immune cells chow through glutamine at rates equal to or higher than glucose, showing the body's preference for glutamine as immune fuel.[185]

Cysteine also becomes essential if you have chronic inflammation. That's because cysteine is necessary for your body to manufacture glutathione (an incredible antioxidant your body makes), and without cysteine you won't be able to make enough glutathione to meet your needs. This may be why supplementation with cysteine (N-Acetyl Cysteine, or NAC) has been shown to increase glutathione levels and reduce oxidative stress in a variety of contexts.[186] Research has even shown supplementing with NAC to be beneficial specifically to endometriosis sufferers, not only increasing fertility but actually shrinking endometriomas.[187] In fact, supplementation with NAC stopped *endo-ing* in these participants much more than hormonal treatments have been observed to do.

Luckily, both cysteine and glutamine are pretty widely available in both animal and plant proteins with careful selection, so you should be meeting your mark as long as you eat enough whole foods-based protein sources. For example, glutamine is found in animal sources such as beef, pork, eggs, chicken, milk products, and fish, but also in decent levels in cabbage, beets, and other plants. For cysteine, good sources include pork, beef, and lamb but also quinoa and split peas. If you're eating a diverse range of protein-rich whole foods and aiming for your own (higher) protein needs, you should be close to meeting your daily glutamine and cysteine needs.

Glycine is an amino acid that takes a little more care to consume enough of, but worth the effort. Glycine is vital for fighting inflammation, protecting against LPS, hypoxia, free-radical damage, and inflammatory cytokines, *and* is an immunomodulator.[188] So yes, it's *incredibly* important on numerous fronts for those of us with endometriosis.

While the body may be able to make up to 3 g of its own per day, a healthy 150-pound person needs around 10 g/day (although you may need more when faced with inflammation).[189] This means that if you have an inflammatory condition like endometriosis, you need to make sure you're *directly* consuming abundant amounts in your diet or you won't have enough to meet your needs.

Because glycine is essential for collagen formation, you will find it concentrated in the collagen-rich tendons, ligaments, organs, and skin of animals. This means you will get plenty of glycine if you prioritize the bits we often neglect: meat on the bone, rough cuts or roasts (like pulled pork, brisket, or pot roast), rich bone broths, chicken or fish *with the skin left on*, seafood, organ meats, or even collagen powder (easily stirred into your tea). It goes back to ancestral nutrition, when our ancestors ate from snout to tail, all of the animal, and in this way easily consumed plenty of glycine. You can also see how many of us may be deeply deficient in this inflammation-fighting super nutrient if we only consume muscle meat, or no meat at all.

While you may have heard glycine is abundant in plants, it's unfortunately not. You would have to eat an enormous amount of plant-based glycine to meet your minimum needs per day (a daily allotment of 10 cups of beans or 2 cups of spirulina, anyone?). This is where animal products come in handy to easily meet your increased glycine needs.

When considering quality, choose wild-caught fish and grass-fed meat if you can. If you're looking for grass-fed meats or organs, check with local butchers, ranchers, or farmers' markets. Often these more direct avenues will offer you more affordable cuts than looking at boutique health food stores, although you can look there, too. If this is all new to you, start with a simple Google search like "grass-fed meat _____ [insert name of your town or city]" and see what pops up. If you can't afford or find grass-fed options, don't worry, just do the best you can within your means. Look for chicken on the bone, rough cuts of brisket or rump roasts, and organ meats—they're usually the cheaper options anyways, which makes it a win-win for budgeting. Remember that every small change you make can make a big difference in how you feel.

BOOSTING YOUR DIGESTIVE MOJO FOR PROTEIN

One of the biggest issues that arise for those with endo who are looking to increase their protein intake is that some of us have a very hard time digesting it. I had one client who would quite literally vomit after eating animal protein because her body wouldn't—couldn't—break it down. In a less extreme example, I remember years ago reintroducing animal protein and feeling my meal slosh around in my stomach more than two hours after I'd eaten; it took *that* long to empty. In these cases, it doesn't mean animal protein is evil; it more often means the stomach is so weak that it doesn't have the digestive mojo to break down such complex proteins.

If your stomach feels raw, on fire, or unable to process protein, I recommend starting with meat broths, soups, stews, slow-cooked meats, or even just supplemental collagen powder for a while, as your stomach slowly rehabilitates and heals. Glycine-rich bone broths are fabulous, and they do the heavy lifting for you—pre-digesting your food, so to speak—by cleaving the proteins into amino acids so your own stomach doesn't have to. Chicken, turkey, and fish are other easier-to-digest options if you simply can't tolerate red meat yet. Supplemental collagen powder stirred into tea or soup can also be very helpful.

However you do it, aim to get enough protein, especially if you suffer from painful joints, muscle weakness, exhaustion, shortness of breath from simple stairs, back pain, or muscle aches—as these can be signs your body may be mining your muscles for the protein it needs.

HEALTHY FATS

Fats act as delivery mechanisms for fat-soluble vitamins, offer slow-burning energy to regulate our blood sugar, grow healthy children, and offer the foundational building blocks for each cell in our bodies. Unfortunately, they have also been vilified in more recent years, something that has been detrimental to overall health.

"Fat" is made up of complex chains of fatty acids that together make up the broad categories of saturated, monounsaturated, and polyunsaturated fats we're familiar with. Like protein, fats are an important part of balancing blood sugar by slowing the time it takes for glucose to drip into the bloodstream. It's why eating an apple with peanut butter or smoked salmon on toast will satiate you much longer than just eating an apple or toast alone. Additionally, they are the vehicles that deliver a wide variety of nutrients, such as DHA, EPA, and vitamins A, D, E, and K. Without enough quality fats, you will be deficient in these nutrients.

Truly, we need healthy fats to function. Your brain alone is made up of 60 percent fat, so your cognitive abilities depend on it as much as your fertility, skin, organs, joints, and immune system. Moreover, your body has trillions of cells all coated in something called a lipid-protein bilayer. It's a fatty coating with some protein mixed in, and your cells depend on high-quality fats for this layer to function properly. If there's a fat shortage in your diet, or an overabundance of poor-quality fats like vegetable oils, your cells will directly suffer (imagine Legos being made of powdery chalk).

So what fats should you incorporate to keep "braking" your blood sugar and lend your cells a nutritious, healing hand? Here's a basic beginner's sheet:

- **Saturated fats** are great for cooking. They don't oxidize at high heat (meaning they don't form free radicals), so they're beneficial, rather than inflammatory, for high-heat cooking. When it comes to nutrients, *grass-fed* butter or ghee is loaded with vitamin A, CLA (a type of anti-inflammatory fat), and butyric acid, which helps heal your intestinal lining. Coconut oil contains lauric and caprylic acid, anti-microbial ingredients to help stave off bad yeasts and bacteria in the gut. Palm oil (rainforest- and orangutan-friendly varieties) contains carotenoids, sterols, vitamin E, and antioxidants. If you cook with fats like these, you'll be getting more nutrient bang for your buck. [Note: If you've heard that you shouldn't consume saturated fats if you have endo, that's a myth.][190]

- **Monounsaturated fats** are great for cooking at moderate heat or pouring over salads or veggies. Extra virgin olive oil is rich in healthy fatty acids and antioxidants. Avocado oil or macadamia nut oils are wonderful options as well.
- **Polyunsaturated fats** (think: omega-rich fats) from delicate, cold-pressed nut or seed oils are fantastic for using cold. Good oils include cold-pressed flax, hemp, walnut, pumpkin, almond, or other seeds or nuts from food sources, as well as supplements like fish oil, evening primrose oil, and borage oil.
- **Incredible fatty foods** include (but are not limited to) avocado, egg yolk, oily fish, fish eggs, coconut, fatty meat cuts (preferably from 100 percent grass-fed animals to avoid toxins), full-fat dairy (if you can tolerate it), nuts, and seeds.

The fats we should avoid are the inflammatory seed oils many of us consume in abundance today—a.k.a. vegetable oils with nice names like soy, corn, canola, safflower, and sunflower, or marketed as "vegan butter" or "plant-based spreads." These modern fats we more or less invented in labs, and they dramatically skew the balance of omega 6s to omega 3s in the body and may create a significant interaction between inflammation and endo progression. I'll talk about this in the next chapter.

If you're budgeting on food overall, quality fats are one item I ask you to splurge on because the *quality* of fats is foundational to your healing (old, rancid, or poor-quality fats are often oxidized, which will contribute to systemic inflammation).

For cooking fats, buy a few varieties and cook with different ones throughout the day to offer the body a range of fatty acids without having to think much about it. Use coconut oil, olive oil, butter, ghee, or grass-fed tallow for cooking. Try cold-pressed nut or seed oils like walnut, sesame, macadamia, or flax (look for this in the refrigerated section) for pouring on salads or dressing meals.

JALEEN'S STORY

Simply put, the Heal Endo approach saved my life. For years I had lived under the assumption that my "time of the month" was going to be a constant, agonizing struggle. My cramps, fatigue, and digestive issues were so severe at times that I was having to cancel plans, take time off work, and even felt that getting out of bed was a challenge. At the same time, I was living a fast-paced life, drinking beer (I worked at a bar), and my love for cheese was *real*. I had just never put it together that there could be a connection.

After talking to Katie, and making some moderate changes to my diet and fitness, I feel like a brand new human being. Going gluten-free and dairy-free had once seemed impossible (given my love for things like noodles and beer) suddenly seemed very achievable with some careful planning. And, in my case, it was worth it because after I finally committed I felt so much better! Not to mention her genuine care and concern about my health and well-being made it far easier than any other fad diet or exercise plan I had ever attempted. I was lucky, I didn't have to change my whole life, just weave some new elements into it while kicking a few bad habits to the curb. Two years later, I am happier and healthier than I ever thought possible, all through small, very-achievable shifts. -Jaleen, USA

PUTTING IT TOGETHER

Where to start balancing macronutrients with all this information in mind? Breakfast. The way you tackle this meal alone will set you up for a day of success ... or blood sugar failure. To set yourself up right, I recommend you start every day with a solid breakfast with protein, fat, and fiber—whether it's an egg and veggie omelet, sausage and veggie sauté, or plain Greek yogurt topped with nuts, seeds, and berries. This will mean your body will automatically stay full longer and without an insulin spike first thing in the morning. This lays the foundation for the rest of your day.

How to know if your breakfast is spot on? See how long you can go before you need lunch or a snack. Many of us may find we can't go more than two hours before we need to start munching. This may mean you actually need a lot more protein than you're used to. (In my practice, protein is the usual suspect folks who can't make it more than 3 hours skimp on.) However, you may need more fiber, or perhaps a bit more fat. Play around with it, adding more protein, fat, or even fiber-rich carbs until you can dial in a satisfying breakfast, aiming to eat enough to tide you over for at least 4 hours. The longer you can go without a blood sugar dip, the more you'll begin to retrain your insulin response. Yes, just as cells can become insulin resistant, they can also be re-sensitized to insulin. That is the goal!

If you still feel you need more support in finding your perfect carbohydrate threshold, you may consider a *short-term* blood sugar-control diet, where you remove all starchy and sugary carbs (even healthy whole foods like grains, beans, and fruit), and then slowly reintroduce enough carbs to find your perfect balance. If you need extra support in doing this, I recommend you check out the *Honey Blood Test Workbook* available at my website which will guide you easily through the process. If you need extra support, there are plenty of programs available to help. I like the 21-Day Sugar Detox or Whole 30 as starting options.

As your cells become efficient users of glucose again, you may also find your energy levels increase, your hormones balance, your stress reduces, and perhaps some of your endo symptoms fade away.

WHAT DOES THIS LOOK LIKE?

If you want one hundred inspirational meal photos to tag along with all this information, check out www.healendo.com/food-inspo.

Making a Plate: The Basics

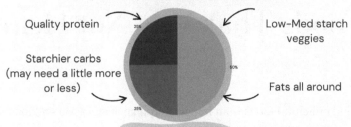

Quality protein → 25%

Low-Med starch veggies

Starchier carbs (may need a little more or less) → 25%

50%

Fats all around

Quality Protein:

While many foods contain protein, this list prioritizes iron, zinc, EPA/DHA, Vitamin A, and glycine:

Beef	Egg yolk	Scallops	Mackerel
Bison	Liver	Clams	Sardines
Lamb	Heart	Mussels	Anchovies
Venison	Kidneys	Salmon	Shrimp
Pork	Oysters	Herring	Fish roe
			Bone broth

Fats

Cook with: **Pour them on cold:**

Cook with:	Pour them on cold:
Butter	Almond oil
Ghee	Walnut oil
Coconut oil	Flax oil
Avocado oil	Hazelnut oil
Olive oil	Olive Oil
Grass-fed butter, tallow, or lard	

Starchier Carbs

White potato	Plantains	All grains
Sweet potato	Most fruits	All beans
Yam	Breadfruit	Cassava
Peas	Taro	Parsnips
Starchy squash		Corn

Plus fermented veggies: Sauerkraut, kimchee, lacto-fermented pickles, etc.

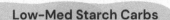

Low-Med Starch Carbs

This shouldn't be boring! Think as many colors as possible for maximum antioxidant intake cover with delicious fats, herbs, spices, and flavors

Green:					Purple:
Broccoli	Collards	Limes	Cranberries	Coconut	Eggplant
Kale	Brussels	Green beans	White:	Yellow:	Radicchio
Spinach	Celery	Pears	Cauliflower	Yellow pepper	Purple cabbage
Chard	Artichoke	Green onion	Turnips	Spaghetti squash	Beets
Zucchini	Peppers	Snap peas	Mushrooms	Summer squash	Kholrabi
Arugula	Bok choi	Red:	Onions	Lemons	Blackberries
Lettuce	Chard	Red pepper	Shallots	Orange:	Blueberries
Cabbage	Parsley	Tomatoes	Garlic	Carrots	
Cucumber		Red onions	Jicama	Orange bell pepper	
				Squash	

Green: Asparagus Cilantro Pomegranate

Chapter 10:

Foods That May Not Help

Removing unhelpful foods is an important pillar of any good endometriosis dietary strategy, although it's often the only one that gets attention. We can all agree we hear recommendations on what to avoid long before anyone recommends what to include, right? Endo dietary confusion is especially prominent here since recommendations on just what to remove will depend on whom you ask.

To cut through the noise, there are indeed a handful of foods that are problematic for just about everybody, endo or not. While I've already touched on high-sugar or high-starch diets that cause blood sugar dysregulation, this list also includes vegetable oils and alcohol. These all create inflammation in some way, either by promoting free radicals, feeding inflammatory infections, damaging the gut epithelial lining, initiating an inflammatory immune response, creating insulin resistance, or more.

Then there is a second tier of foods we often hear are pro-inflammatory but may not be for you. It depends on the source of the food, processing technique, or quantity eaten, and how your body reacts to them. These foods include red meat, dairy, gluten, soy, and caffeine.

As you can see, it's likely there are at least a few foods you may consider avoiding, either completely or as best as possible. Here I will discuss what foods to consider removing, and why.

THE KNOWN INFLAMMATORIES

Vegetable Oils

Vegetable oils, although they may have fancy names like safflower, sunflower, canola, soy, corn, or simply vegetable oil, are actually a not-so-great industrial food product. They are not even made from vegetables. They are made from seeds that have undergone an intense chemical-refining process to make them clear, shiny, flavorless, and odorless.

The processing and refining techniques that turn delicate seeds into cooking oils render them oxidized (i.e., full of free radicals) even before you open the bottle—yes, even organically grown oils. To make seeds into tasteless cooking oils, they are first heated to very high temperatures and then processed with a petroleum solvent to extract the oils. Next, because the oils now taste and smell bad (ever smelled rancid or burned oil?), they are mixed with a chemical cocktail to deodorize them and improve their color (this is why vegetable oils have no flavor). All of this heavy processing creates a toxic by-product that triggers oxidative damage and promotes system-wide inflammation every time you consume them.[191] As you might suspect, over-consuming vegetable oils may directly inflict damage and pain on your endo.

Even more, vegetable oils are chock full of omega-6 fats. As we learned in our Endo-9, we need to consume a lot of two omega 3s (EPA and DHA). But just as important as the quantity eaten is their relation to how much omega 6 we consume. Indeed, omega 3s and 6s need to be consumed in balance to mitigate the relative *intensity* of your inflammatory response.

Think of it like this: most omega 6s turn into compounds that promote in-flammation, while omega 3s most often transform into compounds that are *anti*-inflammatory. If you think a 1-to-1 fight sounds fair, or maybe a 4-to-1 if you were really strong, your body agrees. That's why we find the ratio of omega 6 to omega 3 is perfectly balanced for humans at a ratio of 1:1 to 4:1. But when we have too many omega 6s in comparison to omega 3s, that ratio becomes skewed toward pro-inflammation, and that fair fight suddenly resembles more of a bar brawl (the average American consumes a 16:1 ratio, a highly inflammatory state). That means we are getting too little of the omega 3s DHA and EPA, which are part of the Endo-9, and way, way, way too much of an omega 6 called linoleic acid (LA).

Where is all this LA coming from? Predominantly from … vegetable oils. In fact, while meat gets the biggest blame for excess omega-6 consumption, vegetable oils may actually contribute up to 13 times more than beef, eggs, and dairy *combined*.[192] If you want to see just how this is possible, look no further than nutrition labels, where we see soybean oil has a 16:1 omega ratio, corn oil 46:1, and grapeseed oil 696:1, ratios that are equal to or substantially worse than any factory-farmed steak.[193] Just because some veggie oils are marketed as high in omega 3s, they will *never* be high enough to balance the overload of omega 6s they also contain.

The Omega Scale of Inflammation

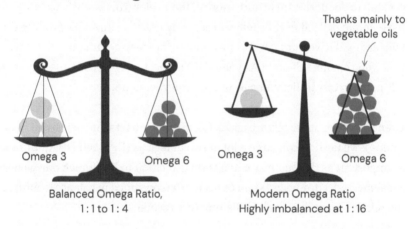

Moreover, once you begin to store excessive amounts of omega 6s in your tissues, you become even *more* susceptible to free-radical damage.[194] This obviously becomes problematic when we're dealing with a disease known for its associated free-radical damage. So while these oils are marketed as healthy, know that excess veggie oils in the diet may contribute significantly to inflammation, perhaps even making endo pain and associated tissue damage worse.

So, quick, run to the kitchen and toss out any of these veggie oils you're cooking with: canola, rapeseed, sunflower, safflower, grapeseed, corn, soy, or simply "vegetable." Make sure to also look at the ingredients in other fats you may have such as margarine, vegan butter, spreads, or olive oil "blends," which often are made up of these oils. Replace them with the oils listed in the previous chapter.

Next, check your pantry. Even if you toss those cooking oils, you will have to address the fact that most of the pre-packaged foods you buy at the store will be stuffed with these oils, as will nearly all restaurant food. Basically, vegetable oils are a cheap ingredient, so if you buy any type of processed food—whether it's Cheetos and French fries, or organic oat mylk and popular meat-free "burgers"—chances are you're consuming vegetable oils. Just another reason to choose whole, unadulterated foods over processed, prepackaged ones.

Alcohol

Drinking alcohol in even low to moderate amounts may dramatically exacerbate your endometriosis symptoms, and may even promote endo-ing. Alcohol is a known inflammation provoker for so many reasons. It's a potent immune disruptor, a nutrient-robber, and is widely associated with mental health issues. Alcohol consumption is also related to premature ovarian failure, infertility, and early menopause, showing that alcohol is truly harmful to the female reproductive system.

And if that weren't enough, alcohol is also extremely toxic when it comes to the microbiome and gut health. It's well understood that alcohol directly causes leaky gut and is associated with aiding and abetting LPS to cross the intestinal borders and get straight into your bloodstream.[195] If you remember just how good LPS is at provoking endo growth and progression, consider alcohol a hostess that escorts LPS directly to the endo table. Alcohol also damages the mucosal layer of the intestinal tract, which is home to your immune system and protectorate of "keeping the insides of your intestinal tract from leaking into your body." Without a hefty mucosal lining, you're only one cell away from leaking undigested food, pathogens, and other particles into your body.

Women are more susceptible than men to the ravages of alcohol, perhaps due to differences in the way we metabolize alcohol. Even moderate consumption of alcohol has been associated with higher levels of circulating estradiol, the type of estrogen you don't want more of with endometriosis.[196]

After all this ranting, is there *any* room for some alcohol on the table? For some of us, yes. I'm no complete teetotaler myself. Yet, some of my clients notice such a huge improvement in their symptoms when they cut out alcohol they decide it's not worth the cost. This is why I always recommend my clients remove alcohol completely for 30–60 days to see if there is an improvement in symptoms. Be aware of both the shift in your specific endo complaints, as well as energy levels, motivation, and mental state. If you find you do tolerate some alcohol, please consider the quality, quantity, and frequency of your alcohol consumption.

GRAY AREA FOODS – TO EAT OR NOT TO EAT?

Gluten

Gluten is a protein found mainly in wheat, and lesser amounts in barley and rye, and thus in all products containing these grains: bread, pasta, couscous, baked goods, flour, crackers, faro, matzo, and spice mixes. It's also hidden in most ultra-processed foods, even if they don't appear to be wheat based (think condiments, sauces, dressings, etc.). This means gluten-containing products aren't just a part of our diets, but often the foundation of them—unfortunate since gluten may be on the endo most-wanted list for many of us. As a known immune trigger (for those sensitive to it), if you have endo pain, endo belly, systemic inflammation, or any other chronic disease issue, you may not be tolerating gluten as well as you think.

As a systemic immune provoker, gluten intolerance can come in the form of rashes, eczema, swelling, joint pain, allergies, inflammation, and many gastrointestinal issues like constipation or diarrhea, bloating, or an inability to lose stubborn weight. Gluten intolerance is a known fertility disruptor, potentially causing hormonal imbalances, ovulatory disorders, or an inability to get pregnant or carry a baby to term.[197] If endo pain is your worst symptom, going gluten-free may help a lot. In one study of women with endo, 75 percent of participants who cut out gluten had dramatic reductions in their pain from this act alone.[198] Another study illustrated how gluten increased inflammatory markers in *all* individuals, not just those with a diagnosed disease.[199]

> **75 percent of participants who cut out gluten**
> **had dramatic reductions in their pain**

Celiac disease is another story worth mentioning since it's an autoimmune disorder associated with endo.[200] Being celiac means anytime you consume gluten—even accidentally or in minuscule quantities—your immune system will mistakenly attack your intestinal villi (the little nutrient-absorbing "wands" that line your small intestine), creating damage lasting up to three to four months. This means if you eat gluten even just a few times per year, your intestines may never be allowed to fully heal. Because of the malnutrition associated with this damage, undiagnosed celiac disease may be a contributor to infertility or miscarriages in the endo population, especially since doctors may delay a diagnosis for celiac by assuming your infertility issues stem from the endo instead.[201] This is why it may be even more important to be diligent about cutting out gluten if you're in baby-making mode.

As a separate consideration when talking under-nutrition, most modern wheat varieties have fewer nutrients and are often contaminated with the toxic herbicide glyphosate.[202] This means if you're filling up daily on products such as bread, pasta, baked goods, etc., you're at risk for body-wide inflammation *and* increased levels of under-nutrition.

All of this is why I recommend at least trying a gluten-free diet for anyone with endometriosis, even if for only a few months, to see if you notice a difference. And, with the Heal Endo approach to eating, there won't be much room on your plate for gluten anyway since you'll be so focused on veggies, proteins, and healthy fats (said an overly enthusiastic nutritional therapist). Of course, change is never easy, and we all love our bread and pasta! So here are a few tips to start.

- **Focus on one meal at a time.** Maybe breakfast would be easiest for you to avoid gluten, so focus on that first. As you feel confident in your food substitutions, add another meal, until all your meals and snacks are carefully weaned.
- **Focus on replacement rather than restriction.** If you're used to grab-and-go snack or lunch items and suddenly cut them out, you may feel starved, although there are plenty of alternatives. Make a shopping list of acceptable alternatives and make sure to have them to hand.
- **Read labels, or at least look for a Certified Gluten-Free logo.** Just because something says it's made with corn or rice doesn't automatically mean it's gluten-free. And even wheat-free labels don't mean gluten-free, since gluten is also found in rye, barley, malt, and brewer's yeast. Gluten is also found in seemingly odd foods, often in condiments like soy or BBQ sauce, snack foods like crackers and chips, or even in candy! If you buy it in a box or bag, check first for gluten-free certification.
- **Aim to avoid replacing gluten with gluten-free processed foods.** This is important. If you need to use gluten-free substitutions as a short-term crutch, that's okay, but since one of our biggest goals is to reverse malnutrition, filling up on gluten-free bread or crackers won't help this cause. Instead, aim to replace a gluten-containing food with a veggie or quality protein. For example, instead of wheat pasta, try pasta sauce over zucchini noodles or spaghetti squash, replace

morning toast with a homemade sausage patty, or replace crackers with celery and nut butter.

- **Don't give up if you don't feel the effects right away!** Some people take 6 to 12 months to fully feel a difference, which makes sense when we think about just how much gluten can disrupt hormones, the immune system, and the microbiome.
- **Go as slow as you need.** There's nothing worse than burnout, so make this change as slowly as you need to make the swaps sustainable. Still, keep the goal the same: to eliminate gluten completely for 3-6 months.

Two Ways to Do Gluten Free

"Gluten Free" Rich in starch, low in nutrients	Also Gluten Free Rich in nutrients, antioxidants, and fiber

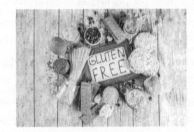 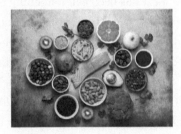

TWO WAYS TO EAT GLUTEN-FREE

When I began to remove gluten, I substituted all of my favorite processed foods with gluten-free alternatives. Gluten-free mac and cheese, crackers, bread, toaster waffles, you name it. Needless to say, I didn't feel *that* much better, and I thought gluten-free wasn't worth the effort. It wasn't until I realized most gluten-free processed foods are still contaminated with trace amounts of gluten, often full of industrial seed oils, low in nutrients, and also spike blood sugar that I decided to try gluten-free again—this time with a Heal Endo approach based on veggies, quality protein, and healthy fats. The results were astounding. So if you've tried gluten-free before (while filling up on all the gluten-free goodies you could find), I recommend you try doing it again in this new, whole foods way.

Red Meat Sourcing

Nutritionally speaking, "red meat" is the umbrella term for meat from animals that is higher in the protein myoglobin. This includes nearly all mammals excluding the white meat portion of chicken (*technically*, the "dark meat" legs and thighs of chicken are also considered red meat since they have a different nutrient profile). This means read meat is so much more than beef, including cuts from just about every farm, forest, savanna, and arctic mammal.

Red meat has been eaten liberally by humans for hundreds of thousands of years. We evolved by hunting and using every part of these animals for survival and health. Yet, red meat has somehow become one of the most controversial foods available today, especially in the endo realm. I too believed this rhetoric for a long time, becoming a staunch vegetarian for 12 years (vegan on and off). The odd thing was that when I hit rock bottom on my endo journey and tried what I call a nutrient-dense "ancestral diet" that included red meat and other animal products, I suddenly started to feel ... better. Much better. And that was hard to believe after everything I had read about red meat and endo.

After my own experience, I began to more fully investigate whether red meat is bad for endo the way we're told. After combing extensively through published research to pinpoint data on where our fear of red meat comes from, I was surprised to find there is no conclusive evidence linking red meat and endo.[203] If you're surprised to hear that, I was too. While the most cited observational study (The Nurses' Health Study) shows an *association* between increased red meat consumption and endo, the participants eating high levels of red meat were also more likely to be smoking, sedentary, and consuming more trans fats and alcohol—a pretty damaging set of lifestyle choices. So can we really blame red meat exclusively, when this overall lifestyle is also problematic for endo? Not exactly. There are other studies too, of course, and while some observe higher meat intake is associated with endo (and again, not looking at the accompanying lifestyles) there seem to be just as many that find no association at all.[204]

As a researcher, my takeaway from this conflicting information is that, when it comes to red meat, context is everything. It may be that if you eat loads of red meat *in addition to* sugars, alcohols, and vegetable oils, with very few veggies, fiber, or omega 3s, you'll be putting yourself in the "risk of disease" category (more likely to be *endo-ing*). Conversely, if you're eating red meat, preferably grass-fed or organic, in addition to loads of fresh produce and omega 3s, with low levels of sugar or vegetable oils, you will start to put yourself in the "protected from disease" category. Nothing is black and white.

The good news is that red meat, when properly sourced, is an incredibly nutrient-dense option for your plate. Red meat, bones, and organs are some of the *best* sources of iron, B vitamins, vitamin A, vitamin D, CoQ10, and zinc. Bone broths are also rich in the anti-inflammatory minerals and amino acids we need. This is why I highly recommend red meat, organs, and bone broths in a balanced endo diet.

Still, there are gray areas that arise from sourcing, processing, and overconsumption, and this may be where you find yourself needing to make some changes. Heavily processed meats such as cold cuts, ham, and bacon products, canned meats, sausages, and fast foods are often infused with excess sodium, sugar, chemical preservatives, and nitrates, and may also be more heavily contaminated with chemicals. Perhaps that's why diets rich in processed meats tend to be associated with increased levels of chronic diseases.[205] Fresh or fresh-frozen meat, on the other hand, is minimally processed, if at all. Eating unprocessed red meat may also be an indicator that folks are eating more whole foods overall (those that require cooking and preparation), rather than a diet based on pre-packaged and processed foods.

"Sourcing" refers to where your meat comes from and does play a role in the quality of our food. For example, 100 percent grass-fed animals in well-managed grazing operations live their entire lives on the range, eating grasses and shrubs, dealing with the elements, absorbing the sun, and sequestering carbon for us. The meat from 100 percent grass-fed animals has a healthier fatty acid composition (including more omega 3s), as well as more beta-carotene, vitamins D and E, B vitamins, and antioxidants than factory-farmed beef.[206]

Organically raised meats are a second-tier recommendation, the difference being that these animals are fed organic grains, although they're still often housed in indoor feeding operations rather than having access to fresh grass and pastures. Still, these animals benefit from eating food without pesticide contamination, have access to the outdoors (according to the USDA organic program), and the animals aren't dosed with antibiotics and synthetic growth hormones. Organic meat may even be more nutritious. A 2019 study analyzing the differences in nutrient content between organic and factory-farmed beef found that organic has 170 percent more omega 3, 24 percent more vitamin E, 53 percent more beta-carotene, and 34 percent more CoQ10 (an antioxidant).[207]

Lowest on the recommendation totem pole are factory-farmed meats (also known as "conventionally raised"). These meats are the least nutritious. They're also more likely to be contaminated with chemicals, pesticide residue, and antibiotics. The industry also adds more chemicals into our environment (chemicals that will provoke endo in the next generations).[208] Indeed, the Environmental Working Group estimates it takes 167 million pounds of pesticides per year just to produce livestock feed for these animals, all contributing to an increased environmental burden.[209]

However, as much as I wish we could eliminate the recommendation of all factory-farmed meats for animal welfare and environmental impact control, it is not a reasonable option for everyone. Many people living at or below the poverty threshold can't afford organic or grass-fed meats or don't have access to them. And meat is often replaced with heavily processed starch and sugar-laden foods, which actually leads to more serious health complications and intensifies under-nutrition. Again why nothing is black or white.

To prioritize based on finances and access, I like to recommend meat consumption to everyone using this priority scale:

- Purchase 100 percent grass-fed meat as the first priority, or organic as a second priority.
- If you can only budget for conventional meats, then buy the best *fresh* or *fresh-frozen* options within your means, with the lowest fat content (fat is where the toxins are mostly stored). Trim off all excess fat, and drain fat from the pan.
- Do your best to rotate cuts (bone-in roasts, chucks, flank steak, etc.), organ meat varieties, and bone broths to diversify the amino acids consumed. Glycine-rich cuts are usually the cheapest, which is a win-win!
- Avoid ultra-processed options like cold cuts, hams, sausages, hot dogs, and spam.
- Don't make meat the centerpiece of your plate, no matter which meat you purchase. Focus on fresh veggies first and foremost.

TOSHA'S STORY

My endometriosis started when I was 16, I'm now 34. I had blood in my urine and painful periods and I was put on the contraceptive pill and codeine for years. Sometimes the codeine would have no effect and I would need to go to the emergency room for morphine. Despite all of this my doctors never once said they suspected endometriosis, just painful periods. In December 2020 my symptoms changed; I started to experience blood in my stools and constipation that forced me to the ER. Finally, I was referred to a gynecologist with suspected endometriosis that night.

My gynecologist said there were no other options but to operate. When I booked my surgery I was told there was a waitlist of a year, so I began doing research to assist me while I waited. The more I learned the more I realized there were women being able to control symptoms with diet.

This is when I stumbled upon the Heal Endo approach and began to eat a diet consisting of about 80 percent nose-to-tail animal products accompanied by seasonal fruits and fermented vegetables and the occasional soaked and sprouted grain (per the recipes in the 4-Week Endometriosis Diet Plan). While I saw zero results initially, about 6 months in I was shocked to get my first pain-free period since I began menstruating at 16. Two months later, I fell pregnant, which I was told would be very hard for me without the surgery.

Although I sometimes still experience blood in my stools, it is very rare (and may need to be resolved after I give birth), and my pregnancy has been a dream. I know I will continue eating this way forever. -Tosha, Australia

Dairy

If tolerated, dairy is an incredible source of calcium, iodine, A, D, K2, and B vitamins. You could get even more of a bonus if you eat dairy from 100 percent grass-fed animals, which is shown to have more omega 3s, antioxidants, and vitamins A and K2.[210] Fermented dairy offers a smorgasbord of probiotics that can help aid the gut microbial communities, and consumption of fermented dairy has been observed to lessen certain inflammatory markers and increase certain beneficial microbes within the intestinal tract.[211] This makes properly sourced dairy products a pretty nutritious option ... as long as the body consuming them tolerates dairy, which yours may or may not.

Two potential triggers within dairy are lactose and casein. Lactose is the naturally occurring sugar in milk, which some of us can't digest. If you have lactose intolerance you probably know it, since your symptoms will probably be of the digestive nature when you eat lactose-rich milk, cheeses, or ice creams: bloating, foul-smelling gas, or diarrhea.

Casein intolerance is different than lactose intolerance. Casein refers to a protein found exclusively in dairy, of which there are two types: A1 and A2. A1 casein is found mainly in dairy products from Holstein and Friesian cows (the cows most commonly used for dairy operations in North America, the UK, and Australia) and is perhaps the biggest dairy culprit associated with endo inflammation. The problem with A1 casein is that, for many people, the body turns it into a product called casomorphin, an opioid-like substance that can stimulate inflammation.[212] Casomorphin is also a potent histamine liberator—and histamine is directly tied to endometriosis pain and many endo-related symptoms (perhaps that's why eliminating dairy alone helps some endo cases of pain tremendously).

A1 Dairy	A2 Dairy
From Holstein and Friesian cows (the cows most commonly used for dairy operations in North America, the UK, and Australia).	From goat, sheep, camel, and certain cow breeds such as Jersey or Guernsey.

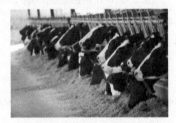

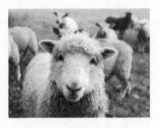

Associated With
- Histamine liberation (allergies or painful periods)
- May stimulate inflammation
- May suppress the absorption of cysteine (which is important to fight inflammation)
- May produce a gut inflammatory response

Associated With
- Increased glutathione (antioxidant) levels
- May help increase cysteine uptake

Not Associated With
- Histamine liberation
- Gut inflammatory response

Conversely, A2 casein doesn't appear to produce the same negative effects. A2 is found in dairy products from goat, sheep, camel, and certain cow breeds such as Jersey or Guernsey. A2 is not associated with histamine liberation, and in a comparative analysis didn't produce the same gut inflammatory response that occurred with A1 consumption.[213] A2 may even be *beneficial* to your antioxidant systems, since A2 consumption has been shown to significantly increase glutathione levels, potentially offering a protective effect against the free-radical cascades associated with endo.[214]

This makes A2 casein a pretty different food, proving to offer anti-inflammatory benefits instead of being pro-inflammatory, immune- and histamine-stimulating. It's also why those who think they are allergic to dairy products may just have an issue with A1 varieties but could tolerate A2 just fine.

Still, because there are so many gray areas when it comes to dairy and the endo body, I believe the best way to understand your own tolerance for dairy is by cutting it out totally for one to three months to see how you feel. Follow your digestive changes as well as changes within your menstrual cycle and pain, since any symptoms may be associated with dairy consumption. After that time, I recommend trying to reintroduce foods one by one to see if you tolerate them without reaction, starting *only* with A2 dairy. If you tolerate A2 then add in some A1 to see if you can tolerate that as well.

If you can enjoy dairy to some degree, seek out organic and 100 percent grass-fed dairy options that are known to be lower in antibiotic and pesticide residues.[215]

Soy

Soy was on the endo-enemy #1 list when I was first reading about the "endo diet" over a decade ago, right up there with red meat and dairy. So it's interesting that, like red meat and dairy, soy is also in a gray area. Instead of being wholly damaging, it turns out its ability to damage your body (or not) is dependent on sourcing, processing, and overall quantity.

The original theory on why soy was bad for endo was based on a class of phytonutrients (called phytoestrogens) that resemble estrogen to a certain degree, so it was assumed they could "feed" our endo growth. Phytoestrogens are *highly* concentrated in soy. Yet, ongoing research has uncovered that phytoestrogens may actually be *anti*-estrogenic, leading to a lower overall concentration of estrogens available.[216] This may be why a Japanese study found that diets higher in phytoestrogens were associated with a reduced risk of advanced endometriosis.[217]

Still, there's more to the soy story than phytoestrogens. Soybeans are one of the most highly concentrated sources of phytates in our diets, containing over 10 times more than rice![218] Remember that phytates are known as "anti-nutrients" because they rob you of the minerals in the food you eat. Our ancestors knew this, why ancestral populations rarely, if ever, ate soy non-fermented. This is why foods like soy sauce, tempeh, tofu, miso, and natto look and taste so different than fresh soybeans—because they have changed so much through fermentation. Today, the art of fermenting soybeans has dropped precipitously, especially in the West, with most of the soy we eat quickly prepared and with the phytates wholly intact. Soy milk, soy cheeses, soy sauce, soy burgers, soy protein—most of these foods are fast-produced without any fermentation. So even though soy is marketed as rich in calcium and iron, you may not be getting nearly as much as you think unless the phytates have been dissolved (namely through fermentation).

Then there's the issue of production, since it's estimated that 94 percent of soy in the United States is genetically modified to be resistant to the herbicide Roundup (glyphosate), which farmers liberally spray on soy crops to prevent weeds. Indeed a 2013 study found non-organic soy to contain high levels of residual glyphosate, less protein and zinc, and more omega 6s.[219] Comparatively, the organic soybeans contained no glyphosate or other agrochemicals, higher levels of nutrients, and a healthier fatty acid profile.

With all of this in mind, we can take a step back and learn from our ancestors who enjoyed soy as part of their healthful diet, eating it fermented and in moderation. We can also purchase organic varieties that prohibit the use of chemical herbicides like glyphosate. These fundamentals, when taken together, can turn an inflammation-provoking and nutrient-robbing food into something quite different: a food full of flavor, nutrients, and beneficial phytoestrogens.

Non-fermented soy products to consider avoiding include soy nuts or flour, soy milk, most commercial tofu, and highly processed soy "things" (like soy cheeses, fake meats, etc.). Traditionally fermented products you may want to include are tempeh, miso, soy sauces, natto, and *fermented* tofu or *fermented* soy milk (of course, always read labels to make sure they're fermented since many are not).

Eggs

Eggs are an incredibly nutritious food, especially the yolk. Rich in choline, vitamins A, D, and E, and EPA/DHA (if the hen was fed an omega-rich diet), eggs offer many of the exact nutrients we need in our endo bodies—why I highly recommend eggs for all who tolerate them.

Unfortunately, they are in the gray area for some of us. While egg allergies, in general, are on the rise, those of us with endo may react more because of an enzyme called lysozyme found in the egg white. Lysozyme has the innate ability to quickly slip through the gut barrier, which doesn't usually create problems in healthy individuals.[220] The problem can arise when they stick to problematic particles in our gut (such as LPS), and *then* transfer across the gut barrier into the body, prompting a big inflammatory immune response for some of us (perhaps aiding in the "great migration").

It may also be that many of us can tolerate the yolk but not the white, which is annoying but still beneficial for the nutrient-minded. If this is you, consider eating fried eggs (with the whites removed), hard-boiled eggs (minus the white), and mayonnaise made with just the yolk. If you tolerate eggs just fine, please don't remove them from your diet.

SHOULD I TEST FOR FOOD ALLERGIES?

Unfortunately, there is no test available that can measure the *many* immune responses our bodies can have for food. Instead, the best way to see if you have a food intolerance is through an elimination diet protocol. To do this, remove the food in question completely for 2–4 weeks, taking care to note specific symptom improvements/changes. After that period of time, reintroduce with a solid serving of that food, and wait two days while observing symptoms. Be watchful not just for tummy upset, but for any symptom of an inflammatory response (anything from joint pain and headaches to pelvic pain or anxiety). If you experience negative symptoms, you may indeed be reacting to this food. If you don't, try to eat a serving every day for a handful of days. Experiencing any new negative issues? If not, then you should feel confident in reintroducing this food. Remember, the more foods you can eat the better since diversity is key for a healthy microbiome, mindset, and nutritional availability!

Caffeine

Ah, caffeine. Whether it be a special cup of coffee or tea to start our day, a soda with lunch, or an afternoon energy drink, we look forward to that little java jolt to pick us up. But is it good for our endo? Like other gray area foods, it all depends on you.

Caffeine is a stimulant that increases blood flow to the brain and muscles that make some of us feel great, others nervous, and worsens some endo symptoms. It's very much a gray area food for these reasons, as well as because of other physiological changes that can happen when we consume too much or abuse its "magical powers of energy."

If you find caffeine gives you a slight buzz of anxiety, it's because caffeine elevates your cortisol, the stress hormone we really don't need any more of. In fact, if you're already a worrier, caffeine may make it even worse. In one study we see that caffeine intake without stressful situations didn't appear to affect cortisol much, but when taken in stressful situations, caffeine caused a "robust elevation in cortisol," indicating just how much caffeine intensifies the stress response.[221] For this reason, if you're stressed at all, I recommend staying away from caffeine.

Increased caffeine consumption also appears to affect estrogen metabolism, since both caffeine and estrogen are metabolized by the same liver enzymes, which may lead to increased estrogen levels.[222] Caffeine is also known to affect natural energy levels and sleep quality, two things many of us with endo lack. Researchers have consistently found big-time coffee drinkers to be more tired in the morning, leading to more caffeine intake, leading to poorer sleep quality, which takes us back to being more tired in the morning—known as the "coffee cycle."[223] If you're an endo sufferer who is really, really tired and relying on caffeine to get through the day, understand that your caffeine habit may be making the problem worse.

That being said, if you know you don't tolerate caffeine well, don't drink it. Not even that organic green tea overflowing with antioxidants. You can get antioxidants elsewhere without anxiety. If you love coffee and don't feel it poses a threat to your health, stick to one cup (preferably before noon) to avoid any issues with digestion, increased estrogen, or sleep problems. If you want another cup, try reaching for an herbal caffeine-free tea or decaffeinated coffee instead.

For those of you dealing with chronic fatigue, caffeine may seem like the only way to get through the day. Believe me, I was there! Instead, aim to use this book as a guide to start regaining lost energy and simultaneously work slowly to wean yourself off caffeine. You may be surprised to find natural energy slowly starting to creep back when you balance blood sugar, remove stressful triggers, infuse your cells with nutrition, and start moving your body more.

If you decide caffeine fits into your life, I simply recommend following the "golden rules" of consumption: no more than 1–2 cups per day, preferably before noon, preferably organic, and avoid the sugar-laden varieties, which include café-blended coffee/tea or energy drinks.

Chapter 11:

The Joy of Food

Food should be delicious, fun, rewarding, and bring people together. So how do we prepare tasty meals without the buzzkill of nitpicking over the Endo-9, macronutrient balance, or dietary triggers? I believe the best way is with a sprinkling of curiosity for new flavors, a hearty dollop of preparation, all mixed together with a willingness to learn.

Imagine a life in which the majority of your meals are made from whole, unprocessed foods. Cue a Pinterest-perfect video with inspirational music playing in the background, shooting a well-stocked pantry with jars of beans, spices, coconut milk, honey, and freshly ground flours. The refrigerator is opened to highlight the grass-fed meats, wild-caught fish, pastured poultry and eggs, a rainbow assortment of fresh veggies (preferably local and seasonal), and fermented foods in jars. On your counter you see an assortment of healthy oils one could rotate through for cooking, perhaps coconut and extra virgin olive oil or avocado oil and grass-fed butter or ghee. There's probably a bowl on a table with fresh fruit and another for onions, garlic, ginger, and turmeric. You feel inspired and ready to cook!

Of course, reality is a little different than perfect Pinterest-worthy images, so I hope you're ready for some "Pinterest-fails" along the way (if only I could show you all of mine). It will also take some bravery for those of you who turn away at the mere thought of reducing reliance on sweet and starch-rich foods while focusing more on veggies and proteins that include (gulp) organ meats and cold-water fatty fish. But with time, patience, bravery, commitment, and a sense of humor, I know you can get there.

Because this is a lifestyle swap, the goal is to integrate new nutritional habits into your life for the long term. I know too many folk who started a short-term whole foods diet, felt so much better, but then jumped ship after 30 days claiming it was way too hard, strict, or boring. That is the type of attitude you want to shift away from when incorporating changes to your normal, everyday eating. Your average daily diet should not resemble a medical diet, a 30-day challenge, or anything super restrictive (which could be anything from popular carnivore and keto diets to vegan or raw diets).

Instead, you want to learn to eat a wide variety of whole, unprocessed foods the majority of the time, and feel like your food choices are building you up (rather than holding you back). Learning this will take time and patience as many of you may need to learn how to cook meals mostly from scratch, impart flavor through herbs and spices, and stock an incredible pantry that makes the process inviting. Helping these habits stick will be the difference between enjoying your new dietary plan and forcing yourself to endure it (which isn't a healthy habit, but a mental prison). Over time what you'll find instead is the joy in cooking. Here are some steps to get you started.

PREPARING YOUR PANTRY

Being well-stocked is the absolute key to success when it comes to cooking whole, unprocessed foods. If you don't have the ingredients, you can't make the food, and you will instead open a box of whatever cereal you stashed away for moments like this. If that happens a few times as you're learning, no big deal. If you realize you do this often throughout the week, it's time to be better prepared. Here are some of the basic ingredients I recommend you have available.

Fresh produce: The foundation of any endo-supporting diet is really fresh produce, with an overarching emphasis on the varieties lower in starches and sugars. Shop accordingly: fresh produce should take up the majority of space in your shopping cart. If you have access to a local farmers' market, shop there. Local produce has more nutrients and forces variety into the diet (as food availability flows with the seasons). If you're afraid of new flavors, instead aim to buy different varieties of produce you know you like, such as different colored cauliflower or different varieties of tomatoes, apples, etc. Farmers' markets also allow you the opportunity to make friends with growers who may be willing to sell you "ugly" produce that is still very tasty at a discounted price. Because of the perishable nature of fresh produce, you'll have to get in the habit of shopping weekly for these food staples. If you don't have access to fresh produce, frozen or canned will suffice. If you can afford it, prioritize organic.

Meat: Getting enough quality protein is important for healing from inflammation. *If you can afford it,* purchase 100 percent grass-fed, or organic. Focus on collagen-rich cuts, organ meats, meat on the bone (with skin on), and bone broths. Luckily, because these cuts are often less prioritized (mostly because they require longer cooking times to make them melt in the mouth) they are usually the cheapest cuts—so it's a win-win. If you shy away from the unique flavor of organ meats, I recommend you try "hiding" them in meat mixes. My favorite is a mix of equal parts ground beef, bacon, liver, and heart. Put together in a food processor and pulse until the mix resembled ground beef. Season accordingly, and use in chili, tacos, or plain old burgers for a secret nutrient infusion that even your kids won't notice (of course, if you're *extra* squeamish, start with 1–2 tbsp of liver in this mix and increase as you feel ready).

Seafood: For EPA and DHA, seek out cold-water fatty fish such as salmon, mackerel, or herring. Canned anchovies make salad dressings delicious, while canned salmon and sardines are a tasty, fast, and often affordable option for salads or sandwiches. Oysters are a wonderful source of iron and zinc and are made more affordable if you find smoked and tinned varieties. Because of ocean pollution and overfishing, we need to be careful of larger mercury-accruing species such as swordfish, shark, and large tuna.

Eggs: If you tolerate eggs seek out 100 percent pastured eggs, which means the chickens are kept on pasture similarly to grass-fed cows. You will often find these types of eggs at farmers' markets, although they are available in grocery stores as well (such as the Vital Farms brand). The more sun, bugs, and grass a hen gets, the more nutrient-dense the egg, which is why egg yolks from free-roaming hens are a much deeper shade of yellow or even orange (thanks to the increased levels of vitamin A) compared to the eggs from hens kept indoors and fed grain (which have pale-yellow yolks). If you can't afford pastured or organic, conventional eggs are still a good source of nutrients and protein, so do your best to stock what's in your means without self-judgment.

Fats: Cook with fats that fare well under high heat, such as organic coconut oil, avocado oil, sustainably harvested palm oil, grass-fed butter, or ghee. Lightly sauté with olive oil, or drizzle it on salads. Pour cold-pressed nut and seed oils such as flax or pumpkin on salads, veggies, or even in smoothies. I recommend having 3 to 4 varieties and rotating among them. Please, do not be afraid of fat.

Beans and grains: If you like beans and grains, the best way to purchase them is dry so that you can soak and sprout them at home (to dissolve phytates). Plus, it's more affordable. Soaking before you cook is not hard, it just takes forethought and thus will be a new habit to fold in if you feel best eating these foods. Ask yourself each evening if you plan on eating grains or beans the following day, and if so soak them overnight to dissolve some of the phytates. (Of course, if you want to use cans in the meantime while you get into the groove of soaking and cooking, by all means, do so.) Switch up your varieties regularly rather than, say, always buying black beans and white rice. Consider teff, amaranth, oats, buckwheat, lentils, black-eyed peas, garbanzo beans, kidney beans, and more. I recommend these foods as a side addition to your meals rather than making up the bulk of it, since they are often high in starch.

Nuts, seeds, and nut butter: Like beans and grains, nuts and seeds have phytates in them so require soaking to release nutrients for absorption. Luckily there are many more brands that sell pre-soaked and dried options of both whole nuts and seeds, as well as nut butters. Seek out brands that say "sprouted." You can also make them at home by purchasing nuts raw (sunflower seeds, almonds, cashews, Brazil nuts, macadamias, etc.), soaking them for 8 to 24 hours, and then dehydrating them at a low temperature (around 115 degrees) until crispy. If your oven doesn't go that low, place it on the lowest setting possible and stir frequently until crisp. Let cool and store in airtight jars. Remember to eat nuts and seeds in moderation (limit them to 1/4 cup per day). If you find yourself constantly craving oily nuts or peanut butter, it may signal a fatty-acid deficiency—try eating more cold-water fatty fish, avocados, and/or cooking with more fats.

Pantry staples: These include bottled, canned, and other options that allow you to make your food taste great! Consider a variety of vinegars, including apple cider, balsamic, and white wine. Jarred tomato paste, whole or diced tomatoes, or pasta sauce is helpful for quick meals. Look for tomato products in glass jars if possible, since more BPA can be leeched from canned varieties due to the acidic nature of tomatoes.

For baking, consider a few staples to start with, such as tapioca flour as a thickener/starch, plus any baking flours you may need to replace wheat flour. I personally like oat or teff flour. There are some excellent new gluten-free flour blends on the market that make it easy to replace wheat flour in all your favorite recipes. Baking soda, baking powder, chia seeds, dark or semi-sweet chocolate chips, and 100 percent pure vanilla extract will be required for many baking recipes, so it makes sense to have these on hand if you're an avid baker.

Flavor requires spices, but buying more than 1 or 2 at a time can get pricey. If you're budgeting, I recommend purchasing what you need for one recipe at a time and slowly building up your spice rack. Always have unrefined sea salt and black pepper on hand.

Honey and maple syrup are great sweeteners for baking and other recipes. Coconut sugar works well as a placement for table sugar. Please remember that just because these options are healthier than refined table sugar (as in they contain more nutrients), they still spike blood sugar, so keep use to a minimum.

Produce, Pantry + Provisions

Stock your pantry and fridge to the max before you endeavor to change what you're eating. This will prevent you from feeling hungry or deprived, and make it so much easier for you to start cooking!

PROTEINS

- Beef or Bison: ground, roasts, etc.
- Wild game: any/all varieties/cuts
- Pork: pork butt, bacon
- Eggs
- Chicken: thighs or whole
- Salmon: smoked, fresh, or canned
- Sardines: canned or fresh
- Organ meats & sausages
- Traditionally fermented tofu or tempeh

FATS

- Coconut oil
- Extra virgin olive oil
- Palm oil (sustainably harvested)
- Grass-fed butter, lard, or tallow
- Sesame oil
- Cold pressed flax, almond, macadamia, walnut, pumpkin seed

VEGGIES, EAT THE RAINBOW

- Green: broccoli, kale, spinach, chard, zucchini, arugula, lettuce, cabbage, cucumber, asparagus, collards, brussel sprouts, celery
- Yellow: yellow bell pepper, spaghetti squash, summer squash
- Orange: carrots, orange bell pepper, squash
- Purple: eggplant, radicchio, purple cabbage
- Red: red bell pepper, tomatoes, red onions, beets
- White: cauliflower, turnips, parsnips. mushrooms, onions, shallots, garlic

LOW-SUGAR FRUITS

- Berries
- Lemons, limes, or grapefruit
- Avocado

HERBS AND SPICES

- Basil, arugula, cilantro, marjoram, rosemary, etc.
- Unrefined sea salt, pepper, paprika, chili powder, garlic powder, onion powder, cayenne, etc.
- Don't be afraid to spend some extra money stocking up on spices! These will be the flavors that make your whole foods cooking enjoyable, not boring.

FLAVOR MAKERS

(read labels to make sure no sugar)
- Salsa
- Hot sauce
- Unrefined sea salt
- Honey
- Full fat Coconut milk
- Curry paste
- Mayonnaise (avocado, olive, or coconut oil only, NOT made with seed oils)
- Mustard
- Apple Cider Vinegar
- Red Wine Vinegar
- Seaweed + nori wraps
- Sauerkraut, kimchee, and all other fermented veggie options.
- Raw cacao powder
- Nutritional yeast

NUTS + SEEDS

(eat in moderation)
- Almonds, walnuts
- Cashews, brazil nuts
- Macadamias, pumpkin seeds
- Chia seeds, flax seeds
- Nut butters

MAKING FOOD

The biggest hurdle for some of us will be learning how to cook, as well as the time management to do so. This will include not only creating a well-stocked pantry and fridge but also learning how to easily throw together simple whole food meals without opening boxes of pot pies, pizza, pasta, or whatever else is easy. If this seems overwhelming, please take your time, and try to relax and enjoy the process. As you continue to learn, focus on making changes at a steady (not frantic) pace that will become lifelong habits. Most importantly, the more changes you make, the better your body will feel.

To begin, I recommend getting some cookbooks to help inspire you, such as my own book *The 4-Week Endometriosis Diet Plan, 75 Healing Recipes to Relieve Symptoms and Regain Control of Your Life,* available on Amazon. It is designed to make it very easy for you to change your eating habits to start healing in the exact ways you just read about. It includes a 28-day meal plan to help you create simple yet nutritious meals that meet the *exact* requirements laid out in this book (gluten and dairy-free, rich in veggies, and planned to meet or exceed your Endo-9). It shows you how to reduce your time in the kitchen by batch cooking and it even provides shopping lists to get you started.

To learn how to cook from scratch (and, how to cook in general) I also recommend *Salt Fat Acid Heat*, by Samin Nosrat. I don't think there's a better, or more beautiful, book out there that so simply gets the points across about how to cook from scratch. Samin's simple tips and advice help us see that cooking doesn't have to be hard.

Time, of course, is one of the biggest considerations when we start to cook like this. Not only do we have to do a bit more planning, but also extra washing, chopping, cooking, and cleaning up. With three meals a day it can seem daunting. Add kids and a hungry partner to the mix (like me) and it can be downright overwhelming. The best strategy to adopt here is, in my opinion, batch cooking. Aim to spend 1–2 hours a day, 3–4 days a week prepping food. This means you'll be making the kitchen dirty three times per week rather than three times per day. For me, this means ensuring I have an extra hour after the farmers' market to wash and stash my produce, and an extra 2 hours on some days to make two food items for the week, like a casserole, pulled pork, or stew. I also use that time to throw some veggies in the oven so they're already roasted and ready to go, such as roast carrots, fennel, beets, yacon, green beans, or more. Now when my family is hungry in the future, there are easy options *already made* in the fridge, and I don't have to be cooking a fresh meal every time we need to eat.

If finances are an issue, please know this dietary approach is not for the elite only. While it's best to prioritize organic produce and pastured or grass-fed meats I'm giving you the green light to continue without these options if you can't afford it. A diet based on non-organic whole foods is still light years better than one based on processed, refined fare. I'm also here to remind *a lot of you* who say you can't afford better food to consider rearranging your budget (i.e., cutting out that online shopping habit!) for the sake of healing. You will be glad you did, especially when you start to feel better.

Of course, being too strict with your diet isn't good for your mental health, and we need to strike a balance when it comes to nutrition and what brings us joy. If you say goodbye to sugar and vegetable oils forever, you probably will never eat out at a restaurant again. This is where the 80/20 rule can really shine: eat well 80 percent of the time, and relax a bit for the other 20 percent. Does this mean you can include some chocolate cake and French fries? Sure. When I was changing my diet from mac and cheese to liverwurst, I made sure to include some homemade flourless chocolate cake almost every day as a stepping stone (I even put the recipe in my aforementioned cookbook). Eventually, I was able to get to the place where I really *enjoy* my nutrient-dense meals, both in flavor as well as the feeling of vibrant health they give me (something my chocolate chip and banana sandwiches weren't).

Until you can get to a place where you're really content eating nutrient-dense foods, the 80/20 rule allows you to eat incredibly well most of the time but still leaves you wiggle room to have fun going out to restaurants or friends' houses. This is not about leading a lifestyle of deprivation for the sake of health, but understanding that we *should* prioritize the foods we know have the ability to heal us, at least most of the time. But friends and community heal us too, so don't let perfection stop you from enjoying some French fries from time to time with your bestie.

Of course, if you react terribly to certain foods, you probably need to stay away from them 100 percent of the time. For me, this is gluten, conventional dairy, wine, and egg whites. For you, it may be soy, caffeine, or [insert food here]. Or you may be on a strict, short-term medical or gut-healing diet like low FODMAP or the Paleo AIP that doesn't leave wiggle room. If you're stuck in this predicament, work hard to not let it affect your ability to go out with friends or family and continue to enjoy their company (i.e., don't let your diet isolate you). There is often *something* on a restaurant menu you can get, and friends are most often accommodating enough to work with you to find a place you all can enjoy. And when all else fails, it never hurts to eat before you go out. Remember, community = immunity, so don't self-isolate!

And while this book isn't big enough for recipes, here are some *very* basic meal ideas to help you begin to visualize just what a nutrient-dense, blood sugar–balancing diet looks like (and also to show you that it's not too hard), and a pantry-stocking list to get you started. I also have a page on my website at www.healendo.com/food-inspo with an incredible assortment of meal images highlighting what the Heal Endo approach looks like in my own everyday life.

Egg-free Breakfasts

- Veggie + ground beef skillet, emphasis on the veggie. You can do a kale + basil pesto skillet with chicken, red peppers + onions + grass-fed Kielbasa, or sweet potato + spinach + ground beef. The sky is the limit with combinations.
- Homemade sausage patties made with hidden liver and heart, with a heaping serving of sautéed veggies on the side.
- Berry, zucchini, cucumber, avocado, coconut milk, and collagen powder smoothie.

- Leftovers from the night before (breakfast doesn't have to be "breakfast food").
- Smoked salmon, avocado, and thinly sliced red onion on sweet potato "toasts" or gluten-free sourdough bread.

Egg-based Breakfasts

- Omelets or scrambles with any veggies. Top with sheep or goat cheese.
- Scrambled, topped with guacamole and salsa, side of fajita-style onions, spinach, and peppers.
- Boiled or poached over roasted potatoes and wilted greens, such as chard, kale, or spinach drizzled with olive oil and sea salt.
- Vegetable-rich frittata.
- Eggs baked over veggies in tomato sauce. This is one of my favorites!
- Fried in butter or coconut oil, served over spinach and squash with a pesto sauce.
- Egg baked in half an avocado, with thyme and rosemary.

Mighty Big Salads (get a BIG bowl for your salads, and fill it up)

- Lettuce, arugula, hardboiled eggs, nuts + seeds.
- Spinach with a variety of chopped rainbow veggies, sardine salad, and balsamic vinaigrette.
- Radicchio salad with pear, bacon, and honey mustard dressing.
- Caesar with romaine, shredded carrots and beets, eggs, or chicken.
- Rainbow salad with lots of veggies and salmon salad.
- Taco salad with ground beef, avocado, shredded carrots, and bell peppers.
- Dressings: olive oil with balsamic vinegar & sea salt; Creamy Garlic with avocado oil, red wine vinegar, mayo, garlic, and shallots; Tahini Herb made with tahini, sea salt, water, apple cider vinegar, and two large handfuls of green herbs (I like mint basil, and cilantro); or simple

Honey Mustard made with flax oil, honey, stoneground mustard, and a little water.

Mains

- Old-fashioned, melt-in-your-mouth pot roast with veggies.
- Roasted chicken legs on a sheet pan with fennel, onions, celery, and carrots.
- Chili with ground beef, "hidden" liver or heart, tomatoes, greens, cauliflower, and sweet potato.
- Chicken, beef, or pork fajitas with sautéed peppers, and onions. Side of sprouted and cooked black beans.
- Grass-fed steak with mashed squash and roasted cauliflower.
- Sardine salad (like tuna salad, but swap in sardines) in lettuce wraps with red onions and mayo.
- Hearty slow-cooker stew (made with rough, glycine-rich cuts) with veggies.
- Herbed Thai coconut soup with shrimp, chicken, or pork, bok choi, broccoli, onions, lemongrass, ginger, Thai basil, and green onion.
- Tempeh and veggie curry made with bone broth and coconut milk, over cauliflower rice.

Basic Smoothie Makeover

- A base of berries (a low-sugar fruit, high in antioxidants).
- Add any: handful of greens, beets, celery, zucchini, cucumber, avocado, etc.
- Protein: 1–2 scoops collagen powder or nut butter.
- Liquid: full-fat coconut milk or nut milk.
- NO extra sweetener.

Sauces

- Quick dairy-free cream sauce: put a can of coconut milk in the fridge. When it's cold, skim the cream off the top. Simmer with any spices you prefer (think curry, cumin, cayenne, paprika, etc.) and sea salt. Great over meats, veggies, or eggs.
- Italian tomato sauce.
- Herb Sauce: grab a few handfuls of fresh herbs such as basil, cilantro, and arugula, and blend with olive oil, lemon juice, and sea salt. You can easily change the flavors depending on which herbs you use.
- Nut cheese: soak raw cashews in water overnight. Drain. Blend with nutritional yeast, sea salt, apple cider vinegar, and just enough water to create a thick "cheesy" spread. Can swap out nut varieties for different flavors.

Easy Snacks

- Hardboiled or deviled egg with red pepper slices.
- Sliced turkey and cucumber with mayo wrapped in lettuce.
- A small handful of nuts or cheese with apple slices.
- Hummus and cucumber or carrots.
- Nut butter on celery.
- Salmon salad with avocado on rice crackers.
- Avocado with sea salt and salsa.
- A popsicle made from your leftover smoothie.
- Sardine salad lettuce wraps with your favorite sandwich fixings.

Sweet Ideas

- Chocolate avocado mousse sweetened with a small bit of honey.
- Coconut cream poured over or blended with frozen blueberries.
- 80 percent dark chocolate, the real deal.

Part IV:

Beyond Nutrition – An Endo-Healing Life

While nutrition is one key aspect of addressing an inflammatory condition like endometriosis, it's only one factor of many that might need to be addressed to combat this multifactorial disease. This is where additional inputs really shine. To bring a body back to health we may need to move more, move better, address bacterial overgrowths, remove chemicals and stress, increase sleep, and/or work with endo professionals to get to the root cause of some of our worst symptoms—exactly what we'll cover in the following chapters. Healing like this reminds us just how much endo is a full-body issue more than it is a period problem, often requiring multiple changes to both our diet and lifestyle (as well as working with surgeons, and specialists when needed) in order to heal in the way we deserve.

Chapter 12:

Move More and Move Better

We all know that physical activity is important for health (cue eye-roll), but turns out it also is very effective in decreasing endo-associated pain.[224] In fact, according to some research, it may be even more effective than painkillers![225] Thanks to increased movement, inflammation caused by low oxygen levels in your tissues (hypoxia) is reduced.[226] So you can see that moving more is an important strategy for healing your endo.

Yet, this chapter is not about exercising. Rather, it's about becoming committed to *moving more* and moving *better*. This is critically important since, to reduce your endo pain and lower inflammation, you need to increase blood flow to your glutes, abdomen, and pelvic floor—all of which requires more activity. Not only that, but you need to strengthen your deep core, which will require a new approach to how you move and breathe.

MOVE MORE, SIT LESS

When I first stumbled upon the idea that moving more (and sitting less) could help quell pelvic pain I was skeptical, to say the least. But my curiosity was piqued after reading an article by biomechanist Katy Bowman on how a 10-day hike had eliminated her menstrual pain (through bringing back blood flow to the core muscles and pelvis), with follow-up comments from other women who had similar results.[227] Empowered with knowledge, I immediately added more movement to my life to try for myself. I aimed for one 5-mile walk per day, in addition to constant and regular movement *throughout* the day: sitting on floors instead of chairs, standing desks, squatting, setting a timer every 30 minutes, and walking around my property. The results of this new movement attitude were stunning (more energy, less stress, increased muscle length and strength, and *far* less pelvic pain to boot), leading me to be an endo-movement convert, as my clients will attest.

Truthfully, most of us are quite sedentary, as abundant public health campaigns remind us. We wake up and sit for breakfast, sit driving to work or school, sit at work or school, sit driving home, sit eating dinner, sit on the couch, and go back to bed. It's estimated we only average a *total* of 1.5 to 2 miles of walking per day, with *less than* 1 in 5 women getting the minimum amount of recommended exercise per week.[228] For the folks who are active for an hour a day (what most of us refer to as "working out"), Katy Bowman calls this *active sedentary*, reminding us that even if you work out 1 hour per day, 7 days a week, that's still only about 6 percent of your waking hours! For the rest of the 94 percent? Most of us are probably... sitting.

Too much sitting is a public health crisis, but it's a specific problem for endometriosis because it restricts blood flow to the pelvis. Restriction in any blood flow is harmful to the functioning of your body since *all* of your muscles, tissues, and cells need consistent blood flow. (Ever had your leg fall asleep from sitting the wrong way? That's what happens.) There's a scientific word for this, *ischemia*, which occurs when there's low to no blood flow to an area.

Although most of us don't have ischemia of this level too often (where a limb falls fully asleep), you probably have lower levels of ischemia more frequently than you realize. That's because your body will naturally reduce blood flow to muscles and tissues when they're either (a) not being used, or (b) being consistently squished. When we spend 8 to 12 hours a day in a sitting position, we're not using the entirety of our musculature, and we're also in a constant state of "squishing" our glutes, hamstrings, and even our genitals. In fact, because sitting decreases the oxygen level of the glutes *quickly*, this directly reduces pelvic blood flow since they share the same arteries.[229]

To add insult to injury, chronic muscle tension (like sucking in your stomach too much, or trying to hold Kegals) is another form of "squish." When a muscle is stuck in a contraction it can't fully function, leading to less blood flow in that area even if something isn't physically pushing on it (like a chair seat).

This means a tense and underused body will end up with some *chronic* ischemia, which is especially problematic in the case of endo. Ischemia causes an intense inflammatory reaction as the body continuously tries to repair and rebuild tissue to increase blood flow without much success (because you're still not using the muscle).[230] In this way, inflammation that is supposed to be short-lived actually becomes another chronic inflammatory trigger because the muscle or tissue being repaired never seems to "come back to life." And now this inflammatory reaction will recruit many of the same inflammatory immune factors associated with endo.

Think about it like this: Ischemia = less blood flow, leading to decreased oxygen (hypoxia), which increases inflammation, that is all associated with endometriosis establishment, progression, inflammation, and pain. This is why your goal of reducing inflammation begins with the simple acts of moving more, and sitting less.

Use Circulation... or Lose It

Weak, Atrophied, or Tight Muscle   **Well Used Muscle**

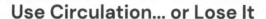

Very little circulation means increased inflammation

High levels of circulation means oxygen, nutrients, and lymph, and less inflammation!

Unused muscles will have fewer blood vessels. This means less access to oxygen and nutrients, so an increase in hypoxia (inflammation).

Well-used muscles have much more circulation and thus vastly increased access to oxygen and nutrients. Wake up sleeping muscles by using them, reduce squishing your tissues, and release any longstanding muscle tension.

When you need to sit, make it your new sitting culture to get up and move frequently. Research shows it only takes 15-30 minutes of sitting to create ischemia in the pelvic region, while it only takes 2 minutes of movement to bring the blood back.[231] With that in mind, consider setting a timer for 20–30 minutes of sitting, followed by 2 quick minutes of movement—simply walking around your home or office will do. It may even increase your mental focus when you return. Win-win.

> **Research shows it only takes 15–30 minutes of sitting to create ischemia in the pelvic region, while it takes 2 minutes of movement to bring the blood back.**

I also encourage you to explore other ways to integrate more movement into your *regular* activities, to keep ischemia at bay. These movements add up over the day and will start to rehabilitate your body, develop a stronger cardiovascular system that infuses your tissues and organs with more oxygen, activate the lymphatic system, and deliver nutrients to every cell in your body.

If you're interested in learning more about moving more in our sedentary world, I highly recommend following the work of Katy Bowman, who helps people like us (the chronically sedentary and tight kind) retrain our bodies to move naturally again. If you have chronic back, knee, shoulder, or wherever pain, check in to see if you can fix it by moving more throughout the day. You can find the basics at www.nutritiousmovement.com.

I'm also a big fan of Pvolve.com for rehabbing the glutes, hips, and overall movement patterns. So much more than doing squats, this program helps wake up the entire pelvic musculature (all three gluteal muscles plus the hips and core need to be activated, lengthened, *and* strengthened). And there's no easier way to do it than in the comfort of your living room.

ENDO TIPS: MOVING MORE
IN A SEDENTARY WORLD

- Walk or bike instead of driving.
- Take frequent breaks from sitting and walk or jog around your house or office (outside if you can). Go for walks with friends instead of coffee or breakfast dates.
- Find a hill and walk up it. Or walk up a flight of stairs several times a day.
- Dance in the kitchen to an oldie mix while you are cooking. Puts more joy in cooking, too.
- Instead of simply lying on the couch, do small exercises, mellow stretching, or glute activation exercises while bingeing on Netflix.
- Park your car at the far edge of the parking lot and walk to your destination.
- Keep light weights in plain view and do small, frequent repetitions throughout the day.
- Do gentle stretching exercises to lengthen and strengthen atrophied muscles.
- Play active games with your kids—they'll love it, too. Frog jump, ninja kick, the sky is the limit!
- Surf a wave (or boogie board).
- Hike, swim, dance, make it fun!

DIANA'S STORY

Like many women with chronic pain, I was able to present a put-together façade to the outside world. No one knew that I would sometimes have to pull over on the highway during my drive to work and throw up from the pain, or that I had a constant feeling of a burning ache in my pelvis; it was simply a matter of getting through each day, no matter what. Thankfully, I was able to conceive when I was 24 years old since the later damage became too severe for more pregnancies. At 35, to prioritize pain control over *anything* else, I had a second excision surgery and oophorectomy to remove the endo implants, and a full hysterectomy to remove the adenomyosis.

During one of my pre-op appointments, my surgeon told me that "surgery was the easy part, but that healing is the challenge," as well as "healing is a lifelong process and unfortunately endo is a lifetime (chronic) disease." Basically, my work fighting endo wasn't done, even without my uterus.

In my post-op research to build a healthier body, I stumbled on the *Heal Endo* approach. My own biggest takeaway was the importance of alignment and proper movement. This was reinforced when my surgeon stood against the wall near my hospital bed and demonstrated how to start standing correctly post-op. I had been told by previous surgeons that my fascia looked like "microwaved saran-wrap" while my physiotherapist said my right glute was atrophied, my core/pelvic muscles were unengaged, and my stance was slightly collapsed and twisted. To heal this dysfunction, I've been working with movement therapists, taking photos of my progress, and *feeling* the progress in my body, has been so encouraging.

At this point, I'd say I'm 75% improved from where I was before – which is a lot better than passed out on the floor or puking beside the highway. Healing is a long-term daily process, and I'll continue to do the work, whatever that looks like. As Christiane Northrup said, "Every woman who heals herself helps heal all the women who came before her, and all those who come after her." - Diana Dearden, Canada

MOVE BETTER, AS IN, ADDRESS YOUR CORE DYSFUNCTION

Another critical component to healing endo pain is moving *better*, and that starts with your core. Your core musculature is so much more than your abs, and actually includes your transverse abdominis, obliques, glutes, pelvic floor, inner thigh, back muscles, and *many* more. Basically, it is the muscles that make up the central core of your body. These muscles rely on teamwork to communicate and fire properly.

But being too sedentary means we're not using the muscles of our core enough. This leads to atrophied muscles, which become stiff, inflexible, and weak—altogether unable to function correctly. We're also often telling our core what to do rather than letting it work as it should. We suck in our flab, flex our abs, hold in farts, hold Kegels, and, in order to get that perfect picture, we stand in strange-though-flattering positions that shove our ribs out of alignment and tweak the pelvis. Not to mention chronic pain itself can cause incredible tension in the pelvic floor. Now your core musculature isn't just weak, it's confused. *Core dysfunction* ensues. When this happens, your core musculature is no longer working together properly.

What Is The Deep Core?

The deep core consists of these four factors below. They need to activate properly when pressure increases, as it naturally does many times throughout the day.

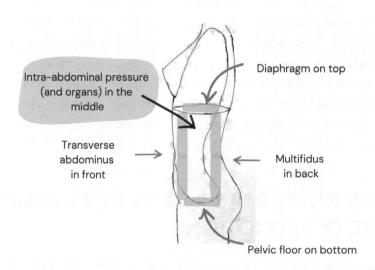

Intra-abdominal pressure (and organs) in the middle

Diaphragm on top

Transverse abdominus in front

Multifidus in back

Pelvic floor on bottom

Core dysfunction is especially problematic within the *deep core*, the should-be strong musculature that acts like a corset around your abdomen and pelvis. When dysfunctional, the deep core becomes confused about when it should brace—such as when you cough, sneeze, or pick up items off the floor (leading to back pain, pelvic pain, prolapse, and more)—or when it should relax—like when you're breathing (leading to shallow breathing and anxiety), having sex (leading to pain), or when you are pooping (leading to constipation). In all, core dysfunction can lead to pelvic pain, pelvic floor dysfunction, digestive problems, sexual dysfunction, disk herniation, prolapse, and more.

When core muscles become confused and weak like this, it can also lead to an issue called *mismanaged* intra-abdominal pressure (IAP), and vice versa. IAP refers to the natural, slight pressure that exists inside your abdomen. Think about it, there are no direct holes in or out of your abdomen (like when you're really bloated, extra "stuff" doesn't pop out of your belly button or vagina to make room). Rather, your abdomen is an airtight container that houses your vital organs, so when something happens to take up more room inside (like bloating or inhaling air), the pressure in your abdomen increases rather than organs falling out. When this pressure is correctly managed (with the proper expansion of your ribs and firing of your deep core muscles), this is not a problem. But when you add core dysfunction to the picture, that internal pressure can quickly become a *big* issue for endo.

If you have core dysfunction, your ribs might not budge while you are breathing. This means that as your lungs fill up with air, your diaphragm will be forced to descend deeper than it should into the abdomen, pushing your organs (including your reproductive organs) down with it. And, if your deep core is inactivated or confused, it won't properly brace, allowing your organs to be pushed into the lower belly and down onto the pelvic floor. This is *mismanaged* IAP, something you can visually see if, when you breathe, sneeze, cough, yell, or sing, your lower belly pushes out with each breath (no, your lower tummy does not have air in it, those are your organs).

It is obviously problematic for our endo when the brunt of 11 pounds of organs are continuously being pushed down onto the uterus, ovaries, cysts, and endo lesions. It may be why you have a painful endo flare during exercise (or simply getting up quickly off the couch). It's how an hour of yoga, cross-fit, Pilates, or HIIT *combined with* core dysfunction can cause damage at the cellular level, perhaps even bursting cysts or provoking your endo misery. It may be why you have a bloated-looking lower tummy that won't "flatten" no matter how many crunches you do. Not to mention that constant battery like this may be contributing to an inflammatory pelvic environment without you realizing it. That's why retraining core function and decreasing the pressure on your organs is a foundational need of the endo body.

How Do You Inhale?

When you inhale, about a pint of air (here shown as a pint jar) has to go somewhere in your body. Where does it go?

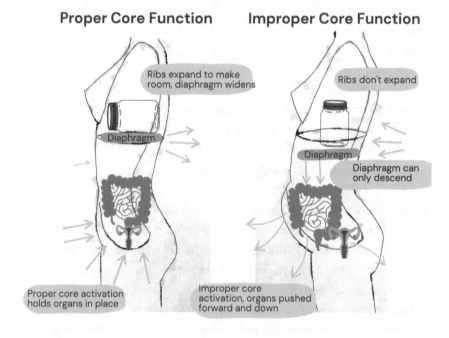

Proper Core Function

Ribs expand to make room, diaphragm widens

Diaphragm

Proper core activation holds organs in place

Improper Core Function

Ribs don't expand

Diaphragm

Diaphragm can only descend

Improper core activation, organs pushed forward and down

Core dysfunction is obviously problematic for our endo when the brunt of 11 pounds of organs are continuously being pushed down onto our uterus, ovaries, cysts, and endo lesions.

FOUR TESTS FOR CORE DYSFUNCTION

Core dysfunction is actually quite common, and there are a few simple tests you can do at home right now to find out how your core is faring:

1. Put one hand on your lower tummy, below the naval, just to observe what it does. Now, take a breath in and .... forcefully blow out imaginary birthday candles! Did you feel your lower stomach slightly suck in or brace (yes!), or did it poof out (uh-oh)? If it poofed, it shows your deep core isn't correctly activating when IAP increases, and instead of supporting your organs upwards they are being pushed *downward*. If this happened with an exhale, it probably also happens with coughing, sneezing, running, planks, etc.

2. Look in the mirror while you inhale deeply. Notice if your ribs relax and open wide side to side (yes!), or do they not budge at all and the only way you can take a "deep" breath is if you allow your lower belly to balloon out (uh-oh)? Your ribs should not be locked in a static position... ever. They are the key to reducing mismanaged IAP.

3. If you lie on your back and do a crunch or double leg lift, do you see a bulge that resembles a "bread loaf" poof out of your tummy? That bulge simply should not be there, as it's a direct visual of your organs bulging *out* and *down* rather than being supported by correctly functioning core musculature.

4. Do you often queef or feel air bubbles come out of your vagina? Do you sneeze pee or leak urine when you run or jump? Does your tampon fall out? Or maybe you can't insert it all the way because your uterus is *that* close to your vaginal opening? These are all signs of pressure pushing your organs south, signs of poorly managed IAP and core muscle dysfunction.

Do You "Loaf"?

Correct core activation: When lifting legs (or doing a crunch, plank, etc.), no "loaf of bread" in stomach.

Incorrect core activation: When lifting legs (or doing a crunch, plank, etc.) you see what resembles a "loaf of bread". This is really your organs pushing forward and down.

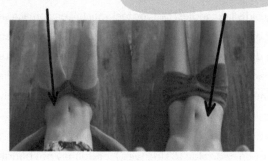

If one or more of these tests challenged you, you probably have some poorly managed IAP, the common denominator that leads to core dysfunction (and vice versa). The problem is that chronic and repetitive IAP causes your amazing and dynamic core musculature to become *stuck* in contraction—frozen, if you may—as it tries desperately to hold your body together.

THERE ARE 5 BASIC STEPS TO START REHABBING YOUR CORE:

Because I am not a movement specialist or doctor, I consulted with Dr. Angie Mueller on the best ways to begin rehabilitating a core with significant dysfunction. Dr. Angie has a Doctorate in Physical Therapy, a Bachelor's in Health and Exercise Science, and specializes in pelvic health, spine and core rehabilitation, prenatal/postpartum training, and manual therapy. Basically, she's a core function specialist (www.corerecoverypt.com). Here's a summary of what she told me (and please see Appendix 4 for explicit details and healendo.com/coredysfunction for visuals).

Step 1: Posture Is Everything

The starting point for retraining the deep core is through proper spinal position. *It is an absolute necessity.* Correct posture means your spine should resemble a beautiful elongated S curve—not to be confused with an exaggerated S-shape (with rounded shoulders and an arched lower back) nor an "army solute" type posture that juts the ribs forward (for people who are usually trying to hide bad posture).

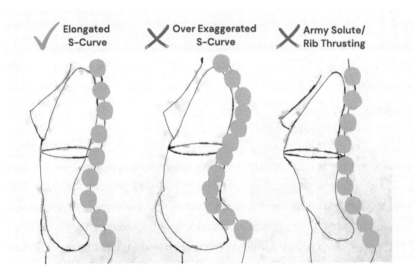

Maintaining proper spinal elongation like this is what creates the perfect amount of core activation. That's because the *only way* to elongate your delicate spine and keep it in the proper position is through properly utilizing the musculature that holds it up—the deep core. If you're flopping over a computer or phone all day, or arching your back in pretend posture, your deep core will simply not engage the way it should.

To start reigniting the strength within, imagine you are pushing away a small weight on the top of your head, growing tall. You can even put something light on top of your head to help navigate this feeling of elongating *up* (like a bean bag or a small folded kitchen towel). Now, try to remember to do this throughout the day rather than slouching in chairs, leaning on desks, resting your hips on countertops, hunching over your phone or meals, or jutting your ribs. Doing so, you should start to feel your deep core instinctively begin to engage.

Step 2: Activate Your Ribs and Diaphragm

The second step to retraining the core is through waking up your proper breathing musculature. Because most of us take shallow breaths in the upper chest, we deactivate the deeper breathing muscles that we should be using *all the time*: the muscles between the ribs, known as the intercostals, and the diaphragm. As a result, these weakened muscles can no longer expand to accommodate our breath. You may realize just how atrophied yours are if you look in the mirror while inhaling and realize your ribs don't budge. I was in this boat myself, with a ribcage so atrophied it felt like I was (ironically) suffocating when I first tried to breathe with the correct breathing musculature.

Luckily, like other body muscles, your breathing musculature can come back to life with proper training. Through specific breathing techniques that force you to use your breathing muscles (see Appendix 4), you can strengthen the intercostals and retrain the diaphragm to expand wide when breathing rather than forcing your diaphragm to descend too low and forcing "belly breathing." [By the way, deep belly breathing can be great—when lying down. So please save the deep belly breathing for the end of yoga, before bed, or when you're watching Netflix.]

By elongating your spine upwards (Step 1) while breathing naturally with a relaxed rib cage (Step 2), your tummy should naturally begin to regain function and brace when needed. If you diligently work to stop sucking in and instead focus on these two factors alone, I know you'll begin to see improvement.

Step 3: Retrain Your Deep Core Through Proper Breathing

You must know something about your core muscles: they are primarily involuntary muscles! Involuntary muscles are those that work by reflex rather than you thinking about contracting them. When your autonomic nervous system (a.k.a., subconscious) picks up clues, it shoots your involuntary muscles a "text," so to speak, telling them to contract or relax without waiting for orders from your brain. You can imagine your involuntary muscle fibers at work when you get scared of noise in the bushes and reflexively jolt away without thinking.

Similarly, your deep core muscles are governed by reflex in all they do for our bodies: spinal support, posture, balance, keeping our organs centered and lifted, managing the pressure in our abdomen, helping us take in and expel air, bladder and bowel function, and supporting sexual function. Yes, they should do this without you consciously "making them." Because of this difference, we have to retrain them using different methods than we would for muscles that respond well to conscious contractions, such as sets of squats or bicep curls. It's why consciously contracting the core muscles through "sucking belly button to spine" or "doing Kegels" is ineffective for rehabilitating core dysfunction. Instead, to retrain the deep core, *we must trigger a reflex,* and that reflex is breathing—the direct link to these involuntary muscle fibers.

To do so, Dr. Angie recommends hypopressive breathing for 15-20 minutes daily. This practice triggers your deep core to reflexly brace when necessary (while also strengthening the diaphragm and intercostals). It's a bit tricky to understand at first glance, so remember to check out www.healendo.com/coredysfunction for a visual.

Step 4: Activate Your Glutes

Your glutes are a collection of three muscles that also include what we commonly call the "hips": the gluteus maximus, medius, and minimus. In addition to being a soft place to sit, this group of musculature is the biggest and (should be) strongest in the body. It should propel your body forward like an engine, keep your knees from pulling inward, stabilize your ankles, push you up from a squat, or simply off the couch.

Correctly firing glutes are also necessary for healthy pelvic floor function. Because they're such a huge core muscle (sitting right next to the uterus and pelvic cavity), the circulation the glutes create for the pelvis is vital for pelvic health! In fact, sitting *quickly* decreases the oxygen level of the glutes, which directly creates pelvic blood flow problems since the same arteries that supply blood to the butt also deliver it to the pelvis. Thus, atrophied glutes will also mean decreased blood flow to the pelvis.

Glutes that perform poorly are often referred to as "dormant" or "lazy," so named because they stop activating when they need to (which is basically for all your daily movements). Dormancy often starts from too much sitting, which doesn't just atrophy the derriere muscles but also shortens your hip flexor in the front. This is problematic because the front of the leg needs length in order to properly extend behind you when walking. Without proper leg extension behind your body, your glutes physically aren't allowed to fully activate, leading to (you guessed it) even more of a dormant butt.

AT HOME TEST: ARE MY GLUTES DORMANT?

It's good to check in since many of us don't realize this key musculature is compromised at all. To check in, we can ask a few questions to start:

- When you walk up stairs, do your knees align over your toes (good!), or are they pulled at a diagonal inward (uh oh)?
- Do you have chronic knee or ankle pain that is exacerbated by running or hill climbing?

- When you do ten squats, do you feel burning coming from the front of your thighs (uh-oh) or maybe even your knees (super uh-oh), or from your butt (good!).
- Stand up. Now, can you wiggle your kneecaps? If your kneecaps won't budge (uh-oh), don't worry, they're not broken! This actually means they're *already* lifted because your quads are engaged instead of your glutes. This is usually referred to as Quad Dominant, and happens when your glutes are turned off. To *release* them, stand with your back leaning against a wall with your feet a foot or so away. You should now be able to wiggle your kneecaps as you feel them release. See? Slowly move your feet closer to the wall as you consciously work on letting go of the iron grip holding them up.
- If you feel like your hips are *always* tight and that no amount of stretching seems to relax them, it indicates that your glutes (which *are* your hips) are weak. While stretching and foam rolling can help alleviate symptoms of this tightness, no amount of stretching like this will fix the root issue. For that, you need to strengthen.

Rehabbing the glutes is more than doing squats, but instead waking up the *entire* musculature. As mentioned previously, I recommend P.volve to help get there, as well as Dr. Angie's online course which also offers glute-specific guidance. Depending on how much help your muscles need, you may also need professional guidance in retraining your glutes. If you have really painful knee, hip, or ankle problems, a skilled physical therapist will be able to help diagnose your specific strengths and weaknesses and get you on a plan to start the glute-activation process.

Step 5: Help Your Pelvic Floor

Dr. Angie reminds us that your pelvic floor may need professional attention on its own, especially if you've been dealing with a chronic pelvic pain condition like endometriosis.

If you're one of the many who view this as an option only for those with a "broken vagina" post-childbirth, know this is certainly not the case. First, may I remind you that your pelvic floor is not your vagina but a complex set of musculature that sits like a bowl at the bottom of the pelvis. As an essential part of your deep core, this musculature reflexively tenses when you're nervous, angry, sad, scared, or emotional in other negative ways, not to mention *when you're in pain*. That's how chronic pelvic pain (combined perhaps with scar tissue, adhesions, and cysts) can disturb the healthy functioning of your pelvic floor, leading you to clench this group of musculature habitually. To make matters worse, many of us have been misinformed about what pelvic floor health really means (as in, it should be both strong *and* supple) and instead aim to overly «tighten» it by performing 100 Kegels per day, leading to even more clenching.

Where is my pelvic floor?

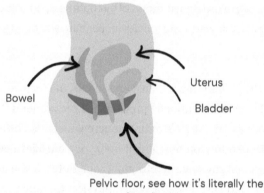

Bowel

Uterus

Bladder

Pelvic floor, see how it's literally the "floor" of your core?

An overly tight pelvic floor is one that is weak, inflexible, atrophied, and unable to perform the full range of functions it should—such as bracing when you cough, sneeze, or do a yoga plank, or releasing to poop, pee, fart, have sex, or live without pain. It's why pelvic floor physical therapy has nothing to do with "fixing a broken vagina" and everything to do with reclaiming your life after years of pelvic pain and tissue damage. Instead, like any muscle group, it may need massage, pressure release, and special exercises to rehabilitate it back to normal.

Luckily, pelvic floor physical therapy does just that! By addressing the pelvic floor muscles directly (internally) as well as everything that may impact the pelvic floor (external muscles, fascia, joints), this form of PT can be life-saving for those of us suffering from pelvic pain, incontinence, pee-sneezing, chronic constipation, painful sex, and more. If you have any of these symptoms, go see a pelvic floor physical therapist who specializes in treating these issues. For a plethora of information on this topic, make sure to check out www. pelvicpainrehab.com. You can also find a list of pelvic floor PTs specializing specifically in endo care at www.icarebetter.com.

One Last Piece of Advice: No More Traditional Core Exercise Until Your Core Functions Correctly. That includes crunches, planks, jack-knives, pilates, strenuous running, or biking. Don't do these core-centric moves until your core functions well again. If you don't pass the core function tests (loafing, tummy poofing when blowing out imaginary candles, etc.) then you won't be doing your body any favors by doing these exercises. In fact, this may be why you have flairs or burst cysts with exercise, or low back or knee pain never seems to improve. So fix your core function first, and only then consider more strenuous core exercise if you need it. In the meantime, Dr. Angie recommends walking, swimming, hiking, hypopressive breathing, or other more gentle movements.

From working with clients and my own experience, I can testify that improving your core function is worth the effort and may provide you with some genuine and unexpected relief from your endo pain. Rehabbing your core could be its own book and requires videos and diagrams to help you understand what to do. (Don't worry, once you get it, it is easy.) To give you a head start on this important journey, remember to read Appendix 4, which includes a *very detailed description* of how to start rehabbing your core, along with great resources and specialists that you can follow up with when you are ready. I cannot recommend enough that you work on retraining your core as part of your endo-warrior toolkit.

KRITHIKA'S STORY

I started the Heal Endo approach after a professional excision surgery with one of the top endo surgeons in the nation. He painstakingly removed all of my endo and, although it helped my pain tremendously, five months later I was still dealing with food and stress-triggered pelvic and abdominal pain, digestive, and urinary problems. Not to mention I had terrible lower belly-bloating that was getting in the way of my career (at the time a model in London). Comprehensive stool tests didn't pick up any big reason *why*, and I was stumped.

After working with Katie, I discovered my bloated tummy was actually an issue of improper musculature use, with additional pain stemming from a partial organ prolapse (caused by increased IAP). By learning to retrain the core musculature and breathe correctly through hypopressive breathing, I was able to lift my organs back up, combat my bloated tummy, adhesion pain, prolapse, and even resolve my lingering digestive and urinary problems. If I had continued to only focus on diet, I would never have found the traction I needed! -Krithika, USA

Chapter 13:

Mending the Microbes

As detailed in Chapter 5, bacteria may be endo's secret little BIG trigger. Dysbiosis in the gut and/or reproductive tract may in fact be triggering the inflammation surrounding your endo as we speak. On a bright note, by implementing the diet and lifestyle strategies detailed in this book, your own unique dysbiosis patterns may be tipped back into balance. Indeed everything from increasing fiber, omega 3s, phytonutrients, and movement, to decreasing sugar, inflammatory triggers (like sugar and alcohol, or foods you react to such as gluten and dairy), chemicals, and stress can have a profound impact on your microbial health.

Still, there is a large number of endo sufferers who will need deeper interventions than a balanced diet alone to address the microbial imbalances we face. If you are one of them, you may have just read the previous nutrition chapters and shockingly realized you can tolerate few of the foods recommended (perhaps instead surviving on crackers, toast, and ginger tea to keep your gut issues at bay). Or, perhaps after dialing in diet you still have a myriad of symptoms remaining that, even if not digestive in nature, may still be related to dysbiosis; issues like eczema, insomnia, anxiety, histamine intolerance, allergies, depression, acne, rashes, joint pain, headaches, and more. If so, this chapter is for you.

While it will be up to you to determine at what level you'll need guidance, in this chapter we'll discuss microbial support at its basic level: digestion, short-term dietary strategies, and when to reach out for help.

DIGEST YOUR FOOD, SUPPORT YOUR MICROBES

Digestion is the process by which your new favorite nutrient-dense meals (wink wink) get broken down into itty bitty nutrients for your body to absorb. Leftover fiber will feed your gut microbial communities. If your carbohydrates, fats, and proteins aren't properly broken down, your microbes may be *reacting* to your meals instead of benefiting from them. This alone can lead to an inflammatory imbalance of bacteria due to poorly broken-down foods in your intestinal tract. In these cases, you may have low levels of beneficial bacteria, and high levels of pathogenic and/or opportunistic bacterias and yeasts. You may suffer from excessive gas, bloating, abdominal pain, heartburn, acid reflux, constipation and/or diarrhea. Yes, a variety of symptoms many of us suffer from. And, if this is your case, the way to reverse it will rely on how well you digest your food.

Proper digestion begins with your main digestive organs: the mouth, stomach, pancreas, and gallbladder. Each produces its own unique digestive juices that aid in the breakdown of your meal into the tiny nutrients our bodies were designed to absorb. Supporting these organs to function properly can offer many of us profound relief in symptoms, as well as a first step in rehabilitating our gut microbiome. To do this, we simply need to be chewing, salivating, and enjoying our meals in stress-free environments. Here are some tips to get you started:

Salivate, chew, enjoy, repeat: Saliva is a digestive fluid, one that starts breaking down carbohydrate-rich foods before they even hit your stomach. This is why you should be salivating with every bite. But often due to stress, bland food, and fast eating practices (like, did you even taste that meal?), many of us barely salivate, nor do we chew.

To help you reconnect to the "lost art" of salivating, first consider just how flavorful your meals are. If they're bland, try adding more variety, such as spices, herbs, citrus, and/or vinegar that will immediately help you salivate. For additional help, you may consider sipping on a few dashes of herbal bitters throughout your meal to remind yourself to reconnect with flavors and produce more saliva as you eat. Similarly, two teaspoons of apple cider vinegar or lemon juice in a 1/2 cup of water sipped a few minutes before or after your meal can help stimulate saliva and gastric juices as well. Really try to chew your food to smithereens before you swallow, which will take an enormous burden off your stomach.

Take a digestive enzyme: *Digestive insufficiency* occurs when you don't produce enough digestive juices. This may be due to nutrient deficiencies, blood sugar dysregulation, inflammation of your stomach lining or small intestine, ulcers, gallbladder problems, the list goes on (and many of us have at least one of these issues if we've been poorly digesting for years).

While your digestive capabilities should naturally increase with time as you heal, you can support your body in the meantime with some digestive aids. High-quality digestive enzymes taken with each meal can dramatically help some of us process carbohydrates, fats, and proteins. Some people may not realize just how much this can help. I like Digest Gold by Enzymedica, but there are a number of good options out there.

Space Your Meals: Aim to have three meals per day, at least 4 hours apart, with no snacking in between. This is one of the best things you can do if you have a sensitive tummy or weak digestion. If you're always snacking or sipping on coffees, sweet teas, sodas, juices, or other things you need to digest, you will never give your body a break for time to repair.

If waiting at least 4 hours between eating seems near impossible right now, don't force it. Rather, make it an eventual goal and work toward it. It may take a few weeks (or even months) to get here since it will involve proper blood sugar regulation and a tummy that can handle a big enough meal to tide you over. If your stomach is so sensitive that it can't handle more than a small plate at a time (so you find yourself hungry quickly), work slowly to eat a little more bit by bit, and start by making it to 2 hours, then 2.5, 3, etc. It may take some time, but with nutritional support and digestive support (like enzymes), it should become easier.

Drink 8–10 cups of water a day … away from meals: If you're guzzling cups of liquid with your food you are simply making more work for your digestive system. Sip if you're thirsty during meals, otherwise make sure to drink 8–10 cups of hydrating water in between meals. The basic rule of thumb is 20 minutes before a meal, or 1 hour after.

SARAH'S STORY

Many people congratulated me on my pregnancy and then felt very embarrassed when they discovered I wasn't expecting a baby. Pain in my belly was so normal, I am only just beginning to discover that it's not. Most nights have been sleepless nights in which I toss and turn to find some kind of position that will relieve the bellyache. And my periods are usually a multi-day hell during which I often hope to die. Hot water bottles and ibuprofen are just not cutting it anymore.

Discovering the Heal Endo approach has been such a beacon of hope for me. I had already discovered the magic of Mayan abdominal massage & Chi Nei Tsang recently, which has changed my relationship to my abdomen and I highly recommend it to anyone struggling with Endo! It's so much easier to relax all the tension and breathe into these areas now. Whenever I have a quiet moment lying in bed, I massage myself and loosen all the hard knots.

I have also taken on the mission to eat slower than my boyfriend, chewing, chewing chewing… I am cutting out little snacks and sticking to three meals, and I am still figuring out how to ensure I drink enough between meals, instead of with my food. I am trying out digestive enzymes with big meals and so far this seems to be reducing the burning in my stomach. After being mostly vegetarian for twenty years I have had mixed feelings about eating meat again but have taken to making bone broths and having the occasional steak or sausage. When I stick to these recommendations, I experience much less pain and bloating. My last menstruation was still painful, but shorter and I had the sense that somehow there was a different quality to the experience. I look forward to seeing how this evolves as time goes on. So far I feel a whole lot better already! I know that I will be referring back to this knowledge for the rest of my life."-Sarah, USA

Elimination Diets: When a Balanced Diet Isn't Helping

The previous nutrition chapters set us up for a healthy, balanced approach to body ecology. However, if you have some serious dysbiosis or leaky gut, you may need to consider extra dietary support while you heal. This is especially worth mentioning for those of us with endo who react terribly to certain foods—although we're not sure exactly which ones. You may be nearly unable to tolerate fruits or vegetables (and probably fainted at my recommendation of 6-9 cups per day). Or you may feel like some foods wire you into stress, or fatigue you into depression. It's all so hard to pinpoint.

This is where a *short-term* (i.e., a few months only) elimination diet may help. You may even consider them "medical diets," not something you want to be on long-term nor one you should undertake lightly (especially if you suffer from disordered eating habits or body image issues), but diets worth mentioning since they have been shown in research to improve symptoms for those of us really suffering.

Elimination diets come in handy by removing potential triggers to allow the intestinal tract to heal and symptoms to abate, followed by a period of food reintroduction to discover once and for all what you were reacting to. When this happens, you will be able to go back to eating a much more balanced diet while feeling much more in control.

Here are two elimination diets to consider:

Low FODMAP: If you have serious gut issues, such as painful bloating or bowel movements, diarrhea, constipation, extreme bloating like a balloon, gas that smells like sulfur, or IBS, a low FODMAP diet may be worth considering.

FODMAP is an acronym for a group of *highly fermentable* carbohydrates, including monosaccharides, disaccharides, oligosaccharides, and polyols. These carbohydrates are contained in a wide variety of foods (which can seem quite random), including everything from dairy and gluten to cabbage, beans, garlic, avocados, and beets. If you react to high FODMAP foods, you may be so bloated you look pregnant, have constant diarrhea, constipation, or a combination of the two. It's because high FODMAP foods exist across many food categories that you may also feel like you can never pinpoint what's giving you digestive distress as you try every diet from vegan to paleo to the Standard American Diet.

So intertwined are FODMAP reactions with endo, that there are studies demonstrating that women with both endo *and* severe GI complaints who use a low FODMAP diet can relieve both digestive and endometriosis symptoms.[232] We also know there's a large overlap between IBS (irritable bowel syndrome) and endo, with many women getting either misdiagnosed or dual diagnoses. A low FODMAP elimination approach is the gold standard to start identifying IBS triggers. I've known folk who followed a low FODMAP diet for their IBS and "miraculously" had their endo symptoms minimized as well.

A low FODMAP approach may also help endo sufferers by reducing histamine levels up to eight-fold.[233] Histamines are potent immune factors, creating inflammation and the allergic responses we commonly know—sneezing, swelling, pain, etc. Because endometriosis lesions have excessive levels of mast cells (cells that *make* histamines), those of us with endo may both *have more of* and *react to* histamines, altogether contributing to systemic inflammation and chronic allergies (food, environmental, or otherwise). By reducing the amount of histamines in the food you will also reduce your body burden, which may help your symptoms.

For this short-term approach, you cut out all high FODMAP foods for 2–4 weeks (see image for examples). If you notice improvements in either your digestive or endo symptoms, it's reasonable to assume you're reacting to one or more of the categories. After those 2–4 weeks, you slowly reintroduce the foods category by category to see what you can tolerate and what you can't. You may be surprised to find that only one or two categories of food are big triggers for you (such as wheat and dairy, for example), rather than this entire list.

Conversely, if you can't reintroduce any foods without reaction, I recommend working with a gut specialist for further testing. It's common that someone unable to tolerate few if any high FODMAP foods will have SIBO (an overgrowth of bacteria in your small intestine).

You may also consider working with a professional if you're just plain confused about what foods to remove and when to reintroduce. You never want to stay on a low FODMAP diet for long because it will actually harm the gut by removing prebiotic-rich foods that are important to your beneficial microorganisms. A quick Google search will uncover an abundance of low FODMAP nutritionists or dietitians, many of whom work on Zoom or Skype.

Some Examples of FODMAPs

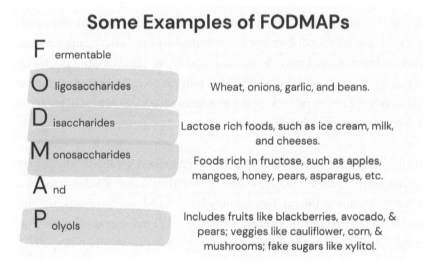

F ermentable

O ligosaccharides — Wheat, onions, garlic, and beans.

D isaccharides — Lactose rich foods, such as ice cream, milk, and cheeses.

M onosaccharides — Foods rich in fructose, such as apples, mangoes, honey, pears, asparagus, etc.

A nd

P olyols — Includes fruits like blackberries, avocado, & pears; veggies like cauliflower, corn, & mushrooms; fake sugars like xylitol.

Paleo AIP Diet: If, rather than serious digestive complaints, you suffer from autoimmune conditions, high levels of inflammation and associated symptoms (insomnia, joint pain, headaches, chronic fatigue, etc), and/or a lot of symptoms that you can't pinpoint the root cause of, the Paleo Autoimmune Protocol Diet may help.

The Paleo AIP is a research-backed approach to addressing inflammation at the gut level. Over the course of 3 to 6 months, you will remove any *potentially* inflammatory triggers such as grains, beans, dairy, eggs, nightshades, and alcohol (yes, that's a lot of foods!) and replace them with lots of veggies, bone broths, grass-fed meat and organ meat, fruits, and plenty of fats. It's a nutrient-dense feast that removes potential triggers while beginning to reverse under-nutrition. Like a low FODMAP diet, the elimination period is followed by a gradual re-introduction, where you test foods to determine your personal tolerance.

The AIP has some serious scientific leverage these days when it comes to lowering systemic inflammation and even reversing some aspects of autoimmune disorders. Recently two studies have been released demonstrating how this approach achieved measurable results (meaning more than just "feeling better"). In one, participants with the autoimmune disease Crohn's who followed the AIP diet experienced an overall reduction in symptoms, better endoscopic results (meaning they actually had some beneficial *structural* changes in the gut), and an overall decrease in inflammatory markers.[234] Another study analyzed participants with the autoimmune disease Hashimoto's thyroiditis who undertook the AIP diet and felt not only an overall symptom reduction but also had a measurable decrease in inflammatory markers and, for some, a decrease in needed thyroid medication.[235]

While there's no science connecting AIP and endometriosis specifically just yet, we can see that a dietary strategy like AIP that's been clinically shown to lower inflammation, heal the gut, balance blood sugar, and reverse under-nutrition may indeed be helpful for an endo body that didn't feel enormous gains from shifting to the basic endo diet discussed in the previous nutrition chapters. It may be that you're reacting to something else—something like pepper or egg whites—and by removing all the *potential* triggers and reintroducing them one by one, you might be able to finally pinpoint the issue you're dealing with.

ENDO TIP: EASY STEPS FOR OPTIMAL GUT HEALTH

Increase fiber... without excess starch: Your microbiome thrives on fiber, less so on starches and sugars. Achieve this by basing your meals around low- to medium-starch veggies.

Eat the rainbow: Studies have demonstrated that a diet rich in polyphenols can reduce or reverse dysbiosis, another reminder to eat a diet as diverse in plant foods as possible.[236]

Don't forget ample amounts of omega 3s: These healthy fats are a microbiome's food of choice! So much so, that supplementation with the omega 3s EPA and DHA has been shown to increase microbiome health and diversity in as little as 14 days.[237] It has been shown to increase beneficial bacteria that produce *butyrate* (an anti-inflammatory compound), maintain intestinal wall integrity, increase bacterial diversity, and support mucosal health.[238]

Eat probiotic-rich foods frequently: If cow yogurt doesn't agree with your endo body think outside of the box: goat, sheep, or coconut yogurt, or raw sauerkraut, kimchi, or other fermented vegetables you find in the refrigerated section (not canned on shelves; these won't be living ferments). If live ferments are too pricey, they are easy and incredibly cheap to make at home (see Further Reading). If your digestion is suffering, introduce these foods *slowly*. Consider 1 tsp a full serving size when you start out and slowly increase from there.

Remove chemicals: Household chemicals, body care products, non-organic foods—all of these can have a negative effect on your microbiome.

Avoid all *unnecessary* antibiotics: This includes pharmaceuticals, plus anti-bacterial soaps, sprays, and disinfectants (unless of course they're *absolutely* necessary, and have been recommended by your doctor).

Wash your hands and brush your teeth: Sounds simple, but many of us don't do this enough. Brushing your teeth after each meal has been demonstrated to reduce candida levels in the gut, while washing your hands after having a bowel movement may be key to preventing contamination of your small intestine with bacteria from your colon.[239]

If you've "done it all" and are still suffering, remember the importance of testing: If you have a gut infection, you'll want to get treated or else nothing you do will make much of a dent in your gut health. Eradicating something like SIBO, *Strep*, or *E.coli* once and for all will dramatically shift your health to the positive. Don't guess, test.

TEST, DON'T GUESS: WORKING WITH PROFESSIONALS

If you have tried changing up your diet, dialing in digestion, or even some of the elimination diets without success in addressing your symptoms, consider working with a professional for testing as the next best step. Please, do not begin the "restriction cycle," where you cut out more and more foods without ever pinpointing what is triggering you. It may just be you have a serious microbial imbalance or infection that needs to be clinically treated. *Truly, I cannot recommend enough working with a gut specialist if you are not seeing results through diet and lifestyle shifts after three or more months.* Proper testing and working with a professional can get you where you need to be in approximately 3 to 6 months, as opposed to crying on the bathroom floor in frustration after years of "trying everything" and cutting out more than half of food groups (been there, done that).

To drive this recommendation home, I'd like to give three examples of how you may need professional help to get the gut-healing gains you need.

One of my clients in Australia ate just about the most incredibly nutritious diet possible. She lived on her own farm, ate nearly 100 percent local produce and meat, fermented her own veggies for probiotics, had relatively low stress, and could not figure out why her digestion was so awful—consistently painful bloating, diarrhea, and foul-smelling gas. And this poor client had these symptoms for over a decade. After testing we found she had a significant SIBO infection that needed to be treated by a doctor with three (yes, three) rounds of antibiotics. After six months of gut work (eradication, digestion, discovering dietary triggers) she was feeling so much better, and she *never* would have gotten to that point with diet alone. She needed testing and professional help.

Another client came to me complaining of SIBO-like symptoms. She had extensive and painful bloating, foul-smelling gas, an inability to eat much at meals, and heartburn. She had tried just about every diet under the sun with little to no help. Yet, the SIBO test was negative. Instead, a GI-Map stool test revealed a pretty substantial *H. Pylori* infection, something that can damage and inflame the stomach lining. After a treatment protocol with a naturopath, and relearning how to digest her foods, she was back to normal, with healthy digestion, and no more bloating, pain, or indigestion. But to get there, she needed to eradicate the *H. Pylori*.

I'd like to offer my own story as the last example, to bring home how mysterious gut infections can be (as in they don't always come with digestive symptoms). As a background, I dealt with nearly 3 long years of unexplained infertility before finally conceiving my firstborn—needless to say getting pregnant was a long endeavor. Two years postpartum I was dealing with some odd inflammatory symptoms, including eczema. I did a stool test, which revealed that I still had a *serious* gut overgrowth of an antibiotic-resistant strain of bacteria. I was following a protocol that was successfully addressing this extensive overgrowth when, 6 weeks later, I started to feel painful pelvic cramping. I was terrified the endo had come back! It turns out that pain was implantation cramps. I was surprisingly pregnant. Another big reminder of how treating your dysbiosis can affect systems far beyond digestion, including fertility. If you've been in this boat too, suffering from either lingering digestive issues or any other mysterious symptoms, you're probably ready to work with a practitioner.

To start uncovering your own type of dysbiosis, I recommend seeking out a naturopath or functional medicine doctor who specializes in the microbiome. Functional medicine doctors are classically trained M.D.s who have completed additional training so they can better evaluate the "whole body," rather than addressing issues individually, symptom by symptom. To put this in perspective, there was once a meme I saw of a patient drowning while the doctor high-fived her to tell her the test results were "all normal." Needless to say, the patient drowned. I can relate, and I bet many of you can too since this situation all too often sums up our experiences at the doctor: a boatload of symptoms, seemingly zero issues found on testing, so zero solutions.

This is where someone trained beyond the general mainstream understanding of (a) what to test for and (b) how to interpret results can be beneficial to your case. Understanding both becomes imperative since symptoms of one type of overgrowth may mimic others and you need to know exactly what you're dealing with in order to address it. Truly, stool testing may be the biggest "secret" to gut health we rarely hear about, which is unfortunate since I do have so many clients arrive at my doorstep having self-diagnosed for years, implementing everything from self-made "candida cleanses" to rounds and rounds of anti-microbial supplements. This can make things much worse in the long run, and why you will find that testing (with successive treatment for your exact issue) is the best way to feel better, once and for all.

Functional medicine practitioners don't have to be pricey, as many are now available in-network. I recommend checking out the Institute for Functional Medicine search tool (www.ifm.org/find-a-practitioner) to start looking for a practitioner near you. Some tests you may consider asking about include:

Small Intestinal Bacterial Overgrowth (SIBO): Consider testing for SIBO if you deal with more extreme levels of bloating, constipation, and/or diarrhea (although, to be fair, you can also have SIBO without extreme symptoms, referred to as "silent SIBO"). To date, there are three known types of SIBO based upon the type of microorganism overgrowing and what specific gas they expel: hydrogen, methane, and hydrogen sulfide. Hydrogen and hydrogen sulfide varieties of SIBO are often associated with diarrhea, and methane is often associated with constipation, although symptoms can present uniquely.

There is only one test currently available that measures all three varieties at once, called Trio Smart Breath Test (www.triosmartbreath.com). For this test, you drink a sugar solution on an empty stomach and then breathe into a tube three times per hour (over the course of three hours), capturing the gases produced in the small intestine. If you have SIBO, the solution will quickly ferment in your small intestine, and you'll see a quick rise in one or two of the gases within that three-hour period. Depending on which gas rises (hydrogen, hydrogen sulfide, or methane), it will mean you have that specific type of SIBO (important to know since these types will be treated differently!).

Comprehensive DNA Stool Tests (such as GI-Map): While these stool tests won't be able to pinpoint SIBO, they *can* point to a wide variety of other forms of dysbiosis. Because these tests measure DNA fragments rather than the actual "bug," they will give you a much more accurate view of what's happening in your intestinal tract than traditional "culture-based" tests offered at your typical doctor's office. Since a culture-based test requires you to scoop the microbe in your stool sample (which is more luck than anything), you can test negative even if you do have an overgrowth.

Test results are comprehensive, and will show levels of beneficial, pathogenic, and opportunistic microbes, as well as viruses, parasites, digestive markers, intestinal inflammation (measured by calprotectin), and even levels of leaky gut, (measured by zonulin). Such tests can give you an *amazing* overview of what's happening inside. Some issues you may see include:

- Gastritis (inflammation of the stomach lining), perhaps caused by *H. Pylori.*
- Overgrowths of numerous varieties of pathogenic or opportunistic bacteria.
- A big clinical infection with a single issue, such as *Giardia.*
- Undergrowths of beneficial bacteria, such as *Lactobacillus* or *Bifidobacterium.*

- Poor digestive function and lack of digestive enzymes, resulting in partially digested fats, carbohydrates, or proteins in the stool.

Endoscopy or Colonoscopy: If you get a referral to a gastroenterologist, they can diagnose ulcers or gastritis through an endoscopy (where a camera is inserted through the throat to the stomach), or bowel or colon issues through a colonoscopy (where a camera is inserted through the anus to get a visual of the colon or large intestine). Some *may* also be helpful in testing for infections, depending on the experience of your provider.

HEALING THE GUT

After dialing in proper digestion and addressing any infections and/or overgrowths, professionals will help you with your gut barrier integrity. The intestinal barrier is composed of numerous layers, and it's what keeps the "insides" of your intestines from leaking into your body. This barrier becomes damaged from any mix of poor dietary choices, improper digestion, lifestyle factors, chemicals, stress, inflammation, and LPS, combining to create what is known as leaky gut. That's when the tight junctures between your intestinal epithelial cells (the cells holding your intestines together) become injured through inflammation or infection, creating larger-than-normal spaces between them.

The best way to address leaky gut is through something called the 4Rs, and it's a long but remarkable process of rejuvenation a professional can help guide you through:

- **Remove** the foods, infections, chemicals, and triggers that are causing inflammation and creating an environment for bacteria, parasites, and yeasts to thrive. This is where you may employ an elimination diet to find your food triggers or, if you need to, eradicate an infection. You absolutely need to remove the triggers before moving forward or else your intestinal lining will not be able to heal.

- **Replace** any nutrients needed for your digestion to work, such as digestive enzymes, ox bile, or hydrochloric acid supplementation with meals. Proper digestion is paramount here.
- **Repair** the damage that has been done, using targeted amino acids and mucosal lining builders. These could include slippery elm, zinc carnosine, glycine, glucosamine, polyphenols, and many more options.
- **Re-inoculate** the good bacteria with specially targeted probiotics, prebiotics, and fermented foods.

Healing the gut also goes far beyond diet. It's also about focusing on sleep, popping that chronic stress bubble, stepping away from screens, and ultimately creating a life you love. Doesn't that sound kind of fun? Yes! So, I'd like you to start thinking about healing as creating a *better* life, not one that's based on deprivation...even if you find you have to forgo some of your favorite foods for a while.

> **Healing the gut goes far beyond diet. It's also about focusing on sleep, popping that chronic stress bubble, stepping away from screens, and ultimately creating a life you love.**

Finding a specialist to partner with doesn't have to be hard. Remember to check out www.ifm.org to find a practitioner near you.

REPRODUCTIVE TRACT INFECTIONS

For some of us, it may *also* be necessary to address microbial imbalances or infections of the reproductive tract directly. Dysbiosis of the reproductive tract may be just as implicated with "The Great Migration" as dysbiosis of the gut, and certainly more implicated with inflammation of the endometrial lining (see Chapter 5). However, please note there are few doctors who specialize in this area. Because of this, you may have to get a little creative when addressing dysbiosis down south.

To first uncover if you may be dealing with some reproductive tract dysbiosis, I recommend doing an easy, at-home test using pH test paper strips. A healthy vaginal microbiome should be relatively acidic (between 3.9 and 4.5). This is thanks to *Lactobacillus*, the predominant microbe in the genital tract that produces highly acidic *lactic acid* to keep pathogens suppressed. When it is reduced, so is the lactic acid, which makes it homier for pathogenic species to flourish. This is why it's concerning to note that 79 percent of women with endo were shown to be above the healthy pH range (meaning pathogens are allowed to flourish), testing anywhere from 4.5 to a shocking 9.0.[240]

To test, all you need is a pH test paper strip that measures pH from 1 to 10, which is cheap and easily purchased online. To do: insert a clean Q-tip into your vagina to coat it in vaginal fluid, then slide it over the dry pH strip until it's coated. Whatever color the paper turns is your result, and you'll be able to see whether you fall into the healthy 3.9–4.5 range, or in the higher 5–9 category. The farther away you are from 4.5, the more likely that a pathogenic overgrowth is present.

If you see a dysbiosis trend, take a step back and remember body ecology and how all systems in the body are connected. Since the gut will directly seed the reproductive tract, reducing consumption of sugars, excess starches, and alcohol can have pretty immediate benefits for some sufferers with chronic yeast or fungus issues, or recurrent vaginal infections. That's why addressing the problem through nutrition and lifestyle can be immensely beneficial without directly addressing the vaginal microbiome first. If that is unsuccessful, and you still fall in the "probably have some dysbiosis" category (either from symptoms or this simple pH test), you should definitely consider further investigation.

Insurance should cover a test for endometritis (an infection of the endometrium), which can be cleared up with antibiotics (remember nearly half of women with both endometriosis and infertility were found to have endometritis). Or, if you have yeast issues, talk to your doctor about taking a pharmaceutical called Diflucan, which can ax yeast overgrowth, or speak to a naturopath about holistic suppositories.

Reproductive Tract Dysbiosis, Inflammation, and Infertility

If never treated, reproductive tract dysbiosis will lend to chronic inflammation within the uterus, preventing pregnancy, as well as provoke an inflammatory response outside of the uterus thanks to retrograde menstruation.

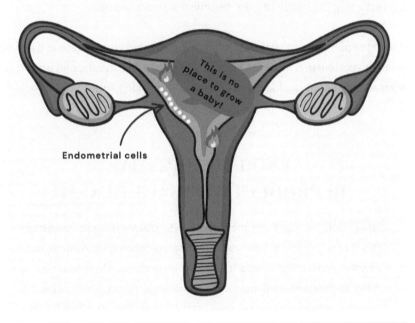

This is no place to grow a baby!

Endometrial cells

> **Nearly half of women with both endometriosis and infertility were found to have endometritis, an infection of the endometrium.**

There are also some incredible new businesses offering vaginal microbiome testing, including Juno.bio and Evvy. After returning a simple at-home test, both companies offer detailed insights into your reproductive tract health, bacteria balance, and proper ways to address any overgrowths. Companies like these may help those of us with endo gain new insights into our disease and our symptoms.

As for a simple but effective recommendation, you may also consider supplementing with a specific probiotic called Fem-Dophilus by Jarrow Research. 75 percent of women taking this probiotic saw significant improvement in vaginal flora composition.[241] Fem-Dophilus may be taken orally or inserted vaginally if extra support is needed, something I actually recommend to many of my clients. One pill inserted vaginally for a month may be incredibly beneficial for restarting the health of your reproductive tract biome.

There are plenty more resources available, depending on the type of dysbiosis you're experiencing, but since each recommendation will depend on you and your unique situation, I leave that for your discussion with a professional.

ENDO TIP: OPTIMAL REPRODUCTIVE TRACT HEALTH

Never douche, use feminine deodorants, powders, or scented menstrual care products: Your vagina is a self-regulating ecosystem, not a sewage system that needs "cleaning" or perfume. Douching and/or using fragranced feminine products can change the pH, wash out healthy bacteria, introduce bad bacteria, and mess up the microbial balance with chemical deodorizers and scents. If your vaginal fluid has a truly bad smell, this can be a sign of yeast, fungal, or bacterial overgrowths and deserves professional attention. To keep your vulva clean, simply wash externally with soap that is chemical and fragrance-free when you bathe.

Always wipe front to back: No exceptions! And if you have trouble getting your rear truly clean (dare I say "skid marks"?), consider using wet wipes. You don't want any skidding on your panties that could rub near your vaginal opening, easily introducing bacteria from your stool to your vagina or your urethra.

Always change out of wet bathing suits ASAP: Keeping your reproductive ecosystem moist and warm is a recipe for disaster, as anyone knows who's had recurrent yeast infections throughout a summer by the pool. The same goes for cleaning up well after intercourse to remove all excess moisture and body fluids, and changing your panties as frequently as you need to keep everything dry.

Keep pH testing: Remember, you want a slightly acidic vaginal canal to keep pathogens at bay. If you find your pH tests keep showing up at high levels, continue working on gut health and consider probiotic supplementation and/or suppositories until you can help reduce the pH of your vaginal fluid to a healthy level. If nothing is budging the pH, it's definitely time to look into more serious testing. (Remember, pH test strips aren't diagnostic, just a fun way to track your progress.)

Chapter 14:

Balancing Your Hormones

As detailed in Chapter 6, hormones play a big part in the story of endometriosis. Indeed, there is an entire endocrine component to this disease! Not to mention that, when out of balance, hormones can act like Bonnie and Clyde—outlaws that create havoc with your emotions as well as your body ecology. Maintaining balance will help keep you grounded, from reducing your endo symptoms to improving your stress resilience, upping your energy and moods while lowering your inflammation.

The good news is that by following the guidance in this book to heal your body and reduce inflammation, your hormones will already be on the road to recovery. That's because, when handed the right ingredients (like a balanced body ecology), hormones will start to balance themselves long before you start micromanaging. As chemical messengers, hormones inform our body what information they pick up, with the body adjusting hormone levels from there. So, while it's common to want to zoom in to fix one hormone at a time (like estrogen), the first step in healing is actually regulating what information your body is receiving by offering it tons of soothing, wonderful inputs. By doing so, you offer your body the opportunity to balance a wide variety of hormones.

As you move forward to formulate your own healing plan, it's also important to remember that no one with endo has the exact same "hormonal blueprint." Having endometriosis means you may or may not have excess estrogen, or that you may or may not have low progesterone. It may mean you have high cortisol and are stuck in an alarm stage, or low cortisol and housebound with chronic fatigue. Maybe neither. Really, contrary to what you may have been told, there is no one-size-fits-all approach for those with endo, so be cautious when applying any old advice you pick up online or from another sufferer since it very well may not apply to your own unique situation.

That being said, there *are* two types hormone imbalances many endo sufferers have been shown to experience to some degree: excess levels of estrogen *in relation to* progesterone, and dysregulated levels of adrenaline and cortisol. Such imbalances may lead to symptoms of heavy periods, PMS, painful periods, hormonal acne, inability to handle normal stressors, fatigue, insomnia, and more. Moreover, they can promote endo-ing in the body.

In this chapter, I will help you begin to address these issues through the lens of fortifying a more balanced body ecology to help our hormone signaling through better sleep and stress management. You will be surprised just how much addressing these factors can bring a body suffering from hormonal dysregulation back into balance in profound ways.

GET MORE SLEEP - EMPOWER YOUR CIRCADIAN RHYTHM

One of the best things you can do to balance *all* your hormones is to strengthen your circadian rhythm, a powerful internal regulator of wakefulness and sleep that helps maintain normal hormone levels. Think of your circadian rhythm like an ocean tide, an invisible force powerful enough to quietly move an ocean back and forth twice in 24 hours. A well-set circadian rhythm will lull you naturally into sleep and then wake you with abundant natural energy, no coffee needed.

If you haven't experienced this before don't feel left out; those powerful circadian rhythms are hard to come by these days. With screens and lights available to us 24/7, our bodies aren't forced to bed with the sunset as our ancestors were, nor do we awake at the crack of dawn with a bright sunrise in our eyes. It's also easy to ignore our body's reminders for rest when we have caffeine, high-stress jobs, or a Netflix binge to continue. This all creates a big problem when we want to balance hormones and regulate energy and sleep. Because our bodies are hardwired to depend on a circadian rhythm, our cells may find themselves feeling a bit chaotic without that safety net, and sleep may start to really suffer.

Unfortunately, poor sleep can lead to chronic inflammation and is associated with a variety of inflammatory diseases.[242] Poor sleep also significantly raises both cortisol and adrenaline.[243] This may be why a 2020 study found that when women with endo have poor-quality sleep, they often experience poorer quality of life, more depressive symptoms, and bladder pain.[244]

As a mom of two young children, I can attest that sleep is imperative for good health. It turns out you can be eating well, moving well, getting outdoors, breathing better—doing all those things to lessen endo symptoms—but without adequate sleep, you may simply still feel terrible. *Even just one night of botched, low-quality sleep can trigger inflammation.*[245] So quality sleep is non-negotiable when healing from a chronic illness like endo.

The first trick to powering back up your circadian rhythm is to offer your body consistency, i.e., consistent wake times, eating times, and sleep times. To start, I recommend making a kind-of-sort-of-strict daily schedule and sticking with it for at least one month. Aim to go to bed at the same time every night and wake up at the same time every day. Aim to eat three balanced meals per day, at the same time, with no snacking in between (if you can't do this yet, just aim to have your snacks at the same time, too). Go outside first thing in the morning (or look out a window for 5 minutes) to let your body know when it's day; turn all screens off by 7:00 pm or 8:00 pm each night to let your body know it's night.

The second trick is to use nourishing habits rather than stimulants to let the power of circadian rhythms take control. As much as you can, eliminate caffeine or sugar to wake up and alcohol or sedatives to calm down. Instead, opt for caffeine-free beverages and offer your body more nourishing meals to allow it to do this on its own.

I know this may sound boring, if not impossible for some. But still, make a commitment to try it for a month. Think of it as a staycation from the powerful pull of screens, stimulants, and fast-paced nightlife, and note how different you feel at the end of the month. It may be the exact thing your body was craving, and you may feel more deeply balanced than ever before, having given your body the basics to regulate its own internal tides. Here are some extra tips to start:

- Do your preferred exercise/movement in the mornings; this will help raise cortisol levels at the appropriate time of day.
- If you need caffeine, limit it to one cup before noon. If you're tired in the afternoon, try a brisk walk instead.
- Get outside! Even if the weather is bad, spending entire days indoors under artificial lights and screens confuses your circadian rhythm. Take as many outdoor breaks as you can to remind your body it's daytime.
- Take a magnesium supplement before bed.
- Spend a few minutes stretching or taking a warm bath an hour before you want to fall asleep. If anything, just get into a good bedtime routine habit that will, over time, indicate to your body that you're going to sleep soon. Reading a good book can be calming and help you forget the day's problems—just stay away from suspense thrillers!
- Try yoga nidra or other sleep meditations before bed to help prepare you for sleep.
- Work on nose breathing throughout the night to limit sleep apnea or snoring episodes, which rob you of sleep. Often, a small piece of tape placed lightly over the front of the lips can be enough to remind your mouth to stay closed, and nose strips to help keep your nasal airways open may be helpful too. Several clients reported great success with this, as strange as it may sound initially.
- Avoid alcohol. Even if it helps you fall asleep, alcohol doesn't allow your body to get the amount of *deep* sleep needed.
- Consider ashwagandha, hops, passionflower, or valerian, all herbs that support healthy sleep patterns without leaving you feeling groggy in the morning. Once your circadian rhythm returns to normal, you should not need to rely on these.

ADDRESS YOUR STRESS

Reducing stress is one of the most important factors to heal your endo, and a significant reason for this is its effect on your hormones. Why? To behave properly, the immune system relies on complex communication between your hormones and your nervous system. When your body is ramped up with stress hormones, your nervous system kicks into *sympathetic mode,* which tells your immune system to prioritize inflammation. This would make ancestral sense since a body in a fight-or-flight mode would *actually* be in a life-or-death scenario (like being chased by a lion), and you may need to heal a wound fast—so having inflammatory immune factors already coursing through the body could immediately help.

Conversely, when you're peaceful and relaxed the flip is switched to *parasympathetic mode*, where healing, rejuvenation, and immune-based repair are prioritized. For endo, we want to stay in this peaceful parasympathetic mode as much as possible to help us heal.

The problem today is that we all seem to be stuck in a deep pit of stress—one without escape. While stress itself is a normal, unavoidable part of life, *chronic stress* is a different story and has become a typical way of life for most of us. In fact, chronic stress has become such a common part of our daily routine that many of us don't even recognize when we're feeling stressed until we're past our tipping point, maybe after a panic attack, chronic fatigue, breathing problem, or the dreaded endo flare. In the United States, a "work until you drop" ethic is rewarded (and expected), leaving many stuck in cycles of burnout and exhaustion—not to mention inflammation.

When we think about ancestral patterns of stress, they are quite different. Certainly, chronic stress must have existed in some instances for our ancestors, such as during a long famine or war, but the more common types of stress were more likely the short-lived fight-or-flight occasions, like being chased by a leopard or a brutal winter storm that destroyed a shelter. When they escaped the leopard or repaired their shelter, our ancestors escaped the stress, for the time being.

Chronic stress is as if the leopard is constantly chasing you...for years. No break, no reprieve, just your brain thinking you're going to have to outrun a leopard for the rest of your life. These "leopards" can present themselves in modern-day life in a number of ways, from ongoing negative self-talk to feeling unable to keep up with daily demands, a lousy boss, poor marital dynamics, or *anything* that causes enduring stress, anger, anxiety, nervousness, tension, jealousy, sadness, loneliness, etc.—all forms of a stressed-out body. Luckily, there are many things that can be done to start to shift our lives away from one of chronic stress, into a world of safety, resilience, and confidence.

KRISTIN'S STORY

I was diagnosed with Endo in 2019 via lap surgery and had most removed except for in sensitive areas. Like most women (sadly), I spent 7 years going from doctor to doctor begging for answers to my pain and infertility. It wasn't uncommon for me to struggle through an 8-hour workday and come home to spend hours laying on the floor in pain. I lost count of the number of doctors that dismissed my reports stating it's just menstrual cramps, it's IBS, it will improve with birth control, or it's just anxiety. Finally, after struggling to conceive for 2 years we found a great RE who found the endo.

After my diagnosis, I researched as much as I could and came across the Heal Endo Approach! I got my husband on board, we got the cookbook, and we did the full 4-week meal plan. I found that I was *not* eating enough veggies and my digestive system was much happier with the upgrade. I honestly feel like my body's inflammation is less after implementing the diet and other stress-reducing measures such as yoga and meditation. I even noticed some physical responses from these changes such as less acid reflux at night and I've stopped grinding my teeth. I've continued to follow the diet and there are a few favorite recipes (like the Moroccan Turkey and Sweet Potato Breakfast Bake) that we eat often!

I rarely have pain anymore. My quality of life is SO much better. My periods are EASY!!! Never thought that would be a thing! I'll soon begin IVF and I know my body is in a much healthier space for this. —Kristin, USA

Feeling Safe in a World of Danger

Once you understand the endo–stress connection you may be ready to finally focus on this elephant in the chronic disease room...but it's hard to imagine solutions when we've been living this way for so long. It can be infuriating and downright confusing when you are in pain and someone tells you to "calm down" or "you need to stop stressing out." I remember years ago thinking that managing stress would be the very *last* thing on my long list of healing to-do's because I was even annoyed (i.e., stressed) at having to think about it. I thought it was a waste of time when I could frantically (ah-hem, more stress) be doing something else to fix my health.

Instead, it really helps to imagine what a world without chronic stress looks like. I have one word that may be helpful here: *safety*. When stress is triggered by your body thinking there is danger, safety is the net that allows us to feel, well, not stressed. Safety tells your HPA axis to take a break and lets your immune system know it can settle down its excess inflammation. Safety happens when you're not being chased by proverbial leopards, when your cells can depend on soothing inputs—basically when you're well-rested and not frantic.

The good news is most of us can (with some time and practice) rewire how we respond to stress and create a life of safety. While we can't avoid all stress, we *can* control (a) how we respond to it and (b) how many stressors we permit ourselves to engage with. This should be something we learn to incorporate into the fabric of our daily lives. It will absolutely help you heal.

Fortunately, there are many ways to offer your body the safety she craves. And before you dive into the mental aspects of stress reduction, there are a number of easy *quick* wins that are within our power to control today:

- **Jettison Caffeine:** If you react to caffeine with any sort of jitters, nervousness, or anxiety, it's proof that caffeine is stimulating your stress hormones. Cut way back and see if that helps. If not, caffeine may be completely off the table for you for a while.

- **Repair Chronic Physical Triggers:** What do chronic knee pain, a chronic toothache, and chronic foot fungus have in common? They're all painful or irritating triggers that never end. If you make a list of the physical issues plaguing you and address them (for example, see a physical therapist for the knee, a dentist for the tooth, and buy new socks and some ointment for the fungus) you will remove a list of annoying stress provokers.

- **Quell Your Blood Sugar Chaos:** Imbalances in blood sugar create wild hormonal swings, and when the famous blood sugar crash occurs (a time of great stress on the body) your stress hormones will surge. This is why you may feel suddenly anxious, angry, and shaky: because you're flooded with fight-or-flight hormones.

- **Pause Your Newsfeed:** When I was a kid the news consisted of the 5 o'clock news hour. Now, the news is 24/7, and it seems its goal is to tear us all apart. If you look up from the news on your phone, you'll probably see really nice people going about their day. Yet, the news would have you think the world is out to get you. We get angry, we get defensive, and all our brain sees is "danger," so stress hormones are released. The truth is, most people are pretty nice (at least face to face), so if the news is making you hate everyone (even yourself), it's time to pause your newsfeed.

- **Take a Social Media Break, Maybe Even Permanently:** Social media can be helpful in many ways, for getting some up-to-date information on endometriosis, hearing from fellow sufferers, getting advice, connecting with friends, and so on. Yet, it's also extremely addictive, polarizing, depressing, and it doesn't heal you. That's right, I'll say it again: no matter how many social media posts on health you read, the best way to get healthy is to drastically reduce your social media or get off it entirely.

Social media stressing you out?

Me: Hi, so you have endo, what have you done so far to try to mitigate your worst symptoms?

Client: So I started vegan but that didn't totally help so now I'm half vegan half keto and part carnivore with a focus on turmeric. I do seed cycling, NAC cycling, luteal phase food cycling, and intermittent fasting plus HIIT during my follicular phase and yoga for my luteal phase. I avoid saturated fat ... except for coconut oil, and not on Saturday which is my cheat day when I eat whatever I want but usually I'm gluten free and dairy free and soy free, except on sushi nights which is part of my 80/20 plan.

Me: Oh, you must be getting all your health advice from social media! And boy, you must be confused.

Client: Yes, very very confused. I feel like I'm doing so much and nothing is helping!!!!

Reduce Your Negative Stress—Solve Small Problems First

You might be surprised to know that you have the magic to reduce negative stress in your life simply by adopting a new, problem-solving mindset. To use an example, let's pretend you're mad at your partner for seemingly never helping with the dishes. At first you're fine, but after a while it starts to really upset you. If you never address the issue then it will start to eat at you, leaving you with growing resentment and distress (i.e. the negative stress we don't want). And sadly the stress will only grow because since, yes, the dishes will continue to need to be washed.

Instead of accepting a new chronic stressor in your life, the new goal is to solve the problem. For example, you talk to your partner about how they need to pitch in 50/50. Or perhaps you both realize your partner is far better at taking out the trash and vacuuming, so you agree to stick on dish duty solo while they help out with other chores. Both of these are solid decisions to close the door on the situation, so it won't linger and keep stressing you out. You turned a stress into a doable task, which you completed, and now you can move forward. Problem solved, stress gone.

If this dish example doesn't vibe with you, I'm sure you can still think up a variety of other types of distress coming from unsolved problems in your own life, both big and small. Some examples may include a parent constantly texting you, trouble paying bills on time, always misplacing your keys, housework you can't seem to keep up with, an overly-complaining co-worker, doom-scrolling too often on the news, or anything else that causes you chronic anxiety, worry, or annoyance. Once you realize you have the power to change your response to the stressor, you can start to dismiss many of the lingering stressors in your life by focusing on solving the problems and moving on stress-free. Want to know more? See the following pull-out for an activity to help you with this.

ACTIVITY: SOLVE YOUR STRESSORS BY SOLVING THE PROBLEMS

For this activity, all you need is a piece of paper and some detective motivation.

Step 1: Notice what you stress about. Be a researcher and, when you're angry, sad, frustrated, annoyed, or anxiety-riddled (all types of basic "stress"), simply jot down *why* on a piece of paper. While some stressors may be big (like a dying family member, marital problems, or financial worries), I guarantee you will notice many distress responses over relatively small issues as well.

Step 2: Analyze your list of distressing grievances and circle what you can address *now*. Circle all the smaller issues that can easily be addressed—too much housework, disorganization leading to overdue bills, overthinking TikTok, or drinking that enormous espresso, for example.

The ones you don't circle are the ones you can't address immediately, such as the "unhappy in the city I live in" if you really can't move right now. Get it?

Step 3: Start small—only address two or three at a time. Choose two or three to address. One at a time, format each stressor into a problem that needs a solution. Next, make a decision to solve it. Always lose your keys? Decide to make a spot in your house to hang them and commit to it. Are bills getting paid late or forgotten? Decide to use a digital calendar to remind you to pay them on specific dates. Set the dates to recur monthly, and you will have reminders for life! Overthinking Tik Tok? Take a social media break. Once you solve the first stressors, keep the momentum going while moving on to the next ones on your list. You get the point. By solving each little problem, you can mitigate a great deal of daily stress in your life. And removing the little stressors gives you more runway to address the bigger stressors.

Step 4: Revel in how much shorter your list is, and how much less stressed you feel. The more solutions you create, the less distress you will have. And while larger issues like unhappy marriages, living situations, or taking care of a sick relative may seem too big to be addressed right now, you may be surprised that as you free up mental space from the non-important stressors, you *can* finally address the big ones. Maybe you finally feel like you have the energy to seek counseling for the wayward marriage (or heck, maybe simply talking about dish-washing duties will help!). Maybe you finally decide to change jobs with a better salary to ease your financial burdens.

Control Only What You Can

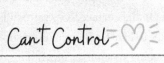

Can't Control ♡

- Having an endo diagnosis
- Other people's emotions
- That I'm broke at this moment
- Life and death
- The weather

Can Control ♡

- I can't stop my endo diagnosis, but I can change the way I respond! Vow to learn more about endo and implement new behaviors to reduce inflammation. Reach out to an endo excision expert. Address excess distress (wink-wink).

- How I respond to other people emotions. Let them roll off of me.

- My ability to not be broke in the future. Listen to financial podcasts, read some books, start a savings account, stop online shopping or eating out, and speak to a financial planner.

- Cultivating deep inner resilience for the natural phases of life, be they birth, passing, relationships ending, moving places, etc. Practice meditation, reading philosophy, and speaking to friends from the heart.

- Ensure my closet is weather-prepared: rain boots and jacket, sun hat, mittens, etc. Now the weather won't bother me.

Stop Being So Darned Perfect

I've had a handful of clients who felt like they were doing everything right and were still not feeling better. On the surface, they were diligently (perhaps obsessively) checking all the boxes to heal their endo: nutrient-dense foods, no chemicals, movement therapy, seeing specialists, etc. But it's often people like this (the do-it-all'ers) who may need to focus more on what makes them feel utterly uncomfortable: letting go of the stress-inducing need to *control*, which is often accompanied by the need to overachieve, whether it is beneficial or not. In other words, stress can be self-imposed, even when following a healing plan.

Paradoxically, sufferers like this may be in the camp that needs to do *less* rather than more: less saying yes to everyone's requests, and less obsessing about doing everything perfectly. They need instead to just say no and focus more on relaxing to let their body heal (believe me, I was there, and it took just about everything I had to stop feeling a need to be so productive). Imagine more walking barefoot, laughing with loved ones, playing music, reading books, doing art, gardening, or simply more time far away from screens. Truly, slowing down (instead of speeding up) may feel difficult and foreign for many of us, yet it is a key component to healing your endo.

So, give yourself permission to do less and be less "perfect." Be present in your activities, and learn the art of saying "no." It will go a long way in helping to break the chronic stress cycle. And it will help you on your path to recovery.

ANGIE'S STORY

My life was like so many people around me; go to bed and get maybe 5 hours of sleep, get up early and eat breakfast as quickly as possible—followed by massive amounts of bloating, gas, and upset stomach—with the addition of caffeine and exercise (as much as possible to try and stay awake). I was tired all day and brain fog was the norm. I had been dealing with endometriosis and gut issues for years, sprinkled in with 2 miscarriages and a ton of stress.

When I started the Heal Endo approach, we took it all on: diet, stress levels, sleep, and over-exercise patterns. We focused on relaxing the incredibly restricted diet I had myself on before starting, increasing the quantity and variety of vegetables, organ meat, and fermented foods I was eating. The amount of sleep I was getting needed an overhaul, so I worked my way up to 7 hours or more each night. I had hidden behind exercise for years, doing more and more intense sessions to cope (which wasn't benefiting me, my stress levels, or my body). Finally, I began to *restore* my body through yoga, meditation, and gentle activities, unwinding the stress. Many of my symptoms pointed to SIBO, which a test confirmed, so I addressed that separately as well. Seven months later, I was overjoyed to conceive (and I now have a beautiful baby boy). Because of my previous miscarriages, pregnancy had once been met with anxiety and fear, but now I embraced this tiny life with confidence and joy. Thanks to this approach, my entire life, as well as my family's, was forever changed for the better. -Angie, USA

Turn That Voice Off

Yes, *that* voice, the one that talks to you incessantly from the cozy interior of your brain, the one that is impetuous enough to use your own voice. Wait, you thought that voice *was* you? It's not, rather it's a collection of your subconscious thoughts put into words—and not all of them are nice, kind, loving, or good. Your thoughts can be your own worst enemy because they're given a voice. Even worse, they're given *your* voice. So if you're feeling down, your internal dialogue may be telling you that you're ugly, stupid, or unpopular. It can convince you that you're not worthy of love, that you'll never feel better, or that no one cares about you. And the more negative thoughts you have, the more this voice seems to badger you. This leads to...yup, more chronic stress.

This voice is so powerful, that it may even make your endometriosis worse. In one study it was observed that women with endo who had less self-compassion (imagine that internal voice who's taken over, and not for the better) suffered more acutely from period pain, back pain, pain with sex, fatigue, and nausea.[246] Conversely, those who had more self-compassion had not only fewer symptoms but also more psychological well-being.

So, work on turning that voice off. Really. When your inner voice starts to be the mean girl (to you or others), change your mental direction. For example, you can focus instead on the soothing environmental sounds outside your head to tune "you" out, be it birdsong, leaves rustling, kids laughing, or even horns honking. Replace that inner voice (not you) with your conscious voice (that's you!)—i.e., talk to your partner, friend, or canine companion about something else. Be sure to tell that inner voice firmly, "I'm not listening to you right now." Seriously, extract yourself from the inside of your head and tell that voice you'll chat later when she decides to be nice.

Instead of Fight-or-Flight, Try to Tend-and-Befriend

If you thought fight-or-flight was a universal approach to dealing with stress, think again. It turns out fighting or fleeing may actually be more of a masculine response (which makes ancestral sense as men were the traditional fighters within groups and tribes), whereas it's been observed that, for women, a tend-and-befriend narrative may better mitigate a stress response.[247] What this means is that, in the face of a threat, women may do better gathering around loved ones or within community, nurturing, tending, caring, and allowing themselves to be cared for in turn.

When we live in a society that is already extremely isolated (social media, the pandemic, so much screen time, having a chronic disease), connecting with other people becomes perhaps the greatest form of self-care possible. This is a good reminder to rebuild community and deep friendships in your own life (however that looks), spending some extra energy nurturing others who will, I promise, come back to nurture you in turn.

Turn on Positive Stress in Your Life

Did you know there is a *good* kind of stress? You probably didn't notice any of it on your bad endo days, but it is a stress that we actually want more of in our lives—something that involves the learning and mastery of new endeavors. This type of stress is called eustress (pronounced "yoo-stress") and is the opposite of the stress we most often think of (known as distress).

Eustress is *positive* stress. It is exciting and motivational but *within your capabilities*. It's when you challenge yourself and are stronger for it at the end, say by training for the 5k, starting that dream business, making an effort to make new friends, or, if you're like me, writing a book with a newborn and toddler in tow. It can be the excitement of learning something new, like cooking from scratch (you're going to need this!), starting a vegetable garden, or volunteering at an animal rescue nonprofit. These tasks may be extra work, difficult, or somewhat uncomfortable at first, but eustress improves our performance and abilities, and fuels our feeling of success and achievement!

Ultimately, this leads to more satisfaction since we, as humans, truly have a deep ancestral and biologic need to keep learning and mastering new things. It's why striving toward goals that involve learning, growth, and mastery is more likely to create feelings of contentment and deep satisfaction.

When we live with a chronic illness like endo, we sometimes retreat into a mental zone that is *too comfortable*, because our stress from the pain and other debilitating systems can seem like too much to bear. We sometimes stop experiencing the joy of living, and the joyful challenges that come with it. This is not good for our mental health... it's stressful.

On the other end of the spectrum are those of us with too many stressors, often the person who wants to "do it all." Big job, high family-life demands, and this person suddenly adds in marathon training or night classes for continuing education. It may be the addiction to overcome adversity that fuels it, but over time this too will take a toll on the body...it's also very stressful.

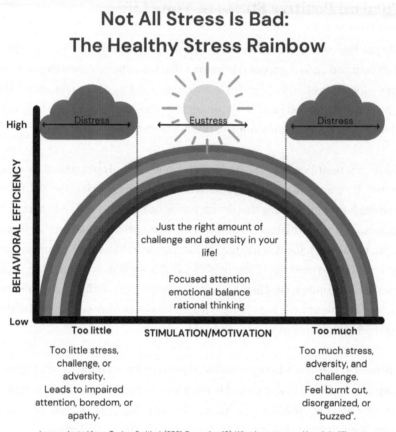

**Not All Stress Is Bad:
The Healthy Stress Rainbow**

Just the right amount of challenge and adversity in your life!

Focused attention
emotional balance
rational thinking

Too little stress, challenge, or adversity. Leads to impaired attention, boredom, or apathy.

Too much stress, adversity, and challenge. Feel burnt out, disorganized, or "buzzed".

Image adapted from: Tocino-Smith, J. (2021, December 10). What is eustress and how is it different than stress? PositivePsychology.com. https://positivepsychology.com/what-is-eustress

The happy medium to find is right in the middle. Not too many stressors that you feel overwhelmed and anxious, and not too little that you feel like you're drifting without a purpose. To get here, what I suggest is that you *first* work at reducing the negative stress triggers in your life (leading to *distress*). Reducing the negative stresses will free up time for you to then turn on your eustress superpower. Find a challenge to tackle, a new hobby to master, or perform somewhere else outside of your comfort zone (be it for better work performances, friendly relations, or overall health) that will help you grow as a person. Not only will this help keep our bodies in the heal and repair mode, but it also helps us feel more in control of our destinies.

When to Get Help

There are many types of stress in this world, anything from the perhaps easier to manage chronic work or home stress to the more potent types of stress that may include anything from childhood abuse or neglect to PTSD from rape or violence. Then there's endometriosis stress, which is directly related to having a chronic disease that your doctors, family, or friends may not seem to understand. Chronic stress and feelings of helplessness can lead to depression or even suicidal thoughts.

No matter who you are and where your stress levels stem from, if they are too heavy to bear on your own, please seek professional help! No one should "just have to live with it." Chronic stress, worry, or fear can truly take over a mind ... and thus take over a life.

Finding professional help in this regard may be covered by your insurance, and it's worth calling to ask. If it's not, and you can't afford private care, there are special hotlines and nonprofits dedicated to helping address mental health on many levels. See the Further Reading for places to start.

APRIL'S STORY

My symptoms started when I was a young teen and worsened in my mid-30s, following a decade of birth control and a post-operative routine tubal ligation surgery. Post-surgery symptoms were painful periods, diaphragmatic pain, chronic fatigue, brain fog, chronic pain in the back, stomach, bowels and vagina, digestion issues, leg pain, depression, anxiety, and neuropathic pain, all exasperated and sent me into a flare-up. The prescribed treatment plan was a medical approach with Lupron, Orlissa, and Visanne.

I began to deepen my holistic healing journey with endometriosis by incorporating a self-management approach focused on quality sleep, diet, emotions, movement, and nourishment. I started my healing journey by doing a complete detox overhaul on my beauty and home products, becoming aware of what our bodies inhale, absorb, and digest. I implemented dietary changes by removing alcohol, gluten, and dairy.

Currently, I focus on what my body needs and it is healing foods that bring down inflammation. My choice of movement is Qi Gong, Tai Chi and nature walks. Products that I use to support me include a heating pad, tens machine, journal, meditation, and nature walks.

We cannot walk this path alone, my path to healing includes God, my family, friends, doctors, healers, nutritionists, endometriosis specialists, naturopathic doctors, acupuncturists, massage therapists, chiropractors, pelvic floor therapists, counselors, and a community of like-minded endo warriors. Today, my symptoms are milder and more manageable. As my endometriosis and stress seem to be exceptionally interlinked, I find that if I'm aware enough to stop the stress cycle before it begins and return to the present moment, I feel much better overall. Pause, breathe, and ask yourself, what do I need? By asking this question, you can return to the present. -April, Canada

BALANCING THE ESTROGEN-PROGESTERONE TEETER TOTTER

No matter where your estrogen or progesterone levels lie (high, normal, or low), we can all aim for healthy levels by first supporting our body's processes that make, absorb, or metabolize these hormones. By following the recommendations in this book to fortify your body ecology, you will naturally target this imbalance. Truly, balancing blood sugar, increasing nutrient consumption, being well hydrated, fostering healthy sleep, movement, and outside time while reducing sugars, alcohol, stress, and bacterial overgrowths can all directly influence your estrogen and progesterone levels!

Moreover, reducing inflammation may have one of the biggest impacts when it comes to the estrogen-dominant microenvironment surrounding your endo lesion. If we could remove the inflammatory triggers, we may have 1/48th of the localized estrogen; and excess estrogen would not be invited to the scene for "wound healing."[248] Not only that, but research has shown that chronic inflammation promotes both progesterone resistance and estrogen sensitivity in normal endometrial cells, meaning these epigenetic alterations may be partially *due to* the result of a chronic inflammatory response.[249] By reducing the inflammatory storm surrounding the cells, you may be able to support hormonal healing in the direct vicinity of your endo. For those who are interested, here are a few more specific tips:

For Healthy Progesterone Levels:

Healthy ovulation is the *main* progesterone-producing event for our bodies. If you don't ovulate (because you're on oral contraceptives or for other reasons), you're missing a monthly surge of progesterone. In combination with progesterone resistance often observed in endo cells, your body may be dealing with a need for extra progesterone. You can help your body in a holistic way with the following support:

- **Reduce stress:** your body will prioritize making stress hormones over fertility hormones. This may be why, after a very stressful time in your life has passed, you may see the return of good-quality cervical fluid at ovulation (one sign of healthy levels of progesterone) or that your cycle regulates itself.
- **Increase nutrients:** You can help increase progesterone levels by ensuring you are getting enough magnesium, zinc, vitamin C, and B6.

- **Work with a practitioner:** If you're concerned your levels are low (as they very well may be), check in with your health care provider on the best next steps. After testing, you may be recommended bio-identical progesterone supplementation. I discuss this more in Chapter 16.

For Healthy Estrogen Levels:

Because estrogen is both healthy and necessary, you want to support healthy levels rather than axing all estrogen (which has its own list of consequences). Here are some specifics to help get you there:

- **Avoid estrogen-mimicking chemicals.** Hidden in our beauty/household/lifestyle/plastic products, these chemicals can dock at hormone receptor sites, creating confusion in the endocrine communication links. I'll talk about this in-depth in the next chapter.
- **Eat more cruciferous veggies.** This includes cabbage, kale, broccoli, and cauliflower. These foods contain Diindolylmethane (DIM), a compound that is known to help the body metabolize excess estrogen.
- **Balance your gut microbiome.** Doing so will also balance the microbes within the *estrobolome* (a funny word for the collection of microbes in your gut that metabolize estrogens, and are essential for balancing estrogen in your body). If your estrobolome microbes are not balanced, your body may be recirculating estrogen when it should be eliminating it into the toilet.
- **Maintain a healthy body weight.** Since body fat makes a certain amount of estrogen, being overweight can create estrogen excess. Weight loss has been shown to reduce systemic estrogen levels.250
- **Consider excision surgery.** Wide excision surgery will remove the endo lesions producing excess estrogen and inflammation.

If you're not seeing the gains in hormonal balance you need by working on the basics, I recommend working with your doctor or naturopath to test levels and formulate a more specific plan. If you're interested in more information on the specifics of balancing progesterone and estrogen levels, see Further Reading for some great book recommendations!

Chapter 15:

Reducing Your Toxic Burden

As discussed in Chapter 3, endo's relationship with environmental toxins is quite intertwined. It's why you may have heard that dioxins *cause* endometriosis. Or, you may have heard that endometriosis happens because our bodies are unable to detoxify—why herbal "cleanses" and liver support are routinely recommended in holistic health circles. While these rumors aren't entirely true, there is indeed some truth behind them, such as:[251]

- Certain environmental chemicals are known to contribute to the creation of an endo-like cell.
- Many of these chemicals also contribute to immune dysfunction.
- Some toxins mimic estrogen in the body—meaning they may be "feeding" your estrogen-hungry endo cells.
- Most environmental toxins cause cellular damage and become a contributor to both chronic inflammation, and immune dysfunction on a mass scale.
- Exposure to toxins is associated with infertility, premature ovarian failure, poor birth outcomes, mental health issues, autoimmunity, and cancer.

This may be why a wide variety of chemicals have been associated with endo. These chemicals are found in common household items, from non-stick pans to cosmetics and body care products.[252] In fact, according to the National Resources Defense Council (NRDC), most of the 80,000 chemicals available for use in the U.S. haven't been adequately tested for safety.[253] This is why there are very *real* reasons why eliminating these chemicals will make you feel better.

Thus, investigating the toxic burden in your own life will be an essential part of your healing plan. And it's a big step, considering how exposed to chemicals we are every day. If this is an overwhelming thought, you're not alone. I have had a very hard time talking about my chemical burden (and Earth's) without feeling a little hopeless. Still, you can be inspired knowing that the changes you make, even just at home, can have a profound impact on your body's chemical load.

A great example of this is in the book *Slow Death by Rubber Duck*, in which the authors, using themselves as guinea pigs, investigate how much *just* the daily products we use affect our toxicity levels.[254] For four days they exposed themselves to everyday items sneakily known to house toxins: canned foods such as beans and soda, personal care products such as shampoos and soap, and common household cleaning products. After just four days of what's considered "normal" chemical exposure, their blood and urine tests revealed that the level of the chemicals in their body had increased by as much as eightfold! Excitingly, they also found that when they removed the products, their chemical load went down as well.

It's clear that what you put *on* your body gets *into* your body. Women using conventional lotions and perfumes had 167 percent higher levels of phthalates in their urine.[255] And phthalate levels in the body may increase 33 percent per body care product used, demonstrating how multiple exposures can add up fast (like, if you use ten body care products before you even leave the house you'll have 333 percent more phthalates in your system).[256] This is a great reminder that even if we can't change all the environmental pollutants we're in contact with, we can make changes at home that can indeed remove an enormous chemical burden from our bodies. There's hope.

Luckily, there is already an abundance of useful information available in books and online to help you reduce your chemical and toxin exposure. This chapter will be a primer to get you started with some easy big wins to reduce endocrine disrupting chemicals (EDCs) that are known to be associated with endo, such as dioxins, phthalates, BPA, herbicides/pesticides, and non-stick chemicals. I'll discuss both reducing overall exposure to chemicals as well as how to support removing unwanted chemicals from the body.

FIRST, REDUCE EXPOSURE

One of the best places to start reducing chemical exposure today is at home, including everything from the food you eat to the cosmetics you use to the way you clean. Because many of us spend the majority of our lives indoors, proper product substitutions can easily reduce our own level of chemical exposure.

Purchasing Food

It can be disheartening to acknowledge that the food we buy at our local grocery stores may be laden with chemicals that affect our endo. But since healthy and nutritious food is the foundation of the Heal Endo lifestyle, it is important to know how to navigate the grocery aisles.

The main culprits are pesticides and herbicides. Exposure to certain pesticides and herbicides may increase endometriosis risk by up to 70 percent.[257] One herbicide of particular concern is glyphosate (commonly sold under the name Roundup) which is chock full of EDCs that are heavily sprayed on crops to prevent weeds. These crops are called Roundup Ready because they're genetically modified to resist damage from the chemical themselves, meaning they can withstand incredibly heavy, repeated applications without dying.

> **Exposure to certain pesticides and herbicides may increase endometriosis risk by up to 70 percent.**

Even more concerning, additional glyphosate is sprayed on some crops such as wheat to dry it out *just before it's harvested* and processed. A 2020 sampling of nearly 8,000 foods found that *nearly half* contained detectable levels of glyphosate residues.[258] Luckily, you can avoid much of this contamination by switching to organic foods, as much as your budget allows. A study that followed four families who ate conventionally grown foods (i.e., with pesticides) and then switched to consuming only organic foods, found that the glyphosate levels in their urine decreased by 70 percent after only three days![259]

It's also important to discuss dioxins, which are highly toxic. Dioxins cause reproductive and developmental problems, damage to the immune system, cancer, and can interfere with hormones, yet they are still used in many popular herbicides sprayed near crops. Additionally, because dioxins sit in the environment for a long time, they blow around with the wind and land in soils and water—ultimately ending up in our stomachs. Unfortunately, they're everywhere. And while we've mainly been told to avoid eating animal products to lessen dioxin exposure, it turns out that both plant and animal products may be equally contaminated (see Appendix 5 for more on this).

Luckily, there are strategies that can help limit exposure to dioxins in food. One way is simply to cook your food, which may reduce dioxins by up to 44 percent.[260] Another way is by supplementing with chlorella, which is a type of seaweed that comes in pills or capsules. When taken with your meal, chlorella may prevent your body from absorbing up to 50 percent of the dioxins in your food.[261] Moreover, chlorella may help your body eliminate the stores it already has. It can help the body excrete nine times more dioxins than those without chlorella, and reduce the amount of dioxins stored in the liver by nearly one-third![262]

Additionally, dioxin damage may be mitigated by adding in more antioxidants to our diets. For example, certain antioxidants found in heart and liver (CoQ10) or cocoa and blueberries (resveratrol) were shown to prevent dioxin damage by offering protection because of their ability to scavenge free radicals.[263] Another reason why diet is a foundational consideration in healing.

Cooking and Storing Food

How you cook your food also makes a difference. Avoiding non-stick pans is a must. Non-stick cookware is made with EDCs from a group called perfluorinated chemicals. When heated or scratched (which you do when cooking), these chemicals are released into the food and air, where they may lodge themselves into your body for 3–5 years.[264] To avoid this contaminant, I recommend switching to cast-iron pans, which not only reduce your chemical exposure but also add a bit of iron back into your food—a supplemental bonus for the often iron-deficient endo body. Conversely, ceramic pans are also a great option. If you microwave, use only glass.

Now that your meal is done and you have some leftovers, don't store them in plastic containers. Plastics contain EDCs, including both BPA and phthalates. In the kitchen, you can find these chemicals in food-storage options such as plastic canisters, cups, or plastic baggies. They are also used to line the cans of foods you have in your pantry, such as vegetables, beans, fish, tomatoes, and even soda. Yes, even if you're a self-proclaimed hippie, you'll find BPA lining your organic almond milk or soy creamer container, and even your can of kombucha.

Kitchen Tips

Safe cookware options include glass, ceramic, stainless-steel or (my favorite) cast-iron pans. Eliminate all non-stick Teflon and aluminum pans.

Get a water filter in your kitchen for drinking and cooking water. Refillable stainless steel or glass bottles for on-the-go are also essential.

Purchase organic whenever possible. If budgeting, try to follow the dirty dozen rule of avoiding the most heavily pesticide-contaminated produce: strawberries, spinach, kale, nectarines, apples, grapes, peaches, cherries, pears, tomatoes, celery, and potatoes.

Store food in glass or metal containers, rather than plastic. And no more plastic water bottles; opt for a reusable metal or glass one instead.

What about BPA-free plastic? These don't get a pass because the industry replaced BPA with BPS, BPAF, or others, chemicals similar to BPA that have already been shown in studies to inflict similar harm.[265] The basic rule of thumb: if it's plastic, it will have unwanted chemicals in it, even if it's BPA-free.

To reduce exposure, purchase and store as much food as you can in glass containers. Many stores sell sets of glass storage containers alongside their plastic counterparts. If these are out of budget for now, consider purchasing simple glass Mason jars with metal lids, or even simply reusing glass jars from spaghetti sauce and such. Instead of soda cans (lined with BPA), try sparkling water purchased in glass containers and add a fresh squeeze of grapefruit or lime. Also because BPA is found lining many pre-packaged foods, you will naturally minimize your exposure when you begin to cook more fresh, homemade meals.

BATH, BODY, AND HOME

We can also make big strides in removing endo-provoking chemicals when it comes to our personal care routines. If you're like me (before I understood just *what* I was putting on my body), chances are you have a bathroom full of incredible-smelling shampoos, conditioners, body washes, lotions, and fragrances. Not to mention a nice assortment of makeup and skincare. Unfortunately, these products are often filled to the brim with endocrine-disrupting chemicals.

To avoid the chemical onslaught, you'll need to actively seek out products that don't have parabens or phthalates. Look for products that market themselves as paraben-free or phthalate-free. If you're unsure, read the ingredient label, searching for words such as "methylparaben" or "isobutylparaben"—or any other word that has "paraben" in it. Similarly, avoid ingredients that have the word "phthalate" in them.

As an important side note, a product can say "phthalate-free," but still have heaps of phthalates in it due to a little-known trick of the fragrance industry.

To keep ingredients secret (so no one knows that special *je ne sais quoi* in your favorite perfume), companies don't have to disclose ingredients. This means even if a fragrance is *rich* in phthalates (which they usually are since phthalates give fragrances staying power), companies don't have to disclose them. Knowing this, you can avoid a product if it has "fragrance" listed as an ingredient, even if all the other ingredients are phthalate-free or the product describes itself as 99 percent plant-based, "organix," or other trendy names. My rule of thumb is that if it smells like perfume—and lasts—then it's probably due to a hidden chemical component.

If you see the word "fragrance" in the ingredients, the product probably has phthalates in it...even if it's marketed as organic or even as phthalate-free.

The truth is, if you don't actively seek out products that are free of EDCs, they will unfortunately be there. If you quickly take a spin around your house, you'll probably see fragrances, phthalates, or parabens hidden in nearly everything from your laundry and dish soap to your lotion and body wash to your perfume and lipstick. This isn't fair, but it's a reality our endo bodies need to face when talking about this new, deeper kind of healing.

Don't feel like you have to toss out everything and spend a thousand dollars on new products today. That feeling of being overwhelmed can leave us paralyzed. Instead, take a breath and know this may be a long journey of substitutions. For example, you may wait until your product is finished and then just replace it with a different one that you researched to be free from EDCs. A great place to do this research is at the Environmental Working Group (www.ewg.org), which has an enormous database of products with safety scores. If you're like me and get easily overwhelmed with too many options, I recommend starting with their pre-made list of EWG-verified products that are all top-rated for ingredient safety. Just pick one product to start, and take it from there

Here's some good news: when talking about cleaning around the home, you can actually *save* money. Vinegar and water work amazingly well for general cleaning. So do alcohol or hydrogen peroxide for sterilizing. There is a lot of information available on how to make your own cleaning products, and it's really easy too.

Cleaning, Home, and Body Care Tips

Basic soap and water or vinegar solutions are great for basic cleaning need. If you need to use heavy-duty cleaning chemicals for any reason, use gloves and a mask as basic precautions.

Because furniture, carpets, upholstery and more may have toxins, aim to keep windows open as much as possible so airflow helps combat dust and debris. Consider HEPA air filtration fans if you spend a lot of time indoors.

FRAGRANCE
FREE

Avoid all products that contain fragrance. Consider laundry products, cleaners, and all personal care products. Yes, there are a lot of products to consider!

Spend time combing through your personal care routine to slowly wean out all products with EDCs. Use ewg.org/guides/ to help.

Laundry detergents are usually highly fragranced, so switching to fragrance-free will be essential. One of the hardest things in my own journey was breaking up with the idea that smelling clean involved smelling like the perfume aisle at the store. I was so obsessed with this idea of smelling "clean" that I had a scented upholstery spray for my furniture, fragrance boosters for the laundry, an assortment of fruity body spray for my body, and scented plug-ins for the whole house. If this is you, please be assured that being clean doesn't have to smell like *anything*. It doesn't smell dirty (think body odor, dirty dogs, or sweat), but nor does it smell like artificial fragrances. If you do like a little fragrance (I still do), I recommend some essential oils and a nice room diffuser.

And although "going green" may sound pricey or challenging, it truly does not have to be! Many books out there can help guide you through the process of turning over a new green leaf, as slowly as you need (for sanity and budget). And while we won't be able to remove all the chemicals in our lives, it's great to have a reminder of how much we can lift the burden on our body by making small changes at home, from the food and beauty care products we purchase to the way we clean.

REDUCING HARM, BECAUSE CHEMICALS ARE EVERYWHERE

While we may not be able to totally reduce our chemical load, there are protective mechanisms that can help us move out the toxins we ingest, absorb, or inhale. By enhancing our own detoxification pathways, we can support the body in eliminating too much chemical buildup.

Sweating is one incredible route to get toxins out of your body, as sweating can remove BPA, PCBs, and phthalates in one fell swoop.[266] That means it's even more important for the endo body to move to the point of breaking a sweat. If moving isn't on the cards right now for any reason (pain, illness, etc.), you can just as easily sweat by gentle walks (or even lying) in the heat of the midday sun, or in an extra-hot bath or shower for 10 to 15 minutes. Make it a goal to sweat every day if you can, even for 5 minutes, making sure that you properly rinse off after you're cooled down so that you don't reabsorb the toxins you just sweated out.

You can also support proper elimination by urinating and pooping well. Your goal is to have at least one fully formed bowel movement per day so that your body doesn't end up reabsorbing chemicals that are ready for excretion. This goes back to recommendations of lots of fiber and clearing up any gut infections that may be preventing you from having a normal bowel movement. As for urine, aim to drink 8 to 12 cups of purified water per day to help flush toxins out. Your urine should be light yellow rather than dark (which means you're dehydrated) or clear (which means you're over-hydrating). Obviously, this water shouldn't be stored in plastic containers, and ideally should be filtered. [For an at-home filtration system, consider a Berkey water filter for countertops, although it is expensive. If you're budgeting, consider a plastic countertop Brita water filter that you use *only* to filter your water, and then store in a glass container.]

Endo Nice List

- Buy as much organic food as you can afford. (Can't afford it? Then don't stress about it, we all have to eat)
- Consider supplementing with chlorella.
- Wash produce before eating.
- Cook with cast iron, ceramic, or stainless steel pots and pans.
- Store food in glass or metal containers.
- Get a water filter.
- Use a glass or metal water bottle.
- Sweat every day.
- Consider HEPA air filtration fans if you spend a lot of time indoors.
- Buy chemical free:
  o Haircare
  o Makeup
  o Beauty products
  o Cleaning products
  o Cooking/kitchenware
  o (Psst, Take as much time as you need doing this)

Endo Naughty List

- Toss plastic food containers.
- Toss plastic water bottles (even BPA-free ones).
- Toss non-stick Teflon and aluminum pans.
- Toss products that have perfume/fragrance listed as an ingredient. Consider these products:
  o Laundry detergent
  o Laundry dryer sheets
  o Cleaning products
  o Beauty products
  o Perfume or body spray
  o Upholstery cleaners
  o House scents
  o Car scents
  o Dish/dishwasher soap
- Avoid touching thermal receipt papers, a potent source of BPA.
- Bring your own coffee cup to avoid BPA-lined paper cups.

DO THE BEST you can for your own circumstances! Every endo body has their own budget to work with. Take this information and apply it to your life and your wallet.

Chapter 16:

Coaching for Your Doctors' Appointments

Because endometriosis is so complex, you may need personalized medical care to help manage your symptoms. This is where contraceptives, hormone therapies, painkillers, and further testing come into the picture. Truth be told, these options can work miracles for some of us, while others may have suffered needlessly from improper use of these aids or because of how their bodies reacted. So let's discuss the most commonly prescribed remedies for endo found at your local OB-GYN office—hormones and pain management—as well as when to consider further testing.

HORMONES

Because endometriosis lesions are sensitive to hormones, estrogen suppression has become a front-line medical treatment over the past few decades, ranging from hormonal birth control pills to medications that induce temporary chemical menopause. Although hormonal suppression is not a long-term solution for endo, it may help manage the symptoms in some women and give the body time to mount its own defenses. However, none of those approaches are without side effects. I believe in full patient disclosure (something I call "meducation").

Hormonal Contraceptives

Hormonal contraceptives (HCs) are potent synthetic hormones, usually a combination of estrogen and progestin (synthetic progesterone), which in most cases prevent your body from ovulating in order to avoid pregnancy. There are a wide variety of brands and formulas, including oral birth control pills, hormonal skin patches, periodic injections, and vaginal inserts like the NuvaRing. They work by dosing your body with enough hormones to override your own hormone loop, essentially taking over your menstrual cycle. In this way, they prevent your body from maturing an egg, releasing it during ovulation, thickening the endometrium lining, and having a true period bleed (one that occurs because of ovulation). In the case of endometriosis, this can work miracles for some in reducing the painful endo symptoms associated with ovulation and menses.

Yet HCs don't work for everyone, and they have side effects, the most common being fatigue, mood swings, weight gain, depression, and loss of libido. But there are additional issues associated with long-term birth control use that are not typically discussed, but are incredibly important to know about, including:

- Nutrient depletion (including B vitamins, vitamin C, and many minerals)
- Gut microbiome changes
- Intestinal lining changes (i.e., leaky gut)
- Mood disturbances (such as anxiety and depression)
- Thyroid dysregulation
- Testosterone dysregulation
- Increased susceptibility to immune dysfunction, autoimmune diseases, and interstitial cystitis
- Increased susceptibility to clotting disorders and stroke
- "Post-Pill Syndrome" (cycle dysregulation for months or years after coming off HCs)

The impact HCs may have on immune dysfunction is very important for the endo sufferer to understand. At a basic level, hormones are cellular communicators, which is why there are hormone receptors on every cell in the body, including immune cells. Estrogen, for example, can enhance antibody secretion, while progesterone has an immune calming effect. Together these hormones act as partners in ensuring the appropriate behavior of the immune system. Thus, when we take potent synthetic hormones to override this delicate system, we may be asking for some immune trouble. In addition, HC-related nutrient depletion can further exacerbate immune dysfunction, since HCs deplete key nutrients absolutely necessary for proper immune function.[267]

This may be why the long-term use of HCs has been shown to significantly increase the risk of developing several serious autoimmune or autoimmune-related diseases, such as Crohn's disease, rheumatoid arthritis, multiple sclerosis, and thyroid disease.[268] Interestingly enough, it's also these *exact* immune-related diseases that are associated with endometriosis. Those with endometriosis are 50 percent more likely to develop Crohn's (a type of inflammatory bowel disease), and long-term HC use may be a potential cause.[269] Another type of immune dysfunction that causes bladder inflammation (called interstitial cystitis) is so linked with endometriosis that it's been labeled her "evil twin." (80–90 percent of endo sufferers also suffer from IC, which is also *highly* associated with long-term HC use.[270])

Whether the increased risk of these diseases is due to a genetic predisposition, to the immune dysregulation that already exists in the endometriosis body, to the long-term use of HCs, or a combination of all three has not yet been studied. I hope that this topic becomes better researched, given that HCs are the most frequently utilized tool offered by doctors to address endometriosis symptoms.

Still, because HCs can be so helpful in overriding the (sometimes radical) monthly hormonal roller coaster that many with endo experience—including relieving symptoms like painful ovulation, life-altering PMS, painful periods, and a heavy flow—they are still a helpful consideration. At the very least, they may be a good short-term option to consider (for a number of months) while you work on addressing other root cause issues. Others may decide HCs are so helpful in managing symptoms that they stay on the pill long term. The most important thing is to trust your own body while understanding the risks.

Progesterone or Progestin Therapy

As an alternative to combined estrogen/progestin hormonal treatments found in hormonal contraceptives, progesterone alone can act as a form of treatment in certain cases, either in the natural form (progesterone) or synthetic (progestins). Progesterone is anti-inflammatory, immunomodulating, and can oppose the inflammatory action of estrogen, something that may be useful when facing endo. This is why progesterone treatments may aid some sufferers in combating some of our most annoying (or even life-altering) menstrual symptoms such as bad PMS, breast tenderness, heavy menses, spotting before menses, and even infertility.

Synthetic progestins will often be those prescribed at a conventional doctor's office, offered in many forms from creams to capsules, injectables, suppositories, or the Mirena IUD. Some can be used for contraception as in the "mini-pill" or IUD, while others like medroxyprogesterone or norethindrone can be used to treat endometriosis symptoms in some by suppressing ovulation and creating a pseudopregnancy.

If you find progestins too tough on your body, you may consider talking to a naturopath or functional medicine practitioner about natural progesterone. Offered in creams or tablets, this type of progesterone may be a more gentle option to balance the systemic estrogen-progesterone ratio or help treat what's known as a luteal phase defect (low progesterone in the two weeks before menstruation). A luteal phase defect will often appear as a shortened cycle since the 12- to 14-day window between ovulation and start of menstruation relies on healthy progesterone levels. If your progesterone levels are too low, you will start spotting or bleeding earlier than you should.

In addition, low progesterone during this time interferes with mood, increases PMS symptoms, can prevent conception (if your luteal phase is too short, a fertilized egg won't have time to implant before menstruation starts), and lead to heavy menses. This is where natural progesterone supplementation may help by lengthening the luteal phase, decreasing problematic premenstrual spotting or heavy periods, lessen PMS symptoms, and/or even support a pregnancy.

When talking to your practitioner about progesterone, understand that different options, and quantities, work differently for each sufferer. For example, one person may do very well with natural progesterone cream while another person may do better with an oral progestin tablet, an injectable, or an IUD. Another person may get anxiety from too high a dose, while another actually needs a high dose to make any impact on her symptoms. That's why I recommend you speak with a *knowledgeable* health care provider who can help you dial in proper dosages and forms based on your own symptoms and goals.

Gonadotropin-Releasing Hormone (Orlissa, Lupron)

Gonadotropin-releasing hormones (Gn-RHa) include types of medication that affect sex hormones like estrogen, with Orlissa and Lupron the brand names us endo folk probably know best. These pharmaceuticals work primarily by shutting down the hypothalamic-pituitary-ovarian (HPO) axis, i.e., the signaling system that tells your body to make hormones like estrogen and progesterone. In shutting down this axis, you induce short-term artificial menopause that lowers estrogen production to post-menopausal levels. This is the method by which this class of medications is thought to help symptoms, as it reduces estrogen to levels so low that the endometriosis won't be stimulated by it.

While you may have been casually offered these treatments by your gynecologist, most specialists will recommend these only as a last resort (if at all) after *no other* treatments are found to offer relief. For these complex cases, this approach may help—perhaps making it worth the side effects that are often associated with it. These medications usually work to temporarily relieve endo symptoms, which, in the context of debilitating pain, is a welcome relief for some. It can also be helpful in preparation for certain in vitro fertilization (IVF) fertility procedures. For example, if a woman with endo is going through the IVF process, her reproductive endocrinologist might recommend a short dose of this medication to "quiet the scene" by calming endo-related inflammation before transferring an embryo into the uterus.

And yet, as many in the endo community who have tried this class of pharmaceutical will tell you, using Gn-RHa meds can come at a *terribly* high price. At the bottom of the list are the symptoms of menopause: mood swings, hot flashes, night sweats, vaginal dryness, painful intercourse, insomnia, bone thinning, joint pain, vision issues, thyroid dysfunction, and more. And there are those who've faced much worse, women who were so negatively affected by this class of medications that they were never able to reclaim their lives long after the drug should have worn off, leading to class-action lawsuits against these companies. Additionally, these drugs are absolutely not safe for long-term use and do not cure endo; rather, they are, at best, a short-term fix to buy time and offer some temporary relief.

My recommendation? Do *thorough* research on the drugs' side effects, as well as others' experiences, before even thinking about committing to them. And if your doctor casually recommends you try them before trying other methods of pain relief or surgery, it's probably time to find another doctor.

SYLWIA'S STORY

I thought that finally getting my endometriosis diagnosis would mean the end of a complex set of symptoms because, knowing the problem, I could now find solutions to it. However, it turned out to be just the beginning of a long journey to wellness. In my case, it wasn't *just* endometriosis; it took time and in-depth investigations to figure out all of my diagnoses. Complex patients are often forced to become advocates for their own well-being and, although healing is rarely linear, the motivation to take care of myself persists.

Even with the complexities at hand, following the Heal Endo approach made me realize how many aspects of my health needed attention, things I had long ignored (or, at least learned to manage) since I was a child. And while healing from a complex symphony of issues is never linear (honestly there've been times I felt worse than ever, and times I

thought I was totally cured), I've come a long way in understanding my body. Even with lingering symptoms, my body's needs are no longer a mystery to me, and that, at least, offers me a feeling of better control.
—Sylwia, UK

PAIN TREATMENT

Pain is the #1 symptom associated with endometriosis. Endo pain can be acute or chronic; it can occur at menses, ovulation, during an entire luteal phase, or all the time. Pain can flare seemingly randomly, with certain food choices, sex, orgasm, stress, bowel movement, or exercise. It can be felt deep in the organs or on the outside of the vagina. It all depends on you. Yet most of us deal with pain regularly enough to at least justify the use of painkillers a handful of times per month...others of us daily.

Common medications like NSAIDs (ibuprofen, aspirin, naproxen, etc.) and opioids (hydrocodone, oxycodone, tramadol, morphine) are widely used in the endo community, and for good reason: they often help. They can make a day, a period, or ovulation bearable or, on a darker note, keep suicidal thoughts at bay. Indeed, some with endo who have also birthed a baby and describe their endo episodes as being *more painful* than childbirth were shamed by doctors for requesting stronger pain meds. Can you imagine shaming a woman who had to go through the pains of childbirth *every day* for needing medical pain relief? Probably not. Likewise, there is no shame in using medications to manage endo pain when needed.

While your long-term goal is to reduce your reliance on pain medication, with some of us finding we can eliminate the need for them at all, the truth is that until you get to the root of your endo symptoms and receive proper care and treatment, you may need to do all you can to address pain. That said, like all medications, pain meds also come with risks. I wish I had been adequately informed when I was diagnosed so that I could have addressed my pain more mindfully.

NSAIDs

The NSAID—non-steroidal anti-inflammatory drug—family includes the most common pain relief medicines in the world, such as ibuprofen, aspirin, naproxen, and others. These drugs can work well for endo pain because they help block inflammatory prostaglandins, one of the common pain triggers for endo. And while taking an NSAID here or there for pain is generally not a problem, long-term and consistent use have been shown to cause significant stomach and intestinal damage, a particularly important point to understand in the context of endo.

It's well known that NSAIDs can cause stomach bleeding and ulcers.[271] This damage to the stomach mucosa will begin to affect your ability to properly digest foods, leading to a cascade of other issues such as intestinal permeability and malabsorption. Researchers observed the effects of NSAIDs on leaky gut and found that "intestinal permeability changes were significantly more pronounced and frequent" in the context of NSAIDs, no matter which variety was taken.[272] A 2011 study examining whether NSAID-related intestinal damage could be avoided found that there's "no proven method of preventing or curing small intestine damage due to NSAIDs. The simplest method is to stop taking the drugs."[273]

Additionally, for those trying to battle endo and achieve pregnancy at the same time, there are links to NSAIDs and increased miscarriage rates. Women who took NSAIDs in early pregnancy were shown to be 4 times more likely to have a miscarriage than those who did not.[274] This information is vital for any endo sufferer in pain who's trying to conceive.

Opioids

Opioids are a class of drugs including oxycodone, hydrocodone, tramadol, and morphine that may be prescribed by a physician for pain management. These are potent painkillers that work by blocking signals to pain receptors throughout the body. While they are effective for suppressing pain, they do come with a high risk of addiction, making them potentially dangerous for long-term pain management.

The highly addictive nature of opioids combined with the over-prescription of this class of drugs in the U.S. has led to a national opioid crisis. This is especially problematic in chronic pain circles where painkillers are consumed more frequently, increasing the likelihood of addiction. In fact, research shows that nearly 1 in 3 people who are prescribed opioids for chronic pain will end up misusing them.[275] This is a dangerous game of Russian roulette to play, especially considering it's estimated that 130 Americans die *every day* from an opioid overdose.

Furthermore, although opioids are great at blocking acute pain in the short term (like a broken arm), they can make your pain much worse in the long term if you're using them to address chronic pain that doesn't go away (like endo). This is called opioid-induced hyperalgesia, when opioids used for pain end up making patients even more sensitive to pain or making chronic pain worse than it was before opioids. This increased pain leaves a patient in need of higher and higher doses to feel better, increasing the risk of overdose.[276]

Beyond the risks of addiction and overdose, it's also important to be aware of the impact opioids have on the immune system. Regular opioid use has been shown to significantly suppress the immune system, decreasing immune response by 20–30 percent.[277] This is why chronic opioid use is associated with increased rates of infection—viral, bacterial, and fungal.[278] Hence, when we see that opiates profoundly disrupt the body's first line of defense against harmful external bacteria, consistent opiate use for endo-related pain may become more of an instigator than a savior.[279]

"COPE BEFORE YOU DOPE": TOOLS FOR PASSING PAIN

Because pain medication comes with risks, establishing some mindfulness around *when* to use them can be helpful. To do this you will need to tune in to your body to better understand when "lasting" pain is coming on versus a "passing" moment when you could potentially utilize other tools to manage it. These passing moments may be a sharp twinge, shooting nerve pain, or pain radiating from within—but that usually passes within a few minutes. If you can relax for a minute, focus on your breath and the noises around you (such as birds, traffic, anything to remove you for a moment from your head), and try to "let the pain pass," you may not need that NSAID after all.

For longer "endo episodes," as I've come to call them, which are marked by long-lasting bouts of pain, medication may be mandatory until further treatment can be accessed. Again, there is no shame in taking pain medication when needed, but it is important to be mindful of what you're taking and how and when you're taking it.

Low-Dose Naltrexone (LDN)

Naltrexone is a pharmaceutical that was first introduced in the 1980s to treat opioid and alcohol addiction by blocking opioid receptors in the brain. Later it was found that subtle blunting of these receptors using low doses (about 1/10 a full dose) could offer some anti-inflammatory and immunomodulating benefits.

While LDN hasn't been well studied in association with endometriosis directly, its benefits of pain reduction have been studied through the lens of pain associated with chronic inflammatory conditions such as ulcerative colitis, Crohn's, and fibromyalgia.[280] Basically, it's been shown to help people with a painful chronic inflammatory disease state, like endo.

I've personally known a few women who were prescribed LDN through their endo surgeon or primary care physician and have exclaimed about the results. With few known side effects (unlike traditional painkillers), the option of a drug that helps reduce stress, anxiety, bloating, and chronic pain would make most endo sufferers ecstatic. Yet, because of the limited information available relating to endo specifically, you will have to think of it as an "off-label" pain treatment, one that you should discuss with your doctor to see if it's a correct fit for you and your symptoms.

Endocannabinoids for Pain Management

The endocannabinoid system (ECS) is made up of a vast network of receptors throughout our bodies. There are two main cannabinoid receptors, CB1 and CB2. CB1 works primarily on neurotransmitters, adding input to the neural feedback loop to help inform the nervous system on how to best behave (and how the "high" of THC can work its effect on the brain), while CB2 primarily works on the immune system cells, which is critical for helping with proper inflammation levels, immune behavior, and pain. These receptors are activated by endocannabinoid molecules that we make in our bodies, but can also be activated by cannabis (i.e., marijuana) since it has a structural similarity. It's quite remarkable, actually, just how easily cannabis can take control of this cellular system to create numerous benefits, one of which is pain control in those with endometriosis, and even in the process of *endo-ing*.

In fact, new research supports the idea that the ESC may directly influence numerous facets of endo, from the creation of pain to the actual creation of disease (inflammation, proliferation, and cell survival).[281] This means helping to regulate this system through external sources may not just help lower pain, but may also offer a pharmacological effect to reduce the establishment and recurrence of lesions. Win-win.

As federal and state limits on this type of "drug" have minimized, it's become easier to access. In most states, you can get a prescription for medical marijuana from a helpful doctor, whereas some states legally allow anyone to access it as long as you're over 18. There are also many varieties of cannabis available, from the original smoking type to edibles (which are helpful if you want to dial in a specific dosage you're comfortable with). There are even options with low- to no-THC for those who would like to skip the "high." If you deal with chronic endo pain and haven't tried hijacking the ESC, it may be time to give it a try. I recommend reaching out to a knowledgeable practitioner who can help you figure out the best variety to try for your specific situation.

PHANTOM ENDO PAIN – AN OVER-FIRING NERVOUS SYSTEM

Endometriosis pain comes in many shapes and sizes, but if you're that en-do-warrior who deals with *chronic, unrelenting* pelvic, abdominal, or really any chronic pain (and you've already had an excision surgery and/or investigated other root causes), your nervous system may be to blame. This happens over time when a body deals with such unrelenting pain that the nervous system can become overactive and/or confused due to chronic stimulation by pain signals—similar to how the immune system becomes confused when faced with too much inflammation.

When the nervous system becomes overactive, it can start to create excess pain, even without actual stimuli (sort of like a stereo system that can play, but only at the loudest level). This is how some people experience "phantom pain": *real* pain but for an unknown reason. Conversely, you may experience incredibly heightened pain with very little stimuli—for example, if someone lightly touches your arm or your bladder is slightly full. This is often referred to as central sensitization (CS) and is a serious issue to deal with if you have it.

CS explains how some of the painful symptoms we feel with endo may not actually be caused by endometriosis lesions, but rather by the impact of an over-firing nervous system. It's how sufferers may still deal with excruciating pain following an excision surgery, or find sex too painful even though doctors have said "nope, nothing wrong." What doctors should be saying instead (after a thorough analysis observing no other pain-causing factors) is that the pain may be thanks to an over-firing nervous system that could be causing you excruciating pain for no reason. When CS takes over, it can send signals of pain to other areas of the body (think bladder, bowel, and pelvic floor), create phantom pain, and make life miserable.

There is a beautifully written example of phantom pain and CS that's written by a pelvic floor physical therapist on Endometriosis.net. In this story, she explains how an endo patient came to her, post-hysterectomy (including her ovaries), with continually severe pelvic pain that no doctors seem to be able to address. The PT did an internal exam, "palpating her pelvic floor muscles, I reached a tender point. I pushed just a little more and she said 'that is my ovary pain' and started crying. She had no ovaries. *It was referred pain from her pelvic floor muscles.*"[282] This story helps demonstrate why you have terrible pain but not "terrible endo," why having a full bladder feels like a belly full of knives, how sex can feel like murder, and how chronic pain can become entrenched with no end in sight.

Luckily, there is a way to address it—you just have to know what *it* is (so when doctors unfamiliar with CS send you away saying nothing's wrong, you now know you have another route to investigate). Successful treatment of CS focuses on the proverbial "soothing" of the central nervous system. In fact, traditional pain medication often won't help these cases. Rather, you work to calm CS through an integrative framework, using any tool from special medication to exercise, to cognitive behavioral therapy and pelvic floor physical therapy (which I've already recommended numerous times, getting the hint?).

Pelvic floor physical therapy is often a must for CS and pelvic pain. This musculature can get tight, spasmodic, or atrophied just like any muscle group, acting as a serious contributor to pain that, unless addressed, can contribute to CS. Moreover, treating pelvic floor dysfunction can also help retrain CS and the over-firing of pain signals. Without calming the nervous system, your pain may truly persist without end.

If you believe that your pain stems from an issue such as CS, you'll need to find a practitioner who understands it (not all of them do). I again recommend checking out the wonderful information at www.pelvicpainrehab.com as a great starting point. Another helpful (and affordable!) baby step may be using a simple app like Curable. Curable is an amazing resource developed to help those with chronic health issues begin to *retrain* the brain to handle stress responses (and nervous system firing) more calmly. There has been an outpouring of beneficial stories from those who have used this app, including clients I have worked with personally. You can find more information at www. curablehealth.com.

BEYOND ENDO: FURTHER TESTING AND CARE

If you don't feel better after employing many of the new techniques described in this book (and you've already consulted with a surgeon), I recommend further testing for issues beyond endo. Truth be told, you may also be suffering from another disease altogether, something like multiple sclerosis, lupus, or fibromyalgia. Or, you could have a virus that keeps taking your energy levels down (something like Epstein-Barr virus), or maybe you have a toxic level of stored lead from contaminated pipes (which one of my clients actually found). Truly, there are many reasons beyond endo that can be making you feel bad. So try to strengthen your resilience and keep seeking. It's not fun to get two diagnoses, but it's better to know what you are dealing with so you can address it, rather than losing hope, thinking that nothing is working.

How do you know what testing to look for? As I mentioned before, I recommend seeking out a functional medicine doctor who specializes in complex cases. Even just finding a physician better trained in *interpreting* results can be life-changing. Using myself as an example, when I dealt with chronic fatigue, no doctor could tell me why, even after many tests. I eventually sought out a naturopath, who explained my ferritin levels at 12 could *definitely* have something to do with low energy (a classically trained M.D. may believe any ferritin level above 11 is okay), and bringing my iron levels back up to what it considered sufficient in functional medicine (50) dramatically changed my life.

Another example I like to give is that of a former client of mine (story below) who had a professional excision surgery from an extremely skilled surgeon and was still suffering. Diet and lifestyle kind of helped ... but she there was something deeper going on, and she knew it. After a lot of sleuthing, she was able to obtain a diagnosis: Lyme disease and mold toxicity. She told me that addressing these issues helped her 10 times more than the surgery did—demonstrating how a hidden health issue can undermine our endo-healing no matter how far removed it seems from our endo lesion. Again, check out the Institute for Functional Medicine, which has a database of practitioners at www.ifm.org/find-a-practitioner.

JESS'S STORY

I've had severe period pain and irregular cycles since age 11. It was a regular occurrence for me to miss school, throw up, and pass out from the pain. And yet, because of a lot of medical gaslighting and a caring, but misguided family, it took me 20 years to get diagnosed with Stage 4 endometriosis and severe adenomyosis. The expert excision surgery I had helped with my daily pelvic pain, but I chose to keep my uterus and had relatively no improvement in my period pain.

When my gold standard excision surgery and diet and gut healing protocols weren't giving me the relief I was looking for, and I was developing full-body chronic pain and fatigue, I dug deeper. In my search to heal the root causes of SIBO, I learned about Lyme disease and mold toxicity. After several years of testing and misdiagnoses, I uncovered the root causes of my immune dysregulation: Lyme disease and co-infections, toxic mold illness, mast cell activation syndrome, parasites, nervous system dysregulation, and trauma. Yes, it was a lot.

As I've been peeling back the layers of my toxic exposures and infections that cause immune disruption, my cycles are regulating and my chronic pain is lessening on its own. I still have period pain and I am still on the journey to the health I want, but I know I'm on the right path. Working to heal my root causes, especially mold illness, has had more impact on my period pain than my excision surgery did! If you are not getting the results you are looking for, don't give up! Keep searching for your root causes because you so deserve to heal. -Jess, USA

Chapter 17:

Removing Endo: Surgery

The removal of established endo lesions is an important step to consider when talking about the "complete treatment" of endometriosis. Endometriosis involves the growth of abnormal tissue that can not only cause significant pain and distress, but can also progress into worse forms of disease with scar tissue, adhesions, and infertility. This is why expert surgical removal of endometriosis is considered the "gold standard" form of treatment—because it fully removes the diseased, inflammatory lesions to offer us a clean slate. It's why surgery is truly an essential tool to have in our endo toolbox.

However, there is a big difference between general surgery and the more advanced type of surgery that someone with endometriosis will need. This specialty surgery is called "wide excision" and must be performed by a skilled surgeon who knows what to look for (endometriosis can hide), as well as how to remove it without causing more damage or leaving any endo remnants behind (which can leave you needing repeat surgeries every few years).

To better understand how surgery can best treat your endo, I reached out to Dr. Andrew Cook, an internationally renowned endometriosis specialist, pelvic pain specialist, and women's health expert, who has devoted his life to helping those of us with complex health problems. In the following Q&A, he helps us better understand why the type of surgical treatment of endometriosis matters.

Q&A WITH ANDREW S. COOK, M.D.

You've been an endometriosis surgeon for over 30 years. Can you give us a little background on your experience?

Since I started learning about endometriosis in 1983, I've seen a gradual unfolding of the conversation around the disease. At that time, endometriosis patients were often isolated and alone in their battle with this disease. Thanks to the internet and subsequent activist movements, endometriosis has now become a household name. Patients with endometriosis are understanding more and more about the disease and how to better treat it. Yet, the most common technique at the time (and unfortunately still today) to remove endometriosis was a burning spot treatment, which usually leaves disease behind untreated. Untreated disease grows back quickly, which often leads women to feel like they need repeat surgeries every year.

My purpose is not to shame or blame general OB-GYNs who are doing their best to treat this complex disease, but rather to help inform patients and doctors alike just how important is the type of surgery performed. While not perfect, a properly performed surgery can be a very effective tool in removing endometriosis and for the vast majority of patients, it provides a huge step in regaining their health. I can't overstate the importance of this.

What is the best type of surgery someone with endo should look for?

"Wide excision surgery" is the term used to describe the complete surgical package used to remove endometriosis. It offers the best tools, processes, and surgical skills needed to provide better outcomes, a lower chance of endo recurrence, and less need for re-operation. It is *far* more precise. It is hard to overstate how important precision is in providing the best-quality surgery. Endometriosis tends to grow on vital structures such as the ureter, bowel, blood vessels, bladder, ovaries, and even the fallopian tubes. In the worst cases, it effectively glues all the organs together in the pelvis and can even eat into the bowel and bladder wall, completely replacing normal tissue. The endometriosis can be a very tough, leathery type of tissue, whereas normal vital organs are soft and delicate. If a surgeon were to pull hard enough on the endometriosis, it would just tear the normal tissue apart. It is often glued or stuck on normal tissue like very strong tape, which is almost impossible to get off the normal underlying tissue.

Vital organs often lie just under the surface of endometriosis. The use of precise instruments that allow the removal of endo implants right off the surface of delicate structures such as veins and the ureter are critical in providing high-quality surgery. My instrument of choice is the Carbon 13 CO_2 laser, the most precise tool available for the removal of endometriosis. I used to have a dollar bill that we would use to laser off some of the ink, leaving the underlying paper undamaged. That is an example of the precision needed to remove endometriosis, as well as the skill of the surgeon to use it.

Ultimately the goal in surgery is to completely remove or correct any abnormalities while minimizing trauma to the surrounding normal healthy tissue, which can be very challenging depending on the case. Precision and skill are needed together.

The Type of Surgery Matters

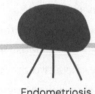

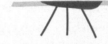

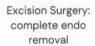

Endometriosis Lesion

Poorly Done Surgery: leaves foundation of endo behind. This can grow back quickly, leading to multiple, poorly done surgeries.

Excision Surgery: complete endo removal

Many of us who had surgeries that weren't wide excision felt the endo "come back" within a year. Can you explain the difference?

If you had your surgery performed by your general OB-GYN, you most likely had *coagulation,* or burning surgery. Burning and spot treatment has long been the most common type of surgery for treatment of endometriosis. It is a relatively easy and quick surgery, using heat to burn the most obvious endometriosis lesions. While it's easy and fast for the surgeon, there are several drawbacks for the patient.

Coagulation or burning surgery is very imprecise, meaning it will destroy some of the disease while also destroying normal tissue. It is virtually impossible to know how much tissue is being destroyed and thus the surgeon has to guess and allow a safe margin to any critical structure such as a blood vessel, ureter, or bowel. This almost guarantees any endometriosis close to vital structures will be left in place and untreated. I have read numerous operative reports stating it was not safe to treat endometriosis because it was too close to a vital structure. This approach commonly results in incomplete removal of disease with excessive damage and inflammation to normal surrounding tissue.

Many studies have shown the presence of endometriosis in normal tissue surrounding visible endometriosis. If skin cancer was suspected, the doctor removing it would cut out not only the pigmented area but also a zone of normal-appearing tissue around it, because of the very good chance that it contained a few cancer cells. This is the best approach for removing all the cancer. The same thing is true with endometriosis. A zone of normal tissue should be removed through a wide excision. In my experience, about two-thirds of normal-looking specimens next to visible endometriosis show microscopic endo when examined by a pathologist. So even if all visible endometriosis is removed, without wide excision, two-thirds of these patients will have microscopic endometriosis remaining after surgery.

Removing only some of the endometriosis is just like pulling the tops off weeds and leaving the roots behind. When the disease stays in the body, even in such small quantities, those cells continue to grow, and the symptoms either persist or come back fairly quickly. This is why many patients get repeat surgeries, since they feel better for a short period of time until succumbing, again, to their symptoms. Unfortunately, these poor outcomes are often blamed on the "hopelessly complex disease" of endometriosis or even on the patient herself, rather than on the type of surgery or the surgeon.

Endo Left Behind Quickly Grows Back

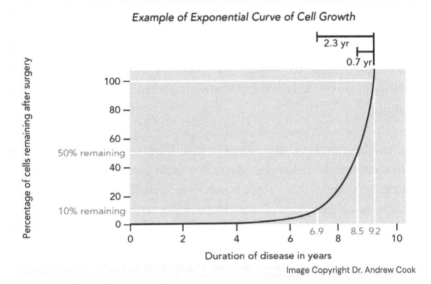

Example of Exponential Curve of Cell Growth

Duration of disease in years

Image Copyright Dr. Andrew Cook

If wide excision surgery is preferred, why is it not the standard surgery offered by most OB-GYNs?

Wide excision takes advanced skill. A non-specialist attempting to perform excision surgery that is beyond their skill set will most likely result in an increased complication rate and injury to the patient. Additionally, wide excision takes quite a bit more time than spot-burning surgery. Unfortunately, insurance companies do not pay for long *or* expert surgeries instead of a quick coagulation surgery, which is much cheaper.

Simply put, for a surgeon to change from spot coagulation burning surgery to excision surgery, they have to take more time, do more complex and riskier surgery for which they have been adequately trained, get paid less, and expose themselves to a higher risk of getting sued.

Besides the skill of surgery, what else can surgeons who specialize in endometriosis offer patients?

While it sounds simple, we can offer an appropriate diagnosis. Sadly, the majority of diagnostic laparoscopies are inadequate, with routine under-diagnosis and even misdiagnosis of endometriosis. Women seeking solutions to their pain may be told they don't have endometriosis because the doctor searching for it hasn't been educated about the many appearances of endo. Endometriosis can be black, orange, red, white, clear vesicles, opacifications, and peritoneal defects or pockets, and some endometriosis is identified indirectly via other findings.

During a laparoscopy, a surgeon creates small incisions to insert a laparoscope to look inside at the abdominal organs. You might think that looking for endometriosis through a laparoscope is similar to opening a door to look inside a room to see what's on the wall. But a better analogy is waking up in the morning with the bedsheets a mess, knowing there is a quarter somewhere in the bed, sheets, or pillowcase. It would be easy to miss if one is not systematic and thorough in looking through everything carefully. So the accuracy of diagnosis is highly dependent on the technique of the surgeon performing the diagnostic portion of the laparoscopy.

What should a patient do if they suspect endo and want a diagnosis, but can't afford or find a specialist near them?

My advice to any woman undergoing diagnostic laparoscopy for endometriosis and pelvic pain is to find a physician who will provide adequate photo (or video) documentation. With modern technology available in nearly all surgery rooms, this shouldn't be a challenge to find. Without pictures, the only information available is the surgeon's *opinion* of what they did, what they observed, and the diagnosis they made—which may or may not correlate with the reality of what was present. If they don't know the wide variety of ways endo can present, they may misdiagnose you. With photos, you can send the images to other specialists who may be able to better pinpoint problems.

Because the cost and invasive nature of the surgery required to obtain visualization of the pelvic cavity is substantial, if we could get every surgeon to take this one simple step—photo documentation—treatment of women with endometriosis and pelvic pain would take a huge step forward.

If you could offer advice to someone diagnosed with endo, what would you share?

Just how different a "conventional approach" to endometriosis is from what I would call an "optimal approach." The patients following a conventional approach are the ones that come to me having managed their endo in a typical fashion: chronic pharmaceutical management of a disease state, along with multiple rounds of poorly done surgeries as needed. Exhaustive use of pharmaceuticals to suppress symptoms may even result in a progressive degradation of health into a chronic condition that becomes much more difficult to treat than the endometriosis alone. Sadly, most of these types of patients have been in the medical system for years with multiple failed treatments, including multiple failed surgeries (an average of 3.4 previous surgeries to be precise) before I see them as a patient. On average, they have been in pain for 11 years.

Following wide excision surgery, this group of women has an average improvement in pain of 75 percent, and the re-operation rate is 17 percent for recurring symptoms. This is not ideal. Because of the track they were on, a number of these women weren't able to get the complete relief they deserved.

The second group of patients has a different profile. I'd consider these patients to be following an optimal approach. They have, for the most part, declined traditional medical treatment, including oral contraceptive pills and generic surgeries, and instead opted to use a more holistic approach as an initial mode of treatment to restore health (diet, lifestyle, integrative care, etc.). After the passing of enough time warranted their holistic efforts weren't effective enough to address their pain, they elected to have wide excision surgery as their *first* surgery. Not only are their outcomes better with an 80 percent overall improvement in pain, but the re-operation rate is only about 3 percent (versus 17 percent in the previous group).

These clinical observations suggest part of the difficulty in the current treatment paradigm is that the severity and gravity of the situation facing women with endometriosis is not treated quickly enough. Some are told to not even seek a true diagnosis since there's little that can be done—something far from the truth. Others are told the only treatment options are surgeries that, as you just learned, are far from ideal, as well as pharmaceuticals to address symptoms (rather than seeking root causes). This process of ignoring the gravity of endometriosis turns a situation that can be addressed into a much worse chronic condition that can be orders of magnitude more difficult to treat.

You mentioned the ideal approach starts with a holistic approach to endo with a properly done surgery considered after that. In your opinion, what is the time frame someone should wait?

It depends on a couple of factors, including how much a woman's quality of life is impacted. When treating patients, in general, we try to start with non-invasive natural treatments aimed at correcting underlying health issues. I believe it is important to work with a good integrative or functional medicine doctor. If over 6 to 12 months, good progress is made and a woman's quality of life is significantly improved, it's possible there may be no need for surgery.

However, if symptoms linger or progress is not made with an integrative approach, then diagnosis and removal of the endometriosis with wide excision should absolutely be considered. I cannot tell you how often I see a patient the day after surgery who feels better than she did the day before surgery. How often I am told the pain of surgery is less than one of their typical menstrual periods. So a properly done surgery is an absolutely essential step for those who need it. It's also important to note that undergoing surgery does not mean stopping integrative treatment; it means adding "removal of disease" to the overall treatment approach.

Based on your observations, how often does wide excision surgery lead to a complete cessation of endo symptoms?

Wide excision as the first step in surgical removal has different ranges in improvement. To use my own clinical observations again, 59 percent of my patients in this "ideal" group have demonstrated *near to complete cessation of pain*. Yet, the average improvement overall was 80 percent, which means a certain amount of patients will need further, integrative care. There are patients who are very healthy overall and, once the endometriotic implants are surgically removed, have almost complete return to good health. At the other end of the spectrum are those patients who have almost complete collapse of their health, often with multiple sensitivities, inflammation, and immune dysfunction.

Again, while surgery removes disease, it does not give vibrant health, so if your body also needs support in the form of nutrition, movement, pelvic floor physical therapy, stress reduction, etc., you may need to address these facets in order to regain the quality of life you desire and deserve. It is my core belief that a holistic approach to health followed in a timely manner with the addition of, when necessary, effective wide excision surgery holds the best hope of restoring health to those with endometriosis.

Can you leave us with some endo inspiration?

Thanks to the wide presence of the endometriosis community of surgeons, researchers, nonprofits, and activists, endo patients are understanding more and more about the disease, how to treat it, and why the type of surgery matters. We are now in the next phase of the unfolding conversation of endo, answering the question of what is really needed to successfully treat the *entirety* of endometriosis. This is exciting because it's apparent that not all women achieve the desired results by wide excision surgery alone as endo can be varied and complex. The missing piece of the puzzle is integrative care, an approach needed to not just remove endometriosis but also to increase the quality of life for those with significant underlying health issues.

The needed changes in the approach to both diagnosis and treatment of endometriosis, I believe, will come about through education and a collective demand from women with endometriosis refusing substandard care. Listen to your bodies. You may not be physicians, but you live with your body and you know what you are feeling. Trust your bodies. Trust that what you are feeling is valid. Demand quality care. The comprehensive information in this book is a great resource for women. There is hope!

AUTHOR'S NOTE ON FINDING A SURGEON

One of the biggest challenges we face in the endometriosis community is finding a skilled surgeon we can afford. As you just learned, there is a big gap between a conventional OB-GYN surgery and one by an expert surgeon who knows how to excise endometriosis! But because insurance companies are terribly behind in what they deem an acceptable surgery, many prominent endometriosis specialists are forced out of network (meaning you'll have to pay out of pocket) in order for their practice to survive. Until there is a national (or international) database differentiating the two, you will unfortunately need to be your own best advocate for finding the care you need and can afford.

Still, there has been lots of movement in the right direction since I started looking at surgery over a decade ago. At that time it was nearly impossible to find endo specialty surgeons covered fully, or even partially, by insurance, so an excision surgery with a specialist was never an option for me. Luckily, doctors have gained significant traction since then, and in researching this book I found more hope when it comes to access to surgery (more than I thought I'd find, actually). Many more doctors are accepting insurance, with some even going to bat *for you* when speaking to your insurance companies and employers. If I ever do need a professional excision surgery in the future, I have renewed hope I'll be able to afford one, so you should have hope, too.

If you're ready to move forward with excision surgery, you will need to do some sleuthing to develop a list of surgeons near you that hopefully are covered by your insurance. Here are some basic strategies you can consider:

1. First, call your insurance company if you have one. Don't guess what they may cover; it is important to call and ask. Also, ask which geographic regions are covered in their network. Is it the city? The state? A region? They should be able to help you generate a list of options far beyond your own OB-GYN. I like to remind my clients that insurance companies technically work for you (you're buying their services), so make sure you squeeze everything out of that service that you can.

2. One of the best ways to uncover the best (and worst) surgeons in your area is by joining a local endometriosis support group. These can be in-person, but more often they're online in forums such as Facebook. Local members can offer beneficial feedback and guidance based on their own experiences with local doctors and knowing which ones take insurance. A colleague of mine found an incredible in-network surgeon in San Diego this way, so there can be immense value in these conversations.

3. icarebetter.com is a wonderful website dedicated to helping you locate an endometriosis specialist. Surgeons are vetted through an application process for which they must submit (among other criteria) three video recordings of surgeries performed as proof of skill. Over half of the listed doctors accept insurance and the ones who don't will assist you in obtaining reimbursements from insurance and/or employers.

4. Once you have a list of potential surgeons, it's important to call them, set up a consultation to meet (virtually or in-person), and ask questions about their services, philosophy, and how they'd approach your case. For a list of beneficial questions to ask, I recommend you check out the endo education site www.nancysnookendo.com/find-a-doctor. Here you'll find a list of suggested questions

about everything from surgery type and tools used to reputation to office location—important details you may not think to ask about.

5. For some of us, interviewing doctors may seem really, really hard. In our society, doctors are often considered elite folk, making it challenging for those of us who are shy or lack confidence to ask questions. If this is you, don't be deterred. Interviewing is *important* and you'll need to muster some strength in order to ensure the best care. I recommend rehearsing before your appointment or, if you know you'll be nervous, bring a confident support person to help. Whether you're shy or not, if a doctor only makes you feel worse (belittled or unheard), that is not the doctor for you. You want a doctor to listen to you as much as you want to listen to him or her.

6. If you can afford the best, make sure they're the best for *you*: just because a surgeon is famous for removing endo doesn't mean she/he will be the best heroine/hero for your story. Interview them just as thoroughly as you would any other surgeon to make sure their philosophy and care methods are in line with your own beliefs and goals.

Chapter 18:

Ten Endo Rules to Live By

Endometriosis is fascinatingly (and frustratingly) complex—a multifactorial, heterogeneous disease, teeming with chronic inflammation and immune system dysfunction. However, a new understanding of the disease—in all its messy glory—is bringing researchers and providers alike to an exciting new frontier. As we begin to better understand endo's truly complex web, we are better able to successfully manage the disease at its roots, rather than just looking at symptoms. By understanding endo as a full-body disease, we can start to tip the scales of health and wellness back in our favor.

Still, *because* of the complexities of endo, it's just important to maintain a healthy perspective when facing a disease with the unfortunate tagline of "there is no cure." Being philosophical in the face of the unknown can help us maintain a problem-solving attitude, appreciate the uniqueness of our case, and better comprehend the many elements that can both contribute to disease *or* help heal. After my own decade of battling endo, years spent working with clients and researching this book, I believe we can all learn to better approach our unique (and sometimes ghastly) situations through ten basic lessons that I hope will be able to help re-center you for the healing journey ahead, starting today:

1. Become the Hero of Your Own Journey

Healing is an action verb, brimming with courage and responsibility. The endo warrior gets her name from finding the strength to face each day, prioritize healing, and act upon it day after day. Work hard to change your perspective from that of someone waiting to be saved to the one that is *actively healing* your own body. Better health, love, deep and meaningful friendships—they are there waiting for you! But just as a horse led to water cannot be made to drink, nor can real changes happen without a willing participant. Don't wait for a hero to save you, rather, become the hero you need.

2. Don't Walk the Path Alone

Even heroes need friends that they count on. Battling a chronic disease can be lonely and depressing. At times it can close the curtains on the friendships and activities we used to enjoy. Fight hard to not let this happen. Leaning into the deep human need for connection and friendship isn't optional on this journey, it's required. Find your strongest voice and explain with clarity to your friends and family how your disease is affecting your life, and tell them exactly what you need from them. Please don't stay quiet, breed resentment, or ghost friends who don't seem to understand. Instead, build partnerships with friends and families to face the journey together.

If you don't find support in your friend circles, reach out to endo-support groups and make new friends! My colleague Jessica Murnane calls these friends *"fri-endos"* because they can directly relate to your experiences. Having other people who understand your experience can be therapy in itself. If you can no longer fill your hours with activities the way you used to, find new hobbies until you are able to heal. Evolve with your disease rather than letting it isolate you.

3. Commit to Nourishing Your Body. Every Day.

This one simple action will kick-start healing. A body steeped in nutrients, movement, joy, and friendship go hand in hand with endo stabilization. Infuse your body with nourishing food, refuel with lost nutrients, remove high levels of circulating blood sugar and insulin, prevent sugar dips that provoke stress hormones, and remove the worst dietary triggers—make these the navigational guideposts of your healing journey. I wish I could express how many thank you notes I have received over the years from clients, blog followers, and book readers who applied the Heal Endo approach and found themselves feeling miraculously better within months, or even weeks.

4. Consult With an Endo Specialist

Sadly, many of us have never been told endometriosis specialists even exist, so we're often treated by people who may know little to nothing about this disease. This may leave us misdiagnosed, not diagnosed at all (at least for many years), or told something such as "back pain isn't related to endo" when we may, in fact, have endo growing in a kidney. Or, told by our fertility doctors that all we need to fork out money for yet another round of IVF when in fact we actually need excision surgery for somewhat symptomless Stage IV endo ravaging the pelvis. So if you're feeling lost, confused, or miserable, I beg of you to consider seeking endo expert help! Even if you think you can't afford surgery, at least seek a consultation. Doing so will put the power back in your hands as you start to unravel the extent of the disease you're facing within your own body.

5. You Must Walk Before You Can Run

If you try to apply everything in this book all at once without mastering the basics, you may contract a sincere case of "healing burnout" three months from now. This is why I repeat that healing from endo is not a crash diet, it's a lifestyle change. And, in order to successfully transition to your new lifestyle, you will need to take the time to master each new skill or integrate new activities into your routine before piling on more.

This is especially true if all of this information is incredibly new to you. Looking at so many new lifestyle swaps can be intimidating, and you may feel "change paralysis" (when there's so much to change, you simply change nothing). Please, don't feel overwhelmed.

Instead of paralysis, start somewhere—literally anywhere—and master one new skill (like learning how to cook, for example) or check off something on your to-do list (such as swapping out chemical-laden cleaning products). Once that skill is mastered (or to-do checked off), you won't even think about it. It will become second nature. Next, move on to another skill while maintaining the ones you previously mastered. In this way, you will master and integrate the many healing skills and tasks that will, over time, have a compounding effect on improving your health.

Simple Steps

Infuse

- Sleep 8 hours a night, minimum.
- Drink 8-10 cups water/day, away from meals to help digest.
- Eat more veggies.
- Eat veggies in the color of the rainbow.
- Be happy when you eat.
- Hang out with friends in real time (texting doesn't count). Make this a real priority.
- Walk 3-5 miles a day.
- Do hypopressive breathing 10 min/day.
- Work on your booty strength and length.
- Stretch, do gentle yoga, or foam roll.
- Eat enough quality protein at every meal.
- Memorize 5 jokes and tell them.
- Turn 5 stressors into problems in need of solving. Now solve them.

- Walk barefoot on grass.
- Be outside without sunscreen just until your skin turns a tad pink.
- Add digestive aids to meals.
- Breathe through your nose when you exercise (and all the time) instead of through the mouth.
- Eat three meals per day, at consistent times, without snacking in between.
- Don't let small things eat you up.
- Consider supplementing with high-quality omega 3's, zinc, magnesium, and Vitamins C and E.
- Find a new hobby that truly lights you up.
- Community! Helping others in need will always help you feel better about your own trajectory.

Remove

- Drink less alcohol.
- Eat WAY less sugar.
- Try going gluten free.
- Try going dairy free.
- Say goodbye to most processed, refined foods.
- Get off social media.
- Limit all screen time.
- Toss vegetable oils.
- Don't heat food in plastic.
- Don't store food in plastic.
- Filter your tap water.
- Don't drink out of plastic water bottles.
- Buy chemical free:
  - Haircare
  - Makeup
  - Body care products
  - Cleaning products
  - Cooking pans and kitchenware

GABY'S STORY

After coming off the contraceptive pill, my periods had been getting worse to the point that I couldn't get off the bathroom floor, or leave bed for those first days. I had a number of scans done and doctors said it was very likely I had endometriosis. Eventually, I was scheduled for surgery. Apparently, it was worse than expected and my surgeon described it as "horrific." A few months post-op I still had pain, bowel issues, and irregular periods, so I felt really frustrated. They did more blood tests and another scan, and I had grown more cysts. I was gutted. I was also told at that point that I had "no chance whatsoever of conceiving" (I have this in writing!).

I decided that couldn't be it, so I researched more and stumbled across the Heal Endo approach and spent my evenings devouring all the amazing information written just for people like me! I changed my diet, incorporated more wild fish, grass-fed meat, and started making kimchi, kefir, and bone broth which I drank daily! I had already cut alcohol and caffeine. I piled on the vegetables and ate liver weekly. I even experimented with reintroducing raw dairy. I started acupuncture, which helped enormously with the pain, and my acupuncturist told me I was like a scrunched-up ball of stress! She told me we needed to work on my stress and my sleep. So we did! I completely reprioritized getting a decent night's sleep, I took Epsom salt baths 3 times a week and I started doing yoga regularly and generally being more conscious of my daily movement. I also went to an Arvigo massage therapist who taught me a glorious massage for the abdomen—great for pain, de-stressing, and also just becoming more familiar with my body. So let's just say I threw everything at it!

I previously was always looking for that single thing that would help, but after months of tweaking my diet and lifestyle I realized that there is no one thing—it's a whole lifestyle that you need to commit to. And once you know what you are doing, scaffolding skills become second nature, it's not hard work. And then…it starts working! It took a while, but a year post-surgery my pain became manageable, no pain killers required(!!) and my energy levels improved significantly. Then, the unimaginable happened, 2 years post-op, I fell pregnant! A complete surprise especially given the previous prognosis of my consultant. I have continued with the same diet and lifestyle—my pregnancy was a breeze, my periods have returned (which I was terrified of) but incredibly, I have zero pain now! Long may it last! -Gaby, UK

6. Cultivate Joy, Release Instant Gratification

If we are honest, we would admit that most of us are addicted to things that give us an immediate sense of gratification (like scrolling our cell phones, social media, caffeine, alcohol—even productivity can be addictive), yet they come with stress. However, life also presents things that make us feel true joy and a long-lasting feeling of contentment. Unfortunately, our society prizes the former, making us believe that a fast-paced, efficient, and insanely productive life is the best reality in which to live. Yet, what really makes us feel lasting joy is quite different, and it involves slowing down, unplugging, and reconnecting with the people and activities that we love. For me this is gardening, hanging out with my besties, walking in the forest behind my house, and playing at the beach with my family, surfboards, and snacks. For you, it may be having coffee with friends, knitting, reading, rock climbing, baking, or making terrariums. So ask yourself, "what am I doing too much of that gives me fleeting pleasure but long-term stress? And what could I replace those activities with that would truly bring me joy?" Then make a commitment to eliminate the joy-drainers and replace them with activities that send your spirits soaring.

7. Ask for Directions When You're Lost

You may need professional help beyond your endo get you on a path to true healing. I myself spent many years battling my poor health by self-diagnosing and self-treating. I was lost, and I spent a lot of time staying that way. I know I'm not alone in this since many of my clients come to my doorstep feeling depleted. They had followed the advice of Dr. Google, social media stars, blogs, books, and every other imaginable way to "heal," many of which were completely contradictory. Not surprisingly, they didn't feel better. Rather, they felt like they had done everything possible, and none of it was working.

An objective professional can help you stop doing this "healing hustle," identify and take control of your symptoms and help you get real *traction*. As a nutritional professional now myself, I'm reminded of this every time I sit down with a new client suffering under a mountain of symptoms. I often immediately identify one or two problematic factors that have been long overlooked (even when they think they have tried it all already) and can start my client's healing process in earnest.

If you're confused about where to start, I recommend you hone in on your worst symptoms and start there. For example, if your tummy issues seem unbearable, seek out a microbiome specialist to address gut infections once and for all; or if you're vastly confused about food triggers (or simply how to eat better) find a nutritionist to help; or if symptoms aren't budging *please* find an endometriosis excision expert to remove that endo once and for all. As in the previous recommendation, just start with one symptom and move forward from there.

8. Nature Isn't Optional

It's easy to forget that we humans are actually animals. Yes, we're complex, but simply having advanced technology has not replaced our biological needs: sunlight, fresh air, outdoor time, walking barefoot, natural movement, feeling the strong tide of circadian rhythms, and a deep connection to other living things. It's why we, quite literally, feel depressed working in cubicles, being isolated, working long hours, and living in concrete jungles.

Nature heals. It reduces our blood pressure, decreases our stress, and it helps us feel more calm and more centered.[283] This is potently visible on Kaua`i, the island where I live. Because on Kaua`i there is, almost literally, nothing to do *except* be ensconced in nature. There are no cities, few restaurants and bars, and more chickens than residents. After several days of being suddenly forced to live in this zone that mimics the ancestral rhythms of nature, visitors start to feel not just relaxed, but content, and safe. I recently saw one couple point to the sky and note "wow, I didn't know you could see the moon during the day." They had gone their whole lives without feeling safe enough to look up to notice the moon, but finally, with a little extra nature time, they could.

The beauty and awe of nature are within our reach to enjoy, but you don't have to be on Kaua`i to enjoy it! Make your great escape in your own hometown: turn away from technology and toward people, find outdoor adventures, watch your neighborhood wildlife, build a healthy and strong circadian rhythm, and perhaps even make it a game to find the moon during the day.

9. Find the Silver Lining

Endometriosis stole my life, or at least a portion of it. For nearly a decade I suffered under the weight of pain, infertility, chronic fatigue, joint issues, hormonal imbalance, chronic stress, and anxiety. And still, even after all of that, I've learned to *thank* my endometriosis. Endo taught me about resilience, and how to stand in the face of terrible adversity without crumbling. It taught me the importance of learning brand-new skills and new points of view. It taught me how to create a new life of abundance; a life better connected to the earth through my gardens and food choices, to my family through my children, and to my new slower pace of life that allows me to enjoy my days rather than rush through them as "productively" as possible. While endometriosis may have taken away the life I had before, I like to think the silver lining is that I was able to create: a new, better way of living.

This may not be your story, not yet or perhaps not ever. It may be that endo took much more than a decade of your life, stole relationships, and the possibility of children. Or, if you're newly diagnosed perhaps your endo story is brand new and yet to be told. Wherever you are, and however this disease has affected you, I challenge you to find the silver lining. I know some folk who became staunch endo advocates, others who went into the health field, found new partners, or changed their lives in some ways for the better thanks (yes, thanks) to endo. So while it can be hard to find a positive spin on something so potentially devastating as endo, changing the *perception* of what we're facing can help buoy the human spirit—and that's an essential ingredient in healing.

HODA'S STORY

Along with the physical symptoms I experienced with endo: sharp, stabbing-like sensations primarily on the R side of my pelvic region and burning sensations that radiated throughout my body, I also felt like a burden on the people I love. I mourned for the life I missed out on because the pain kept me bound to my bed. Being diagnosed at 30 after years of trying to conceive, I remember the despair I felt knowing that we may never be able to start a family. I took the drugs, I had the surgeries, and we tried the fertility treatments but nothing worked.

The temptation to give up led me to find the determination to find another way—I had to address the mental and social impacts of endo alongside the physical. Through the practice of self-inquiry, I listened to my body with discernment to understand its unmet needs. I practiced acknowledging, accepting, and nurturing myself through journaling, monthly FaceTime dates with my dear "soul" friends and family, walking with my daughter hand-in-hand, and moving my body on my yoga mat, just to name a few. I eradicated a SIBO infection. Ultimately, I do my best to take responsibility (my ability to respond) for how I live, for what I put in and on my body, my emotional stability, my psychological growth, and the quality of my relationships.

In my healing journey, endo went from something I tried to get rid of to becoming my greatest teacher. Five years in remission, I feel a deep sense of gratitude toward endo for guiding me to exactly what I needed to grow and heal from. That was my silver lining. -Hoda, Spain

10. Take Care of Each Other

Most of all, please remember that you are not making your healing journey in your own isolated bubble. While your journey to health will be uniquely your own, millions of others are also suffering the effects of endo. They share your dreams, your frustrations, and your pain. Share with them your kindness, your compassion, and your understanding. By helping them, you also help yourself get stronger. Taking care of each other helps us all shoulder a lighter burden and live in a kinder world.

One important thing we can do for each other is to keep advocating for change. Endo research is vastly underfunded; many doctors who are treating us are not educated about *exactly* what they're treating, insurance companies often won't pay for more than sub-par surgeries, and patients may have to know more than their professional care team in order to get the best treatment. The injustice is staggering. But our voices, raised together, can support more medical training about endometriosis, lobby insurance companies to pay for excision surgeries, and support holistic healing recommendations as a complementary line of defense.

Each of us will be an Endo Warrior in our own way, with our own style. It is comforting to know that we face our healing journey together and that we will take care of ourselves and each other.

THANKS FOR READING

Understanding endo as a *process happening within* gives us back control in many ways. When inflammation is the root of the problem, one that drives the disease and the immune dysfunction behind it, we can make some incredible inroads to healing by zapping the triggers. Stop the inflammation in its tracks, and you may be able to slow or stop (or perhaps even reverse) the process of *endo-ing*.

The big question you may have is where to begin—and there's no one-size-fits-all approach to healing. Each reader has her own endo, her own unique circumstances, and her own needs to heal. Not to mention that healing from endometriosis is no quick 30-day plan. It's a long-term lifestyle shift, which you would train for slowly and steadily, incrementally changing your habits and inputs to calm and soothe a body on the fritz. Take your time, re-read this book as needed, and reach out to others for guidance.

And to you, dear reader living with endo: you are a *warrior*. No doubt, if you are reading this book, you have already been through more than most people will ever be able to fathom. Facing this disease head-on takes gumption: standing up to providers and demanding to be heard. Getting through days of pain that you just can't describe until you've lived it, again and again. Learning to *survive* in a world that simply does not understand what you're going through.

As you move forward in overcoming your endo, I hope that you will begin to look at it through a new lens, one that allows you to think about healing as *possible*. Beyond that, though, I hope you can begin to look upon your body with kindness. Give yourself grace as you navigate this wild ride. You are strong, and I am honored to be a part of your endo journey.

Thank you for taking the time to read this book. If you've found it helpful, please leave a review on Amazon (it helps more than you know!), share it with a friend or provider whom you think would benefit from giving it a read, and ask your local library to carry it so that others can read it for free, and be sure to check out the resources I've included in the pages that follow.

Wishing you love, laughter, and good health as you take these next steps. Remember that I'm right here with you, cheering you on. You can find me at www.healendo.com.

FURTHER READING

Find the Author

- Katie Edmonds: www.healendo.com. Instagram @heal.endo, Facebook @Healing.endo

Endometriosis Surgery, Information, Symptoms, and Stories

- *Stop Endometriosis and Pelvic Pain: What Every Woman and Her Doctor Need to Know.* By Dr. Andrew Cook
- *Ask Me About My Uterus: A Quest to Make Doctors Believe in Women's Pain.* By Abby Norman
- *Beating Endo: How to Reclaim Your Life from Endometriosis.* By Dr. Iris Orbuch and Amy Stein, DPT
- *The Doctor Will See You Now: Recognizing and Treating Endometriosis.* By Dr. Tamir Seckin
- *Know Your Endo.* By Jessica Murnane.
- *Endofound.org.* Website of the Endometriosis Foundation of America
- *TheEndo.co.* A nonprofit dedicated to raising awareness, promoting reliable education, and increasing research funding for endometriosis
- *Endowhat.com.* A documentary film about the importance of a properly done surgery
- *Nancysnookendo.com.* An online, patient-centered, endometriosis learning library. Here you will find information about endometriosis and related conditions so that you may engage in truly informed, shared decision making with your health care team.
- *icarebetter.com* is a wonderful website dedicated to helping you locate an endometriosis specialist.

Finding Functional Doctors and Integrative Care

- Association of Naturopathic Physicians: https://naturopathic.org
- Institute for Functional Medicine: www.ifm.org/find-a-practitioner/
- Integrative Women's Health Institute: integrativewomenshealthinstitute.com/provider-directory/
- National Licensed Acupuncturist Directory: https://www.nccaom.org/find-a-practitioner-directory/
- Paleo Physicians Network: www.paleophysiciansnetwork.com

Epigenetics

- *Deep Nutrition: Why Your Genes Need Traditional Food.* By Catherine Shannahan, MD
- *Epigenetics: How the Environment Shapes Our Genes.* By Richard Francis
- *The Epigenetics Revolution: How Modern Biology Is Rewriting Our Understanding of Genetics, Disease, and Inheritance.* By Nessa Carrey

Immune System + Gut Health

- *The Human Superorganism: How the Microbiome Is Revolutionizing the Pursuit of a Healthy Life.* By Rodney Dietert, PhD
- The Paleo Approach: Reverse Autoimmune Disease and Heal Your Body. By Sarah Ballantyne, PhD
- *The Wahls Protocol.* By Terry Wahls, MD
- *An Elegant Defense: The Extraordinary New Science of the Immune System: A Tale in Four Lives.* By Matt Richtel

Nutrition Information, Recipes, and Learning to Cook

- Heal Endo: www.healendo.com
- *The 4-Week Endometriosis Diet Plan: 75 Recipes to Relieve Symptoms and Regain Control of Your Life.* By Katie Edmonds
- *Healthy Gut, Flat Stomach: The Fast and Easy Low FODMAP Diet Plan.* By Danielle Capalino, MSPH, RD
- *Real Food for Pregnancy.* By Lily Nichols, RDN
- *The Art of Fermentation.* By Sandor Katz
- *Wild Fermentation.* By Sandor Katz
- *The Nutrient-Dense Kitchen: 125 Autoimmune Paleo Recipes for Deep Healing and Vibrant Health.* By Mickey Trescott, NTP
- *Salt, Fat, Acid, Heat.* By Samin Nosrat
- *Sababa: Fresh, Sunny Flavors from My Israeli Kitchen: A Cookbook.* By Adeena Sussman

Breathing + Core Function

- *Breathe.* By James Nestor
- *The Oxygen Advantage.* By Patrick Mckeown
- *Corerecoverypt.com.* Website of Dr. Angie Mueller

Stress + Mental Health

- *How to Do Nothing: Resisting the Attention Economy.* By Jenny Odell
- *Do Less.* By Kate Northrup
- *The Joy of Missing Out: Live More by Doing Less.* By Tanya Dalton
- *7cups.com.* A site dedicated to mental health, with caring listeners who are always there for emotional support
- *Psychcentral.com.* A leading mental health website for nearly 30 years, Psyche Central addresses everything from addictions to anxiety mental health disorders, and other mental health topics.

Hormones and Fertility

- *Beyond the Pill.* By Dr. Jolene Brighten
- *Taking Charge of Your Fertility: The Definitive Guide to Natural Birth Control, Pregnancy Achievement, and Reproductive Health.* By Toni Weschler
- *The Fifth Vital Sign: Master Your Cycles & Optimize Your Fertility.* By Lisa Hendrickson-Jack
- *The Period Repair Manual: Natural Treatment for Better Hormones and Better Periods.* By Dr. Lara Briden
- *Fix Your Period.* By Nicole Jardim

Chemicals and Toxins

- *Count Down: How Our Modern World Is Threatening Sperm Counts, Altering Male and Female Reproductive Development, and Imperiling the Future of the Human Race.* By Shanna H. Swan, PhD
- *Slow Death by Rubber Duck: The Secret Danger of Everyday Things.* By Rick Smith

Racial Disparities + Reproductive Justice

- *Endoblack.org.* A stellar organization dedicated to advocating for African American women and women of color affected by endometriosis.
- *EndoFound:* https://www.endofound.org/the-endometriosis-resource-portal-for-people-of-color
- *SisterSong.net.* An organization working to improve policies and systems that impact the reproductive lives of marginalized communities

APPENDIX 1:

Alterations of an Endo-like Cell

There are a wide variety of epigenetic changes an endo-like cell is known for. These changes may be very apparent in some varieties, and less apparent in others (remembering there are many different types of endo). However, here are a few that are often associated with an endo-like cell:

- **Estrogen sensitivity.** Some endo-like cells may have up to 140 times more estrogen (ER*b*) receptors than a normal endometrial cell![284] Since estrogen is a hormone that signals growth, even normal amounts of estrogen nearby can signal rapidly for these cells to grow, grow, grow.
- **Progesterone resistance.** Some endo-like cells have been observed to have nearly *undetectable* levels of progesterone receptors.[285] This is known as progesterone resistance, and a hallmark of many types of endo.[286] Progesterone is the hormone that balances the growth signaled by estrogen, helping to calm growth and soothe inflammation. Without it, there is double trouble in the cell: lots of growth through estrogen, and barely any cooling from progesterone.
- **Aggressive behavior.** Endo-like cells develop enhanced migratory capabilities, increased invasiveness into small nooks and crannies, become much more invasive, and can rapidly produce new cells.[287]
- **Cell abnormalities that lead to infertility.** The Homeobox A10 gene (HOXA10) aids endometrial growth, differentiation, and implantation during pregnancy. Abnormalities caused by this gene are an important aspect of us endo to consider for sufferers dealing with infertility.[288]
- **Inability to take up enough vitamin A (retinoids).**[289] Retinoids are required for proper cell turnover. Without them, endo-like cells are unable to avoid normal cell death (meaning they stick around even when you *really* want them gone).[290]

APPENDIX 2:

Immune Dysfunction of Endo

Part 1: Establishing Your Endo Lesion

One of the biggest culprits in this chronic inflammatory endo environment that has been identified to date is the *macrophage*. Macrophage cells are a versatile type of immune cell responsible for identifying and eliminating (or "gobbling up" like Pac-Man) problematic bacteria and other pathogenic organisms within the body. In one of their many roles, when confronted with a wound site, your little Pac-Man cells will flood the scene, eating up problematic infection-causing germs and then secreting potent growth factors such as vascular endothelial growth factor, or VEGF. VEGF fosters *neo-angiogenesis,* a process that helps grow new blood supply to areas that need it, thereby helping damaged tissue heal. It's a pretty cool process and one that we no doubt need to survive. With endo, however, macrophage cells seem to be a key troublemaker.

When it comes to the wayward endometriosis cells, macrophages (and VEGF) are directly implicated in the "rooting down" of endometriosis lesions, i.e., the establishment of the blood supply, nutrients, and oxygen they need to *thrive.*[291] In fact, macrophages are so implicated in the development of endometriosis lesions that studies have found that by removing macrophages from the scene, endo-like cells were able to adhere and implant to tissue, but never developed into full-blown endo lesions; in other cases, when macrophages were removed from an endo-environment, lesions stopped growing altogether.[292] Caught red-handed.

Although macrophage cells are highly involved in the creation and worsening of endometriosis lesions, they don't act alone. Really, it seems to take an immune village to establish endometriosis, and research shows us there are *many* more immune cells associated with endo pathogenesis, including IL-4, IL-8 IL-10, IL-13, IL-25, IL-33, IL-37, IL-1RaA, TSLP insulin-like growth factor, hepatocyte growth factor, epidermal growth factor, NF-κB, platelet-derived growth factor, and others.[293] That's a lot of immune cells *directly* implicated with the establishment of endo in your body. Here are details on a few other immune factors implicated in the establishment of endo:

Platelets: Platelets are one of the immune system's first lines of defense. When damage is observed by the immune system's "scouts," platelets help slow bleeding and fight infection. Unfortunately, platelets can also induce excess hypoxia, which can provoke endo to create even more VEGF to help them root down. These platelets also activate the production of an incredible amount of estrogen once endometriosis lesions are established.[294]

Neutrophils: Neutrophils are a subset of white blood cells in charge of finding and eradicating microbial infections with short-lived bouts of acute inflammation. Interestingly, neutrophils have been found to be elevated in both the systemic circulation and peritoneal fluid of those with endometriosis. While they are helpful in addressing an acute infection (which is why they may be called to the peritoneal fluid in the first place, during hypoxia), they appear to contribute to endometriosis progression in the context of chronic inflammation. They're even implicated in the early establishment of blood supply to lesions through even more VEGF release.[295]

Tumor necrosis factor (TNF-α): This pro-inflammatory cytokine is secreted mainly by macrophages, which you now know you probably have in abundance if you have endometriosis. TNF-α has been shown to exert inflammatory and angiogenic effects and to foster the invasion and spread of endometriosis lesions by helping to increase the adhesion of endo cells onto collagen and other surface cells. TNF-α also promotes the production of even more pro-inflammatory cytokines (IL-1β, IL-6, and more TNF-α).[296]

IL-1β and IL-6: Elevated concentrations of these interleukins have been found in the peritoneal fluid of women with endometriosis as well as, interestingly, in the blood.[297] Normally functioning IL-6 should inhibit endometrial growth, but in the case of endo, it may do the opposite.[298] If you're looking to place blame for your pain, you may want to start with IL-1β. Although we know that epigenetic changes may increase COX-2 expression (the enzyme that leads to increased levels of inflammatory and painful prostaglandins) in endometriosis, it doesn't seem to be too problematic until you add IL-1β, which increases COX-2 tenfold![299] With no IL-1β saturating your pelvis, you could have 1/10th the amount of pain.

TGF-β1: An anti-inflammatory cytokine secreted by macrophages, platelets, and even certain endometriosis cells. While anti-inflammatory sounds like a good thing, TGF-β1 is associated with helping your endometriosis adhere more tightly to new surfaces, while also significantly increasing its ability to migrate and establish in new and faraway places. It's also associated with increased endo cell survival, attachment, invasion, and proliferation during lesion development. Furthermore, TGF-β1 plays a starring role in scar tissue and adhesion formation as the principal pro-fibrotic cytokine in charge of normal wound healing or, when provoked, adhesion formation. In the story of chronic endo inflammation, it seems to err on the side of adhesions.[300]

Part 2: The Janitor Asleep on the Job

Natural killer (NK) cells are specific types of white blood cells that appear to be both decreased *and* dysfunctional within the peritoneal fluid of the endo sufferer. NK cells have multiple roles, including killing potential tumor cells and pathogen-infected cells. They also play an important role in tissue remodeling within the uterus and are key to a healthy pregnancy. Yet, when NK cells are confronted with endometriosis, they respond with diminished cytotoxic (i.e., tumor-killing or endo-killing) capabilities.[301] Without cytotoxic strength, NK cells lose some of their immunosurveillance, potentially allowing endo cells that should be eradicated to survive in the peritoneal cavity.

Contrary to NK cells, your macrophage (Pac-Man) cells are very *active* within the peritoneal fluid when it comes to endo. While macrophage cells establish blood supply to endometriosis cells in the ReTIAR environment, we see them misbehaving in another way: through dysregulated phagocytosis.[302] *Phagocytosis* is the process in which immune cells like macrophages eat and dispose of dead tissue, red blood cells, and cellular debris. Phagocytosis activity is what we want *a lot* of in endometriosis, as these little helpers essentially chow down on the extra blood, damaged tissue, and endo cells within the peritoneal cavity. Instead, what we often see is a poor phagocytosis capability in the endo body. This may be partly due to an excess of inflammatory prostaglandins (PGE2) in the endo pelvic cavity that suppress the macrophages' ability to chow.[303] It may also be due to dysfunctional immune activity leading to a defective scavenger function, which allows the endo lesions to get away unscathed.[304] In addition, remember that the cells that make up endometriosis may have some built-in epigenetic qualities that make them exceedingly good at resisting cell death.

Part 3: A Systemically Dysfunctional Immune System

The numerous immune components we see misbehaving in certain ways include:

- Macrophages should be destroyed after completing their function, but in those with endo they appear to continue to circulate.[305]
- Macrophages also show reduced phagocytic (Pac-Man) ability.[306]
- IL-6 should prevent and stop the growth of endometrial cells, but that function seems to be lost in endometriosis.[307]
- Inflammatory cytokines IL-1β and IL-6 are both abnormally elevated in the peritoneal fluid *and* blood levels of women with endometriosis.[308]
- IL-13 is an anti-inflammatory cytokine that is shown to be abnormally *reduced* in the endo body. Since it regulates macrophage activation (which there is lots of in endo), a reduction in its levels may contribute to an increased amount of macrophage activity in your pelvis and thus disease progression.[309]

- Levels of body-wide circulating neutrophils (a white blood cell) are elevated in both the systemic circulation and peritoneal fluid of women with endometriosis, and their behavior is dysregulated as well.[310]
- In a healthy body's processes, anti-inflammatory cytokines limit the damage produced by inflammatory reactions. In the case of endo, many of these anti-inflammatory cytokines appear to have either insufficient control over inflammation or to overcompensate in ways that constrain the immune response.[311]

Established endo lesions may even contribute to systemic immune dysfunction in certain ways. For example, some women with endometriosis have been found to have increased levels of immature Natural Killer (NK) cells circulating in the blood (in addition to the peritoneal fluid)—a significant point, as NK cells are required to be in balance for a healthy pregnancy (and thus are associated with infertility when systemic levels are out of balance). In one study, when endometriosis lesions were removed surgically, there was a simultaneous decrease in these immature NK cells in the blood, which suggests that endometriosis lesions may be partly responsible for disrupting the proper development of NK cells to begin with. This may also explain why some of the NK cells had insufficient clean-up function in endo, as well as why removing lesions can help restore fertility.[312]

A Note About Adolescent Endo—The Concern of an Immature Immune System

While we know four immune components that lead to the development and progression of endo, there may be a fifth we learn about in the future: the neuroimmune component. Researcher Dr. Dan Martin speculates that teenagers may be hit with the quadruple whammy of normalization of pain, intimidation by physicians, immune dysfunction, *and* an immature immune system.

As our bodies have periods of development, so too does our immune system, one of which lasts through adolescence until ages 18–25, when it undergoes important and distinct changes. It's maturing, just as your body does. Adolescence is also characterized by the organization and activation of sex hormones such as estrogens and androgens, both of which have profound effects on the immune system. This is why puberty becomes a time when changes in immune function (perhaps stimulated by hormones) can increase risk for certain immune-related disorders, such as the autoimmune diseases lupus or multiple sclerosis, or other immune-related issues such as allergies and asthma. And also potentially endometriosis.

Dr. Martin believes an immature immune system confronted with inflammation and hormone stimulation may play a role in endo pathogenesis of adolescents with endometriosis, and may also be one of the reasons why there is an enormous increase in repeat surgeries for adolescents (whopping 80 percent of those under 18 may elect a second surgery within two years) versus those who are older (36 percent of 19–29-year- olds and 12 percent of 30–39-year-olds go for a second surgery within two years). This is another potential contributor to the endometriosis-immune equation, at least for adolescents.[313]

APPENDIX 3:
Dysbiosis Trains Endo-Immune Behavior

Specifically, dysbiosis may directly "train" the macrophage to improperly phagocyte (chew up) debris. One study found that leakage of bacterial products from the intestinal tract not only resulted in increased numbers of macrophages in the peritoneal cavity but the macrophages had a poor reactivity to LPS similar to their poor reactivity to endometriosis tissue.[314]

Another study observed a neutrophil-associated immune response managed by your gut microbiome may directly *induce* inflammation within the pelvic cavity; unnaturally elevated levels of IL-1β, which are found in the peritoneal cavity of women with endo and are responsible for increasing PGE2 levels and supporting angiogenesis, may be specifically attributable to the gut-microbiome feedback loop; the gut microbiome may over-activate pelvic levels of IL-17, which is a highly inflammatory immune component found in significant amounts in those suffering from minimal-to-mild endometriosis that may lead to the survival, growth, and spread of endometriosis.[315]

Last, macrophages in the pelvis may be influenced by gut inflammation and/or leaky gut, changing their behavior so completely that they may not be able to "see" or clean up endometrial debris.[316]

APPENDIX 4:

Core Dysfunction

A deeper dive into rehabilitating core function:

Step 1: Posture Is Everything

Your deep core consists of the diaphragm and pelvic floor muscles on top and bottom, and the transverse abdominus and multifidus on the front and back. These are *postural* muscles, muscles primarily controlled by our autonomic (subconscious) nervous system, rather than by us telling them what to do. This means that the deep core relies on proper core *activation* more than voluntary exercises like crunches, kegels, flexing, or other forms of mentally forced contraction to re-learn how to behave. That's why the best way to start retraining the deep core is through proper breathing and spinal position.

When upright, the spine needs to retain a beautiful elongated "S" shape (not to be confused with an over-exaggerated S shape, with rounded shoulders and arched lower back). Spinal elongation creates the perfect amount of core activation, without being too much (flexing or sucking in), or too little (atrophy or deep relaxation). *It is an absolute necessity* to elevate the organs and recover core function. The goal is to learn to use the deep core the lengthen upwards. To get here, Dr. Angie has some tips:

- To lengthen up, imagine an alien ship is trying to *beam you up*, with your head moving up towards the sky and away from the lower half of your body. You can even gently grab the base of your neck and lightly "pull" your head straight up toward the ceiling, feeling the spine lengthen as your head drifts up. This will naturally turn on your deep core to draw the belly up and in without you mentally forcing it. Notice how different this is from arching your back in a sort of "military" stance (chest out) to mimic good posture. It should feel like a deep internal lengthening ("beam me up, Scotty!") versus a soldier's call to salute.

- You can also place something light like a bean bag on your head and "push" it away from the ground using your new ability to lengthen your spine. See how your core activates when you do this?

Step 2: Activate Your Ribs and Diaphragm

Due to sedentary and stressful lives, most of us breathe shallowly in the upper chest. Over time this inactivates the deeper breathing muscles we actually should be using, such as the *intercostal muscles* of the ribcage and the *diaphragm.* As the lungs fill with air, these muscles should work together to slightly expand the ribcage 360 degrees (the intercostals widen the spaces between the ribs while the diaphragm expands wide like a trampoline). This is how your body is able to keep most of the air in the thoracic cavity, and most of the pressure out of the abdomen.

When our normal breathing musculature becomes weak, our ribs stop moving and our diaphragm can get stuck, so to speak, no longer able to widen. So now, when we try to take a deep breath, the only way we can do so is by forcing the diaphragm to descend deep into the abdomen, often referred to as deep belly breathing.

Deep belly breathing is great—w*hen lying down.* It's done by totally relaxing your abdominal and pelvic floor muscles, placing one hand on your chest (to prevent you from taking shallow chest breaths) and inhaling deeply. As your diaphragm descends down, it pushes on your organs enough that you see your lower belly rise. This relaxes your deep core and pelvic floor while reminding your body how to let your diaphragm descend (many of our diaphragms are so weak they need help like this to wake up). Yet, because the goal of deep belly breathing is deep core relaxation, it should never be done then you're standing or moving against gravity. With the deep core constantly in relaxation mode, your body will never be able to correctly manage increased IAP. So save the deep belly breathing for the end of yoga, before bed, or when you're watching Netflix.

Instead, rehabilitate a weak breathing pattern through strengthening the intercostals and training the diaphragm to expand side to side (rather than just drop down). If your ribs don't budge then abdominal pressure will constantly increase, and the lower belly bulge will persist. To start, try these tips:

- Inhaling through the nose, force the air in through the back (between and below the shoulder blades). Imagine the muscles in between the ribs relaxing and expanding the entire back and sides of the ribcage as if it's growing twice the size. As you do this, you should also be able to visually see the front of your ribcage spread open from side to side as well.
- You can help do this by visualizing your *strong* diaphragm pushing your ribs apart from the inside.
- If your shoulders are tense while you do this, or you shrug your shoulders as you breathe (often a sign of a shallow breathing pattern), take them out of the equation while you wake up the breathing musculature. Lie on your back with your arms relaxing on the bed above your head; now try.
- *Still having trouble?* Most of us breathe shallowly in the upper chest, so if you find yourself doing this place on hand on your chest for awareness, and now try to *force* the inhalation lower in the lungs and into the back. For now it doesn't matter if you notice you're belly breathing while you do this (as long as you're lying down), just stick with this exercise until your ribs can move more easily and your diaphragm can widen from within. It honestly could take a few weeks if your breathing musculature is very compromised. Whereas before your ribs were locked and your breathing pattern confined to your upper chest and lower belly, you're now on your way to having your ribs and diaphragm to do the breathing work for you as they should!

Two Ways to Inhale

Proper Core Activation

No Core Activation

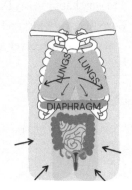

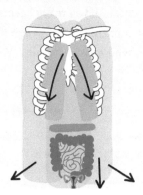

Step 3: Deep Core Activation

Retraining your deep core to correctly manage pressure is what will stop your tummy from "poofing" out when you blow imaginary birthday candles, "loaf" when you do leg lifts or plank, sneeze pee or leak urine when you jump or run, or any other symptoms of increased IAP. Retraining the deep core to fire correctly can also be an amazing help when talking reducing or eliminating endo flairs during exercise.

Remember, deep core activation should be involuntary; it does so on its own without you flexing or forcing activation (i.e., clenching). That's why Dr. Angie recommends a practice called hypopressive breathing to help. *Hypopressive* literally translates to "lower pressure." You can learn to use the power of breath to retrain your entire core to behave in synchronicity, from when you take in a relaxed breath, to when you brace for a plank or sneeze. By doing this technique for only 15 to 20 minutes per day, 3-5 days a week , you will slowly remind your ribs how to breathe and your lower tummy how to brace when under pressure, be it breathing, coughing, or doing yoga. Need a visual? Check out www.healendo.com/coredysfunction.

Having had an incredible level of core dysfunction myself, I can attest to the power of hypopressives. After a few months my deep core was re-trained, and

I've never felt my core stronger. Finding a hypopressive practitioner in the United States is getting easier, so to find one near you try an internet search for "hypopressives [insert your town or state]," or "low pressure fitness [your town or state]." If you're not having much luck, I'm very happy to say Dr. Angie offers an amazing online program called the Core Recovery Method, which includes hypopressive training. You can find her at www.corerecoverypt.com.

If Your Core Needs Support

If you didn't pass the "increased pressure tests", or you notice your butt is inactive or weak (and muscles tight), then stick with the lower-pressure activities until you retrain your core to function better.

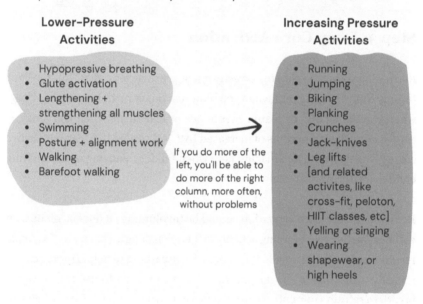

Lower-Pressure Activities

- Hypopressive breathing
- Glute activation
- Lengthening + strengthening all muscles
- Swimming
- Posture + alignment work
- Walking
- Barefoot walking

If you do more of the left, you'll be able to do more of the right column, more often, without problems

Increasing Pressure Activities

- Running
- Jumping
- Biking
- Planking
- Crunches
- Jack-knives
- Leg lifts
- [and related activites, like cross-fit, peloton, HIIT classes, etc]
- Yelling or singing
- Wearing shapewear, or high heels

Movement Through Massage

Maya Abdominal Massage is another tool in the movement toolbox. While relatively unknown, it's a fabulous way to bring oxygen, blood, and lymph directly to where we need it: the peritoneal cavity and uterus. This external technique of abdominal massage developed by Dr. Rosita Arvigo is gentle and slow, yet deeply penetrating into the tissues of the abdomen. It may also help reposition a uterus stuck in an incorrect position (tipped, retroverted, etc.).

While Western medicine doesn't often see a displaced uterus as a problem, women with an incorrectly positioned uterus may present symptoms such as pain with menstruation, irregular periods, dark brown or clotted/chunky blood, menstrual headaches, or back pain associated with their period. Because the most common reason for this misplacement is actually mechanical in nature—usually caused by the weakening or stretching of the ligaments and muscles that hold the uterus in place—Maya Massage may help gently coax the uterus back in place through either lengthening *or* shortening the uterine ligaments in need (each case will present uniquely) and increasing blood and lymph flow to the peritoneal cavity, allowing proper delivery of nutrients, immune factors, and hormones.

Maya Massage is best taught to you by an experienced practitioner. For more info about Maya Abdominal Massage or to find a practitioner near you, go to: www.abdominaltherapycollective.com. You can find a list of certified practitioners at www.abdominaltherapycollective.com, and you can also learn Maya Massage in Dr. Angie's online program The Core Recovery Method (www.corerecoverypt.com).

APPENDIX 5:

Dioxins in Food

Because animals who eat dioxins bioaccumulate them in their bodies—making them a concentrated dioxin food source—we are told to avoid eating animal products to avoid dioxins. However, this isn't totally true, and it's worth understanding if you're avoiding meat specifically because of dioxins (as I believe properly sourced animal products are an incredible addition to our endo arsenal).

It's true that animals eating dioxin-contaminated foods will have more much dioxins on the whole. But not all animals are eating dioxin contaminated foods. For example, a 2015 study sampled hundreds of animals, finding the dioxin range from very low (a steer from Alabama had .08 TEQ, the measurement of dioxins or dioxin-like compounds) to very high (a steer from Iowa had 3.6 TEQ, 45 times more).[317] The difference can depend on anything from where the food is produced, what water is near, what factories, what year, to what wind patterns!

Additionally, plants too can have dioxin contamination. In a 2002 Greece food sampling, rice was shown having 10 times more dioxins than beef.[318] A 2004 study from the Netherlands observed the contribution of dioxins from different foods to be pretty evenly distributed, with 17 percent from vegetable oils, 23 percent from meat products, 27 percent from dairy, 13 percent from vegetable products, 16 percent from fish, and 4 percent from eggs.[319] A 2016 analysis of dioxin consumption within the Italian diet showed that vegetable-based foods contributed more than twice as much dioxins as meat.[320]

This leaves us with a bit of a problem to solve, since it appears dioxins are simply hidden throughout our food supply. But there's good news: dioxin exposure has radically dropped in the past 50 years, with a 90 percent reduction in air emissions.[321] This is why food contamination has become our biggest contributor; the majority of our other exposures have been cleaned up (which is a great thing). Still, there are ways to protect ourselves from the remaining dioxins contaminating our food supply, as detailed in Chapter 15.

ABOUT THE AUTHOR

Katie Edmonds has a BA from the University of California at Santa Barbara. She is a Nutritional Therapist and a Paleo AutoImmune Protocol certified coach. She's the creator of HealEndo.com, a website dedicated to the whole-body understanding of endometriosis, and the author of The *4-Week Endometriosis Diet Plan*. She lives on the North Shore of Kaua`i with her husband, two miracle kiddos, and furry hound.

INDEX

location, 57-58

movement, 56-58

retinoids (Vitamin A) and, 121, 308

endometriomas, 38, 41, 91, 123, 155

Endometriosis Foundation of America, 24

endometritis, 84, 230, 231

Environmental Working Group, 174, 261

EPA. *See* omega 3s

estrobolome, 86, 254

estrogen. *See also* endo-like cell, estrogen
sensitivity and; inflammation,
estrogen and

cell growth and, 92-94

chemicals, 53, 255

diet and, 133, 146, 168, 178-180, 182

dominance, 95-97, 235, 252-254

dysbiosis and, 86

endo trigger, 25, 69, 71, 90

healthy levels, 91-92, 100, 234, 254

immune system and, 66, 69, 310, 314

sensitivity, 48, 49, 51, 59, 308

suppression, 265-267, 269-270

estrogen-mimicking chemicals, 254

eustress, 249-250

Evvy, 231

F

fatigue, 21, 22, 37, 68, 83, 86, 99, 112, 114,
116, 118, 119, 129, 147, 160, 182, 219, 222,
234, 235, 238, 248, 251, 266, 278, 279,

fats. *See also* nutrition, fats

blood sugar and, 140-143, 148-149, 161

fat-soluble vitamins and, 121, 122,

fish, 124, 128-130, 137, 183, 185, 186

healthy, 159-160, 174

monounsaturated, 159

omega 3, 128-130, 154, 165, 166, 173,
174, 176, 223

omega 6, 101, 159, 165-167

polyunsaturated, 159

saturated, 158-159

vegetable oils, 159, 165-167

Fem-Dophilus, 232

fertility. *See also* infertility

amino acids, 155

challenges, 37

dysbiosis, 225

early diagnosis and, 39, 42

epigenetics and, 48, 52, 70

fats, 158

gluten, 169

hormonal balance and, 92, 99

IVF and, 269

nutrients and, 110, 111, 112, 117, 118,
119, 122, 123, 124, 127, 128, 128

preserving, 35, 42

progesterone and, 253

specialist, 295

fermented foods, 176, 179-180, 229, 247

fiber, 78, 89, 113, 140, 141, 143, 148, 149-
153, 161, 173, 215, 216, 223, 263

fibromyalgia, 68, 83, 274, 278

fight-or-flight hormones, 98-99,
238, 241, 248

flavonoids, 132, 134. *See also*
phytonutrients

FODMAP, low (diet), 191, 220-221

*The 4-Week Endometriosis Diet
Plan*, 176, 189

free radicals, 74, 101, 111, 116, 117, 118,
124, 125, 144, 158, 165, 258. *See also*
oxidative stress

full-body disease, 22, 28, 37, 68, 293

G

genetic susceptibility, 49-50

GI-Map Test, 225, 227

glass containers, 187, 259 260, 264

glucose, 101, 140-147, 152, 155, 158, 162

glutamine, 155

glutathione, 125, 133, 155, 178

glute activation, 72, 196, 197, 199, 202, 209-211

gluten, 160, 168-172, 187, 189, 215, 220, 252

glycine, 155-157, 175, 193, 229

glyphosate, 170, 179, 257, 258

gonadotropin-releasing hormone (Gn-RHa), 269-270

grains, 141, 143, 149, 152-153, 161, 168, 186, 222

gut barrier integrity. *See* leaky gut

gut hyper-permeability. *See* leaky gut

gut microbiome. *See* microbiome, gut

H

Hashimoto's thyroiditis, 50, 64, 222

headaches, 68, 83, 86, 116, 119, 181, 215, 222, 321

herbicides, 100, 179, 256, 257, 258

heterogeneous, 24-25, 43, 59, 293

histamines, 70, 177, 178, 215, 220

hops (herb), 237

hormones. *See also specific hormones*
  balancing, 104. 109, 162, 234-254
  contraceptive, 15, 16, 78, 111, 265-266
  definition, 90-91
  imbalance, 28, 95-100, 171, 252-254
  immune system and, 63, 75,
  pharmaceuticals, 265-267, 269
  progestin therapy, 268-269
  sleep and, 235-237
  stress, 97-99, 101, 145-146, 238-250, 294

HPA, 99, 240

HPO, 269

H. Pylori, 225, 227

hydrocodone, 271, 271

hypopressive breathing, 209, 213, 214, 319-320

hypothalamic-pituitary-adrenal axis, 99, 240

hypothalamic-pituitary-ovarian axis, 269

hypothyroidism, 68, 83, 124

hypoxia, 54, 75, 88, 155, 196, 198, 310

I

IAP. *See* intra-abdominal pressure

IBS, 36, 85, 86, 220, 239

ibuprofen, 218, 271-272

IL-1β, 310, 311, 312, 315

IL-6, 310, 311, 312

IL-13, 310, 312

IL-17, 315

Immanuel, Dr. Stella, 33

immune dysfunction. *See also* inflammation; *specific immune factors*
  allergies and, 64
  autoimmune disorders and, 64-65
  cancer and, 65
  chronic inflammation, 22-24, 63-64, 100-101, 106
  definition, 22-24, 64
  dysbiosis and, 77-78, 83, 86, 88
  endometriosis and, 22-24, 62, 64-70, 302, 309-314
  hormonal contraceptives and, 266-267
  insulin and, 91, 145
  nutrition and, 109, 117, 118, 135,
  retraining, 75, 102-107
  stress and, 146
  toxic chemicals and, 100, 255

infertility. *See also* fertility
  alcohol and, 167
  celiac disease and, 169
  cell abnormalities and, 308
  dysbiosis and, 84, 87, 89, 225, 230
  endometriomas and, 41
  endometritis and, 84, 230, 231
  as endo symptom, 21, 24, 32, 34, 36-37, 39, 281
  HPA dysfunction and, 99,
  immune dysfunction and, 313

iron and, 118
mast cells and, 70
natural killer cells and, 313
progesterone and, 268
toxins and, 255
under-nutrition and, 111
vitamin D and, 122-123
zinc and, 117

inflammation. *See also*
immune dysfunction
alcohol, 167-168
blood sugar and, 101, 144, 146
chronic, 22-24, 64-65, 70, 71, 72, 100-
101, 253, 293
chronic vs. acute, 44
cyclic, 74, 83, 106
definition, 22-24, 63
diet and, 104, 109, 115-135,
220, 220-222
dysbiosis and, 56, 71, 77-78, 83, 86,
87-88, 215, 227, 228-232
endocrine-disrupting chemicals and,
52-53, 71, 100, 255,
endometriosis lesion and, 22-24, 28,
59, 66, 69, 71, 94, 100, 254
endo-like cell, 49, 51, 52-59, 253
estrogen and, 25, 71, 90, 92, 94, 253
food triggers, 168-182
free radicals and, 73-75, 101, 111
hormonal contraceptives and, 267
iron overload and, 71, 100
ischemia and, 198
nervous system confusion
and, 276-278
nutrient deficiency and, 101, 111,
112, 115-135
omega 6 and, 165-167
oxidative stress and, 72-75, 101
protein and, 154-156
reduction, 34, 44, 75, 83, 87-89, 102-
107, 150, 196, 220, 228-232, 275

scar tissue, 21, 23, 70, 75, 311
sedentary and, 72, 100, 198
sleep and, 100, 235-237
stress and, 72, 98, 100, 146, 238-251
surgery and, 284
systemic, 65-65, 68, 100-101, 102-107,
159, 169, 220, 222, 234
vegetable oils and, 101, 159, 165-167

insomnia, 78, 215, 222, 235, 270
Institute for Functional Medicine,
226, 279, 305
insulin, 91, 101, 141, 144-147, 150,
152, 161, 294
insulin resistance, 144-145, 148, 161, 164
insurance, 35, 42, 119, 230, 251, 285,
290-291, 302
integrative care, 34, 35, 44, 287, 289, 305
intra-abdominal adhesions, 21, 24, 37, 40,
70, 75, 212, 281, 311
intra-abdominal pressure (IAP), 203, 205-
206, 214, 317-319
in vitro fertilization, 84, 240, 269, 295
iodine, 130, 138, 176
iron (dietary), 114, 118-121, 137, 138, 154,
173, 179, 185, 258, 279
iron overload, 71, 100
irritable bowel syndrome, 36, 85,
86, 220, 239
ischemia, 197-199
IVF, 84, 240, 269, 295

J

Jarrow Research, 232
joint pain. *See* pain, joint
Juno.bio, 231

L

Lactobacillus, 227, 230
lactose, 176
LDN, 274-275

vs. calories, 110

nutrition

80/20, 190

ancestral, 156

balanced, 103-104, 184, 190, 219

body ecology and, 63, 103-104

bone broth, 114, 156, 157, 173, 175, 185, 193, 218, 222, 297

definition, 109

fats, 166

integrative care and, 30, 44-45, 289

red meat, 172

supplementation, 137

under-, 104, 110-114, 169, 170, 174, 222

nuts, 117, 118, 138, 153, 159, 161, 186-187, 192, 194

O

oils, seed. *See* oils, vegetable

oils, vegetable, 127, 158, 159, 164, 165-167, 171, 173, 190, 322

omega 3s, 114, 128-129, 138, 154, 159, 165, 166, 173, 174, 176, 215, 223

omega 3/omega 6 balance, 159, 165-66

omega 6s, 159, 165-166, 179

opioids, 272-273

oral contraceptives, 105, 112, 133, 253, 265-267

Orlissa, 42, 252, 269,

ovarian endometriotic cysts.

See endometriomas

oxidative stress. *See also* free radicals

bacteria and, 88

chronic inflammation and, 72-75, 101, 111

diet and, 101, 111, 116, 117, 118, 119, 125, 133, 155

epigenetics and, 52, 61

endometriosis progression, 70

scar tissue, 70

oxycodone, 272-273

P

pain

abdominal, 85-86, 157, 169, 216, 128, 220, 225

back, 112, 157, 213, 295

bladder, 236

central sensitization, 28, 276-278

chronic, 20, 28, 39, 99, 126, 200, 202, 251, 273, 275, 276, 277, 279

core dysfunction, 201-204, 214

diet and, 111, 116, 117, 125, 126, 129, 133, 143, 147, 165, 167, 169, 177, 181

digestive, 85-86, 157, 169, 216, 128, 220, 225

endo-belly, 85-86, 157, 169, 216, 128, 220, 225

endo lesion, 24, 25, 28, 48, 49, 59, 69, 94-95, 281

inflammation and, 70, 83, 127, 167, 169, 220, 236

joint, 21, 68, 78, 127, 129, 147, 157, 210, 211, 215, 222, 270

medications, 32, 42, 78, 105, 265-276

normalized, 32-33, 43, 50, 143

overactive nervous system and, 28, 276-278

pelvic, 20-21, 42, 87, 196, 212, 213, 279

pelvic floor, 203, 211-212, 277

period, 36, 42, 57, 87, 97, 116, 117, 175, 196, 235, 279

phantom, 276-278

physical activity and, 196-201, 204, 263

sex, 36, 87, 125, 203, 212-213, 248, 270, 271, 276-277

stress, 99, 240-251, 248-249

surgery and, 39, 45, 270, 281-289

symptom, 36, 37, 41, 68, 78, 83, 88, 89, 107, 114, 131, 215, 239, 251, 297, 300, 301

Paleo Autoimmune Protocol (AIP) Diet, 60, 221-222

RAGE. *See* advanced glycation
   end-products
RDI. *See* recommended daily intake
recommended daily intake, 110
red meat, 113, 118, 129, 137, 157, 172-173
regression, endo lesions, 25, 28, 59, 87, 133
remission, 16-17, 46, 61, 75, 107, 301
reproductive tract infection. *See*
   microbiome, reproductive
reproductive tract dysbiosis, 79-80, 85-
   87, 229-233
resistant starch, 152
restriction, food, 15, 113, 170, 224
resveratrol, 132-133, 258
retinoids, 121-122, 308. *See also* vitamin A
retrograde menstruation, 57, 67, 71, 100
rheumatoid arthritis, 267
Roundup, 179, 257

S

salt, 187, 192, 194
Salt Fat Acid Heat, 189
saturated fats, 158-159
scar tissue, 21, 23, 75, 212, 281, 311
screening for endo, 35
seafood, 114, 118, 128-130, 137, 138,
   139, 156, 185
seed oils. *See* vegetable oils
SIBO. *See* small intestinal bacterial
   overgrowth
silymarin, 133 *See also* phytonutrients
sleep,
   caffeine and, 182
   hormones and, 90, 97, 253
   improvement, 27, 148, 235-237,
      247, 252, 297
   inflammation and, 63, 101, 102, 103
   poor, 218, 246, 297
Slow Death by Rubber Duck, 256

small intestinal bacterial overgrowth,
   85-86, 107, 221, 224, 225, 226-227,
   247, 279, 301
   testing, 226-227
sodium, 112, 138, 173. *See also* salt
soy, 153, 170, 178-180, 191. *See also*
   vegetable oils
specialists, endo, 33, 35, 252, 269, 187, 295
stages, endo, 40-41
Streptococcus, 79, 86, 224
stress. *See also* adrenaline; cortisol;
   oxidative stress
   addressing, 45, 89, 102, 115, 131, 148,
      197, 229, 235, 238-252, 275, 278,
      289, 297, 298, 199
   anxiety, 98-99
   body ecology and, 27-28
   chronic, 72, 98-99, 229, 238-240, 242,
      246, 247, 251, 300
   diet and, 104, 109, 110, 111, 112, 116,
      145, 181-182, 219, 241
   digestion and, 216-217
   endo behavior and, 28, 98-99
   epigenetics and, 51
   eustress, 249-252
   free radicals and, 74
   hormones and, 97-99, 101, 145-
      146, 253, 294
   immune system and, 63, 72
   inflammation and, 25, 72, 74, 101
   microbiome and, 215, 228, 229
   social media and, 241-242
substandard care, 42-43, 290
sugar, 63, 98, 102, 140-155, 148-152, 161,
   164, 173, 174, 182, 187, 190, 215, 223,
   230, 236, 253. *See also* blood sugar
superficial endo, 38, 40-41
supplements, 115, 125, 135, 137, 159, 226
surgery. *See also* diagnosis
   adolescent endo and, 314
   asymptomatic endo and, 25

ENDNOTES

1   Koninckx, P. R., Meuleman, C., Demeyere, S., Lesaffre, E., & Cornillie, F. J. (1991). Suggestive evidence that pelvic endometriosis is a progressive disease, whereas deeply infiltrating endometriosis is associated with pelvic pain. *Fertility and Sterility, 55*(4), 759–765. https://doi.org/10.1016/S0015-0282(16)54244-7; Shafrir, A. L., Farland, L. V., Shah, D. K., Harris, H. R., Kvaskoff, M., Zondervan, K., Missmer, S. A. (2018). Risk for and consequences of endometriosis: A critical epidemiologic review. *Best Practice & Research Clinical Obstetrics & Gynaecology, 51*, 1–15. https://www.doi.org/10.1016/j.bpobgyn.2018.06.001; Guo, S.-W., & Wang, Y. (2006). Sources of heterogeneities in estimating the prevalence of endometriosis in infertile and previously fertile women. *Fertility and Sterility, 86*(6), 1584–1595. https://doi.org/10.1016/j.fertnstert.2006.04.040

2   Koninckx, P. R., Ussia, A., Adamyan, L., Wattiez, A., Gomel, V., & Martin, D. C. (2019). Pathogenesis of endometriosis: The genetic/epigenetic theory. *Fertility and Sterility, 111*(2), 327–340. https://doi.org/10.1016/j.fertnstert.2018.10.013

3   Martin, D.C. (2021). Endometriosis concepts and theories. *Resurge Press* (Richmond, Virginia). Accessed February 1, 2021, from: https://www.danmartinmd.com/endo-concepts.html

4   Evers, J.L.H. (2013). Is adolescent endometriosis a progressive disease that needs to be diagnosed and treated? *Human Reproduction, 28(8),* 2023. https://doi.org/10.1093/humrep/det298

5   To note, because of the normalization of pain, it's possible these women had symptoms to some degree but considered it normal. Fuentes, A, Escalona, J, Céspedes, P, Espinoza, A, Johnson, MC. (2014). Prevalencia de la endometriosis en mujeres sometidas a esterilización quirúrgica laparoscópica en un hospital de Santiago de Chile [Prevalence of endometriosis in 287 women undergoing surgical sterilization in Santiago Chile]. *Rev Med Chil, 142*(1), 16-19. Spanish. https://doi.org/10.4067/S0034-98872014000100003

6   Gross, R. E. (2021). "They call it a 'women's disease.' She wants to redefine it." *The New York Times.* https://www.nytimes.com/2021/04/27/health/endometriosis-griffith-uterus.html

7   Drseckin.com. (2021). Petitioning ACOG to change the standards of care for endometriosis patients. *Seckin Endometriosis Center.* Accessed August 8, 2021, from: https://drseckin.com/petitioning-acog-to-change-the-standards-of-care-for-endometriosis-patients/

8   Loveline. (2016). Unofficial Loveline moments: Endometriosis "garbage bag diagnosis" call. *YouTube.* https://www.youtube.com/watch?v=qFbsqsEmxjM

9   Paquette, D., & Andrews, T. (2020). Trump retweeted a video with false Covid-19 claims. One doctor in it has said demons cause illnesses. *The Washington Post.* https://www.washingtonpost.com/technology/2020/07/28/stella-immanuel-hy-droxychloroquine-video-trump-americas-frontline-doctors/

10   Note that because of limited research on *treating* endometriosis and outcomes, most information regarding best practices will be left to personal/professional observation and opinion. For example, there are no long-term studies looking at the differences in outcomes of different approaches as to when or if someone has surgery.

11   For excision surgery as the first step in treatment, this is a recommendation put forth by endo groups who believe that, if you have endo, you should not wait to get it removed. Prompt removal of endo may save quality of life, fertility, and more. See https://nancysnookendo.com/learning-library/treatment/?fbclid=IwAR2mdwyr-g9RV3hvApxdYn26ZizrfFJJw1vq1gC2bqZSzlPEA5S_XTFWYqD0

12   This path echoes thoughts from Dr. Dan Martin, who says, "The natural fight between the body and invader (in this case, endo) *may* actually take care of more cases of endometriosis than surgery.» He notes this «natural fight» is why not everyone with endometriosis needs surgery or has ongoing pain. It›s how some of our worst endo symptoms can subside on their own when managed with diet and lifestyle, anti-inflammatories, antimicrobials, antibiotics, or oral contraceptives. And while having endo «taken care of» doesn›t equate to a cure (because endo lesions may remain, although in a less problematic form), we can at least regain our quality of life.

Dr. Martin proposes the body may "naturally" take care of endo more often than surgery using a general estimation that 10 percent of women suffer from endo, of which an estimated 3.7 percent of women may have infiltrating and painful endo, of which surgery helps about half (near 2 percent). Another estimated 5.7 percent may have incidental endo without symptoms. Thus, we could consider that "nature" (i.e., a healthy and balanced body ecology) may control symptoms in just about 3x more cases than are controlled by surgery. Fuentes, A., Escalona, J., Céspedes, P., Espinoza, A., Johnson, M.C. Prevalencia de la endometriosis en mujeres sometidas a esteril-ización quirúrgica laparoscópica en un hospital de Santiago de Chile [Prevalence of endometriosis in 287 women undergoing surgical sterilization in Santiago Chile]. (2014). *Revista médica de Chile, 142*(1), 16-9. Spanish. https://doi.org/10.4067/S0034-98872014000100003; Koninckx, P. R., Meuleman, C., Demeyere, S., Lesaffre, E., & Cornillie, F. J. (1991). Suggestive evidence that pelvic endometriosis is a progressive disease, whereas deeply infiltrating endometriosis is associated with pelvic pain. *Fertility and Sterility, 55*(4), 759–765. https://doi.org/10.1016/S0015-0282(16)54244-7; Shafrir, A. L., Farland, L. V., Shah, D. K., Harris, H. R., Kvaskoff, M., Zondervan, K., & Missmer, S. A. (2018). Risk for and consequences of endometriosis: A critical epidemiologic review. *Best practice & research. Clinical obstetrics & gynaecology, 51,* 1–15. https://doi.org/10.1016/j.bpobgyn.2018.06.001; Guo, S.-W., & Wang, Y. (2006). Sources of heterogeneities in estimating the prevalence of endometriosis in infertile and previously fertile women. *Fertility and Sterility, 86*(6), 1584–1595. https://doi.org/10.1016/j.fertnstert.2006.04.040

13   Liu, X., Yan, D., & Guo, S. W. (2019). Sensory nerve-derived neuropeptides accelerate the development and fibrogenesis of endometriosis. *Human Reproduction* (Oxford, England). *34*(3), 452–468. https://doi.org/10.1093/humrep/dey392

14   BBC. (2019). Endometriosis: Women 'taking their own lives' due to lack of support. *BBC News*. Retrieved January 10, 2022, from https://www.bbc.com/news/uk-wales-49933866

15   Madjid, T. H., Ardiansyah, D. F., Permadi, W., & Hernowo, B. (2020). Expression of matrix metalloproteinase-9 and tissue inhibitor of metalloproteinase-1 in endometriosis menstrual blood. *Diagnostics* (Basel, Switzerland). *10*(6), 364. https://doi.org/10.3390/diagnostics10060364

16   It's been suggested that an American Fertility Society (rAFS) score of >70 could be used as a Stage 5 for endometriosis. The rAFS scores endometriosis based on points up to 150, with Stage 4 being broken into two scores (4A for 40-70 points and 4B for 71-150 points). Scores higher than 71 are those usually associated with *severe* adhesions, and why certain proponents would like to see a Stage 5 diagnosis exist. Adamson, David, M.D., & David J. Pasta, M.S. (2009). Endometriosis fertility index: The new, validated endometriosis staging system. *Fertility and Sterility, 94*(5), 1609-1615. https://doi.org/10.1016/j.fertnstert.2009.09.035; Canis, M., Pouly, J.L., Wattiez, A., Manhes, H., Mage, G., Bruhat, M.A. (1992). Incidence of bilateral adnexal disease in severe endometriosis (revised American Fertility Society [AFS], stage IV): Should a stage V be included in the AFS classification? *Fertility and Sterility, 57*(3), 691-92. https://www.doi.org/10.1016/s0015-0282(16)54924-3

17   Chapron, C., Fauconnier, A., Dubuisson, J. B., Barakat, H., Vieira, M., & Bréart, G. (2003). Deep infiltrating endometriosis: relation between severity of dysmenorrhoea and extent of disease. *Human Reproduction* (Oxford, England), *18*(4), 760–766. https://doi.org/10.1093/humrep/deg152

18   Guo, S. W. (2020). The pathogenesis of adenomyosis vis-à-vis endometriosis. *Journal of Clinical Medicine, 9*(2), 485. https://doi.org/10.3390/jcm9020485

19   Hansen, K. A., & Eyster, K. M. (2010). Genetics and genomics of endometriosis. *Clinical Obstetrics and Gynecology, 53*(2), 403–412. https://doi.org/10.1097/GRF.0b013e3181db7ca1

20   Yoo, J. Y., Kim, T. H., Fazleabas, A. T., Palomino, W. A., Ahn, S. H., Tayade, C., Schammel, D. P., Young, S. L., Jeong, J. W., & Lessey, B. A. (2017). KRAS activation and over-expression of SIRT1/BCL6 contributes to the pathogenesis of endometriosis and progesterone resistance. *Scientific Reports, 7*(1), 6765. https://doi.org/10.1038/s41598-017-04577-w

21   Tapmeier, T. T., Rahmioglu, N., Lin, J., De Leo, B., Obendorf, M., Raveendran, M., Fischer, O. M., Bafligil, C., Guo, M., Harris, R. A., Hess-Stumpp, H., Laux-Biehlmann, A., Lowy, E., Lunter, G., Malzahn, J., Martin, N. G., Martinez, F. O., Manek, S., Mesch, S., Montgomery, G. W., ... Zondervan, K. T. (2021). Neuropeptide S receptor 1 is a nonhormonal treatment target in endometriosis. *Science Translational Medicine, 13*(608), eabd6469. https://doi.org/10.1126/scitranslmed.abd6469

22   Hansen, K. A., & Eyster, K. M. (2010). Genetics and genomics of endome-
      triosis. *Clinical Obstetrics and Gynecology, 53*(2), 403–412. https://doi.
      org/10.1097/GRF.0b013e3181db7ca1; Moen, M.H. (1994). Endometriosis in
      monozygotic twins. *Acta Obstet Gynecol Scand, 73(1), 59-62.* https://www.doi.
      org/10.3109/00016349409013396; Simpson, J.L., Elias, S., Malinak, L.R., But-
      tram, V.C. Jr. (1980). Heritable aspects of endometriosis. I. Genetic studies. *Amer-
      ican Journal of Obstetrics and Gynecology, 137*(3), 327-331. https://www.doi.
      org/10.1016/0002-9378(80)90917-5

23   Jeffrey Braverman, MD. (2014). Outsmarting endo: Diagnosing silent endometriosis.
      Endometriosis Foundation of America. Retrieved from: https://www.endofound.
      org/jeffrey-braverman-md-outsmarting-endo

24   Bansal, A., Henao-Mejia, J., Simmons, R.A. (2018). Immune system: An emerging
      player in mediating effects of endocrine disruptors on metabolic health. *Endocrinol-
      ogy, 159*(1), 32-45. https://www.doi.org/10.1210/en.2017-00882

25   Shmarakov I.O. (2015). Retinoid-xenobiotic interactions: The ying and the yang.
      Hepatobiliary Surgery and Nutrition, 4(4), 243–267. https://doi.org/10.3978/j.
      issn.2304-3881.2015.05.05

26   Bruner-Tran, K. L., Ding, T., & Osteen, K. G. (2010). Dioxin and endometrial proges-
      terone resistance. *Seminars in Reproductive Medicine, 28*(1), 59–68. https://doi.
      org/10.1055/s-0029-1242995; Koukoura, O., Sifakis, S., & Spandidos, D. A. (2016).
      DNA methylation in endometriosis. *Molecular Medicine Reports, 13*(4), 2939–2948.
      https://doi.org/10.3892/mmr.2016.4925

27   Chou, Y. C., & Tzeng, C. R. (2021). The impact of phthalate on reproductive function
      in women with endometriosis. *Reproductive Medicine and Biology, 20*(2), 159–168.
      https://doi.org/10.1002/rmb2.12364

28   Chou, Y. C., & Tzeng, C. R. (2021). The impact of phthalate on reproductive function
      in women with endometriosis. *Reproductive Medicine and Biology, 20*(2), 159–168.
      https://doi.org/10.1002/rmb2.12364

29   Aldad, T. S., Rahmani, N., Leranth, C., & Taylor, H. S. (2011). Bisphenol-A exposure
      alters endometrial progesterone receptor expression in the nonhuman primate. *Fer-
      tility and Sterility, 96*(1), 175–179. https://doi.org/10.1016/j.fertnstert.2011.04.010;
      Hiroi, H., Tsutsumi, O., Takeuchi, T., Momoeda, M., Ikezuki, Y., Okamura, A., Yokota,
      H., & Taketani, Y. (2004). Differences in serum bisphenol a concentrations in pre-
      menopausal normal women and women with endometrial hyperplasia. *Endocrine
      Journal, 51*(6), 595–600. https://doi.org/10.1507/endocrj.51.595; Signorile, P.G.,
      Spugnini, E.P., Mita, L., Mellone, P., D'Avino, A., Bianco, M., Diano, N., Caputo, L.,
      Rea, F., Viceconte, R., Portaccio, M., Viggiano, E., Citro, G., Pierantoni, R., Sica, V.,
      Vincenzi, B., Mita, D.G., Baldi, F., Baldi, A.. (2010). Pre-natal exposure of mice to
      bisphenol A elicits an endometriosis-like phenotype in female offspring. *General
      and Comparative Endocrinology, 168*(3), 318-325. https://doi.org/10.1016/j.yg-
      cen.2010.03.030

30   Kalluri, R., & Weinberg, R. A. (2009). The basics of epithelial-mesenchymal transition. *The Journal of Clinical Investigation, 119*(6), 1420–1428. https://doi.org/10.1172/JCI39104; Wu, M. H., Hsiao, K. Y., & Tsai, S. J. (2019). Hypoxia: The force of endometriosis. *The Journal of Obstetrics and Gynaecology Research, 45*(3), 532–541. https://doi.org/10.1111/jog.13900

31   Batt, R. E., & Yeh, J. (2013). Müllerianosis: Four developmental (embryonic) Müllerian diseases. *Reproductive Sciences* (Thousand Oaks, Calif.*), 20*(9), 1030–1037. https://doi.org/10.1177/1933719112472736

32   Sasson, I. E., & Taylor, H. S. (2008). Stem cells and the pathogenesis of endometriosis. *Annals of the New York Academy of Sciences, 1127*, 106–115. https://doi.org/10.1196/annals.1434.014

33   The theory of retrograde menstruation is solely one theory of dissemination (i.e. how that endo ended up somewhere else in the body) rather than being "the cause" of endo, as it's often mistakenly credited in the mainstream media and even by certain medical professionals. It posits that if you have an endo-like cell (or a precursor cell) existing within the normal endometrium, retrograde menstruation may introduce this cell into the peritoneal cavity, where it's activated by the immune system into an endometriosis lesion. For researchers who believe in this theory, they know it can only explain, *very specifically*, superficial endometriosis found solely in the general pelvic and abdominal areas. Unfortunately, the misrepresentation of this theory has hurt our treatment plans for decades. Wu, M. H., Hsiao, K. Y., & Tsai, S. J. (2019). Hypoxia: The force of endometriosis. *The Journal of Obstetrics and Gynaecology Research, 45*(3), 532–541. https://doi.org/10.1111/jog.13900; Sourial, S., Tempest, N., & Hapangama, D. K. (2014, February 12). Theories on the pathogenesis of endometriosis. *International Journal of Reproductive Medicine*. Retrieved April 3, 2021, from https://www.hindawi.com/journals/ijrmed/2014/179515

34   Koninckx, P. R., Ussia, A., Adamyan, L., Wattiez, A., Gomel, V., & Martin, D. C. (2020). Correction: Heterogeneity of endometriosis lesions requires individualisation of diagnosis and treatment and a different approach to research and evidence-based medicine. *Facts, Views & Vision in ObGyn, 11*(3), 263.

35   These cells may be more prone to progesterone resistance, Homeobox A10 gene abnormalities (affecting fertility/reproduction), and aromatase production, as well as an enhanced ability to proliferate, implant, and establish blood supply. This may make trouble for proper immune management if these cells "leak" into the peritoneal cavity, which may help to explain why retrograde menstruation is problematic in some cases. The degree of alteration of normally placed endometrial cells has prompted experimentation with new methods of non-invasive endometriosis diagnosis, such as the simple testing of menstrual blood for genetic/epigenetic abnormalities, which has yielded successful diagnostic rates even in the preliminary stages.

Liu, H., & Lang, J. H. (2011). Is abnormal eutopic endometrium the cause of endometriosis? The role of eutopic endometrium in pathogenesis of endometriosis. *Medical Science Monitor: International Medical Journal of Experimental and Clinical Research, 17*(4), RA92–RA99. https://doi.org/10.12659/msm.881707; Nayyar, A.,

Saleem, M. I., Yilmaz, M., DeFranco, M., Klein, G., Elmaliki, K. M., Kowalsky, E., Chatterjee, P. K., Xue, X., Viswanathan, R., Shih, A. J., Gregersen, P. K., & Metz, C. N. (2020). Menstrual effluent provides a novel diagnostic window on the pathogenesis of endometriosis. *Frontiers in Reproductive Health*, *2*. https://doi.org/10.3389/frph.2020.00003; Noble, L. S., Takayama, K., Zeitoun, K. M., Putman, J. M., Johns, D. A., Hinshelwood, M. M., Agarwal, V. R., Zhao, Y., Carr, B. R., & Bulun, S. E. (1997). Prostaglandin E2 stimulates aromatase expression in endometriosis-derived stromal cells. *The Journal of Clinical Endocrinology and Metabolism*, *82*(2), 600–606. https://doi.org/10.1210/jcem.82.2.3783

36   Chandrasekaran, A., Molparia, B., Akhtar, E., Wang, X., Lewis, J. D., Chang, J. T., Oliveira, G., Torkamani, A., & Konijeti, G. G. (2019). The autoimmune protocol diet modifies intestinal RNA expression in inflammatory bowel disease. *Crohn's & Colitis 360*, *1*(3), otz016. https://doi.org/10.1093/crocol/otz016

37   Koninckx, P. R., Ussia, A., Adamyan, L., Wattiez, A., Gomel, V., & Martin, D. C. (2020). Correction: Heterogeneity of endometriosis lesions requires individualisation of diagnosis and treatment and a different approach to research and evidence based medicine. *Facts, Views & Vision in ObGyn*, *11*(3), 263.

38   Koninckx, P. R., Donnez, J., & Brosens, I. (2016). Microscopic endometriosis: Impact on our understanding of the disease and its surgery. *Fertility and Sterility*, *105*(2), 305–306. https://doi.org/10.1016/j.fertnstert.2015.10.038

39   Signorile, P. G., Baldi, F., Bussani, R., D'Armiento, M., De Falco, M., & Baldi, A. (2009). Ectopic endometrium in human foetuses is a common event and sustains the theory of Müllerianosis in the pathogenesis of endometriosis, a disease that predisposes to cancer. *Journal of Experimental & Clinical Cancer Research: CR*, *28*(1), 49. https://doi.org/10.1186/1756-9966-28-49; Koninckx, P. R., & Martin, D. C. (1992). Deep endometriosis: A consequence of infiltration or retraction or possibly adenomyosis externa? *Fertility and Sterility*, *58*(5), 924–928. https://doi.org/10.1016/s0015-0282(16)55436-3; Martin, D. C., Koninckx, P. R., Batt, R. E., & Smith, R. (1997). Deep endometriosis. In Minaguchi, H., & Sugimoto, O. (Eds). *Endometriosis today: Advances in research and practice* (pp. 50–57). Lancashire, UK: Parthenon Publishing Group.

40   Matalliotaki, C., Matalliotakis, M., Zervou, M. I., Trivli, A., Matalliotakis, I., Mavroma-tidis, G., Spandidos, D. A., Albertsen, H. M., Chettier, R., Ward, K., & Goulielmos, G. N. (2018). Co-existence of endometriosis with 13 non-gynecological co-morbidities: Mutation analysis by whole exome sequencing. *Molecular Medicine Reports*, *18*(6), 5053–5057. https://doi.org/10.3892/mmr.2018.9521

41   Yang, M., Jiang, C., Chen, H., Nian, Y., Bai, Z., & Ha, C. (2015). The involvement of osteopontin and matrix metalloproteinase-9 in the migration of endometrial epithe-lial cells in patients with endometriosis. *Reproductive Biology and Endocrinology: RB&E*, *13*, 95. https://doi.org/10.1186/s12958-015-0090-4

42   Qi, Q., Liu, X., Zhang, Q., & Guo, S. W. (2020). Platelets induce increased estrogen production through NF-κB and TGF-β1 signaling pathways in endometriotic stromal cells. *Scientific Reports*, *10*(1), 1281. https://doi.org/10.1038/s41598-020-57997-6

43   Porpora, M. G., Scaramuzzino, S., Sangiuliano, C., Piacenti, I., Bonanni, V., Piccioni, M. G., Ostuni, R., Masciullo, L., & Benedetti Panici, P. L. (2020). High prevalence of autoimmune diseases in women with endometriosis: A case-control study. *Gynecological Endocrinology: The Official Journal of the International Society of Gynecological Endocrinology, 36*(4), 356–359. https://doi.org/10.1080/0951359 0.2019.1655727

44   Rocha, A. L., Reis, F. M., & Taylor, R. N. (2013). Angiogenesis and endometriosis. *Obstetrics and Gynecology International, 2013*, 859619. https://doi. org/10.1155/2013/859619; Delvoux, B., Groothuis, P., D'Hooghe, T., Kyama, C., Dunselman, G., & Romano, A. (2009). Increased production of 17beta-estradiol in endometriosis lesions is the result of impaired metabolism. *The Journal of Clinical Endocrinology and Metabolism, 94*(3), 876–883. https://doi.org/10.1210/ jc.2008-2218

45   Horne, A.W., Ahmad, F.S., Carter, R., Simitsidellis, I., Greaves, E., Hogg, C., Morton, N.M., & Saunders, P.T.K. (2019). Repurposing dichloroacetate for the treatment of women with endometriosis. *Proceedings of the National Academy of Sciences, 116*(51), 25389-25391. https://doi.org/10.1073/pnas.1916144116

46   Kempuraj, D., Papadopoulou, N., Stanford, E. J., Christodoulou, S., Madhappan, B., Sant, G. R., Solage, K., Adams, T., & Theoharides, T. C. (2004). Increased numbers of activated mast cells in endometriosis lesions positive for corticotropin-releasing hormone and urocortin. *American Journal of Reproductive Immunology, 52*(4), 267–275. https://doi.org/10.1111/j.1600-0897.2004.00224.x

47   Hart, D. A. (2015). Curbing inflammation in multiple sclerosis and endometriosis: Should mast cells be targeted? *International Journal of Inflammation*, 452095. https://doi.org/10.1155/2015/452095; Borelli, V., Martinelli, M., Luppi, S., Vita, F., Romano, F., Fanfani, F., Trevisan, E., Celsi, F., Zabucchi, G., Zanconati, F., Bottin, C., & Ricci, G. (2020). Mast cells in peritoneal fluid from women with endometriosis and their possible role in modulating sperm function. *Frontiers in Physiology, 10*, 1543. https://doi.org/10.3389/fphys.2019.01543

48   Kobayashi, H., Higashiura, Y., Shigetomi, H., & Kajihara, H. (2014). Pathogenesis of endometriosis: The role of initial infection and subsequent sterile inflammation (Review). *Molecular Medicine Reports, 9*(1), 9–15. https://doi.org/10.3892/ mmr.2013.1755; Khan, K. N., Kitajima, M., Fujishita, A., Nakashima, M., Masuzaki, H., & Kitawaki, J. (2015). Role of bacterial contamination in endometriosis. *Journal of Endometriosis and Pelvic Pain Disorders, 8*(1), 2–7. https://doi.org/10.5301/ je.5000229; Khan, K. N., Fujishita, A., Hiraki, K., Kitajima, M., Nakashima, M., Fushiki, S., & Kitawaki, J. (2018). Bacterial contamination hypothesis: A new concept in endometriosis. *Reproductive Medicine and Biology, 17*(2), 125–133. https://doi. org/10.1002/rmb2.12083; García-Peñarrubia, P., Ruiz-Alcaraz, A. J., Martínez-Esparza, M., Marín, P., & Machado-Linde, F. (2020). Hypothetical roadmap towards endometriosis: Prenatal endocrine-disrupting chemical pollutant exposure, anogenital distance, gut-genital microbiota and subclinical infections. *Human Reproduction Update, 26*(2), 214–246. https://doi.org/10.1093/humupd/dmz044

49   Klemmt, P., & Starzinski-Powitz, A. (2018). Molecular and cellular pathogenesis of endometriosis. *Current Women's Health Reviews, 14*(2), 106–116. https://doi.org/10.2174/1573404813666170306163448

50   Defrère, S., Van Langendonckt, A., Vaesen, S., Jouret, M., González Ramos, R., Gonzalez, D., & Donnez, J. (2006). Iron overload enhances epithelial cell proliferation in endometriotic lesions induced in a murine model. *Human Reproduction* (Oxford, England), *21*(11), 2810–2816. https://doi.org/10.1093/humrep/del261; Kobayashi, H., Yamada, Y., Kanayama, S., Furukawa, N., Noguchi, T., Haruta, S., Yoshida, S., Sakata, M., Sado, T., & Oi, H. (2009). The role of iron in the pathogenesis of endometriosis. *Gynecological Endocrinology: The Official Journal of the International Society of Gynecological Endocrinology, 25*(1), 39–52. https://doi.org/10.1080/09513590802366204; Van Langendonckt, A., Casanas-Roux, F., & Donnez, J. (2002). Iron overload in the peritoneal cavity of women with pelvic endometriosis. *Fertility and Sterility, 78*(4), 712–718. https://doi.org/10.1016/s0015-0282(02)03346-0

51   Chou, Y. C., & Tzeng, C. R. (2021). The impact of phthalate on reproductive function in women with endometriosis. *Reproductive Medicine and Biology, 20*(2), 159–168. https://doi.org/10.1002/rmb2.12364

52   Scutiero, G., Iannone, P., Bernardi, G., Bonaccorsi, G., Spadaro, S., Volta, C. A., Greco, P., & Nappi, L. (2017). Oxidative stress and endometriosis: A systematic review of the literature. *Oxidative Medicine and Cellular Longevity, 2017*, 7265238. https://doi.org/10.1155/2017/7265238

53   Ngô, C., Chéreau, C., Nicco, C., Weill, B., Chapron, C., & Batteux, F. (2009). Reactive oxygen species controls endometriosis progression. *The American Journal of Pathology, 175*(1), 225–234. https://doi.org/10.2353/ajpath.2009.080804

54   Leonardi, M., Hicks, C., El-Assaad, F., El-Omar, E., & Condous, G. (2020). Endometriosis and the microbiome: A systematic review. *BJOG : An International Journal of Obstetrics and Gynaecology, 127*(2), 239–249. https://doi.org/10.1111/1471-0528.15916

55   Ata, B., Yildiz, S., Turkgeldi, E., Brocal, V. P., Dinleyici, E. C., Moya, A., & Urman, B. (2019). The endobiota study: Comparison of vaginal, cervical and gut microbiota between women with stage 3/4 endometriosis and healthy controls. *Scientific Reports, 9*(1), 2204. https://doi.org/10.1038/s41598-019-39700-6

56   Laschke, M. W., & Menger, M. D. (2016). The gut microbiota: A puppet master in the pathogenesis of endometriosis? *American Journal of Obstetrics and Gynecology, 215*(1), 68.e1–68.e4. https://doi.org/10.1016/j.ajog.2016.02.036

57   Khan, K. N., Kitajima, M., Hiraki, K., Yamaguchi, N., Katamine, S., Matsuyama, T., Nakashima, M., Fujishita, A., Ishimaru, T., & Masuzaki, H. (2010). *Escherichia coli* contamination of menstrual blood and effect of bacterial endotoxin on endometriosis. *Fertility and Sterility, 94*(7), 2860–2863.e33. https://doi.org/10.1016/j.fertnstert.2010.04.053; Khan, K. N., Fujishita, A., Kitajima, M., Hiraki, K., Nakashima, M., & Masuzaki, H. (2014). Intra-uterine microbial colonization and occurrence of endometritis in women with endometriosis. *Human Reproduction* (Oxford, England),

29(11), 2446–2456. https://doi.org/10.1093/humrep/deu222; Koninckx, P. R., Ussia, A., Tahlak, M., Adamyan, L., Wattiez, A., Martin, D. C., & Gomel, V. (2019). Infection as a potential cofactor in the genetic-epigenetic pathophysiology of endometriosis: A systematic review. *Facts, Views & Vision in ObGyn*, 11(3), 209–216.

58 Koninckx, P. R., Ussia, A., Tahlak, M., Adamyan, L., Wattiez, A., Martin, D. C., & Gomel, V. (2019). Infection as a potential cofactor in the genetic-epigenetic pathophysiology of endometriosis: A systematic review. *Facts, Views & Vision in ObGyn*, 11(3), 209–216.

59 Berg R. D. (1999). Bacterial translocation from the gastrointestinal tract. *Advances in experimental medicine and biology*, 473, 11–30. https://doi.org/10.1007/978-1-4615-4143-1_2

60 Khan, K. N., Fujishita, A., Hiraki, K., Kitajima, M., Nakashima, M., Fushiki, S., & Kitawaki, J. (2018). Bacterial contamination hypothesis: A new concept in endometriosis. *Reproductive Medicine and Biology*, 17(2), 125–133. https://doi.org/10.1002/rmb2.12083

61 Endometriosis Foundation of America. (2018). *Is there a link between leaky gut and endo? This researcher thinks so.* https://www.endofound.org/is-there-a-link-between-leaky-gut-and-endo-this-researcher-thinks-so

62 Wang, J., Li, Z., Ma, X., Du, L., Jia, Z., Cui, X., Yu, L., Yang, J., Xiao, L., Zhang, B., Fan, H., & Zhao, F. (2021). Translocation of vaginal microbiota is involved in impairment and protection of uterine health. *Nature communications*, 12(1), 4191. https://doi.org/10.1038/s41467-021-24516-8; Gaiser, R. A., Halimi, A., Alkharaan, H., Lu, L., Davanian, H., Healy, K., Hugerth, L. W., Ateeb, Z., Valente, R., Fernández Moro, C., Del Chiaro, M., & Sällberg Chen, M. (2019). Enrichment of oral microbiota in early cystic precursors to invasive pancreatic cancer. *Gut*, 68(12), 2186–2194. https://doi.org/10.1136/gutjnl-2018-317458

63 Tai, F. W., Chang, C. Y., Chiang, J. H., Lin, W. C., & Wan, L. (2018). Association of pelvic inflammatory disease with risk of endometriosis: A nationwide cohort study involving 141,460 individuals. *Journal of Clinical Medicine*, 7(11), 379. https://doi.org/10.3390/jcm7110379; Lin, W. C., Chang, C. Y., Hsu, Y. A., Chiang, J. H., & Wan, L. (2016). Increased risk of endometriosis in patients with lower genital tract infection: A nationwide cohort study. *Medicine*, 95(10), e2773. https://doi.org/10.1097/MD.0000000000002773

64 Laschke, M. W., & Menger, M. D. (2016). The gut microbiota: A puppet master in the pathogenesis of endometriosis? *American Journal of Obstetrics and Gynecology*, 215(1), 68.e1–68.e4. https://doi.org/10.1016/j.ajog.2016.02.036; Wu, H. J., & Wu, E. (2012). The role of gut microbiota in immune homeostasis and autoimmunity. *Gut Microbes*, 3(1), 4–14. https://doi.org/10.4161/gmic.19320

65 Emani, R., Alam, C., Pekkala, S., Zafar, S., Emani, M. R., & Hänninen, A. (2015). Peritoneal cavity is a route for gut-derived microbial signals to promote autoimmunity in non-obese diabetic mice. *Scandinavian Journal of Immunology*, 81(2), 102–109. https://doi.org/10.1111/sji.12253

66   Cicinelli, E., Trojano, G., Mastromauro, M., Vimercati, A., Marinaccio, M., Mitola, P. C., Resta, L., & de Ziegler, D. (2017). Higher prevalence of chronic endometritis in women with endometriosis: A possible etiopathogenetic link. *Fertility and Sterility*, *108*(2), 289–295.e1. https://doi.org/10.1016/j.fertnstert.2017.05.016

67   Cicinelli, E., Matteo, M., Tinelli, R., Pinto, V., Marinaccio, M., Indraccolo, U., De Ziegler, D., & Resta, L. (2014). Chronic endometritis due to common bacteria is prevalent in women with recurrent miscarriage as confirmed by improved pregnancy outcome after antibiotic treatment. *Reproductive Sciences* (Thousand Oaks, Calif.), *21*(5), 640–647. https://doi.org/10.1177/1933719113508817

68   Khan, K. N., Fujishita, A., Kitajima, M., Hiraki, K., Nakashima, M., & Masuzaki, H. (2014). Intra-uterine microbial colonization and occurrence of endometritis in women with endometriosis†. *Human reproduction (Oxford, England)*, *29*(11), 2446–2456. https://doi.org/10.1093/humrep/deu222

69   Deb, K., Chatturvedi, M. M., Jaiswal, Y. K. (2004). Gram-negative bacterial endotoxin-induced infertility: A birds eye view. *Gynecologic and Obstetric Investigation, 57*, 224-232. https://www.doi.org/10.1159/000076761

70   Maroun, P., Cooper, M. J., Reid, G. D., & Keirse, M. J. (2009). Relevance of gastrointestinal symptoms in endometriosis. *The Australian & New Zealand Journal of Obstetrics & Gynaecology, 49*(4), 411–414. https://doi.org/10.1111/j.1479-828X.2009.01030.x; Wolthuis, A. M., Meuleman, C., Tomassetti, C., D'Hooghe, T., de Buck van Overstraeten, A., & D'Hoore, A. (2014). Bowel endometriosis: Colorectal surgeon's perspective in a multidisciplinary surgical team. *World Journal of Gastroenterology, 20*(42), 15616–15623. https://doi.org/10.3748/wjg.v20.i42.15616

71   Mathias, J. R., Franklin, R., Quast, D. C., Fraga, N., Loftin, C. A., Yates, L., & Harrison, V. (1998). Relation of endometriosis and neuromuscular disease of the gastrointestinal tract: New insights. *Fertility and Sterility, 70*(1), 81–88. https://doi.org/10.1016/s0015-0282(98)00096-x

72   Dukowicz, A. C., Lacy, B. E., & Levine, G. M. (2007). Small intestinal bacterial overgrowth: A comprehensive review. *Gastroenterology & Hepatology, 3*(2), 112–122.

73   Aragon, M., & Lessey, B. A. (2017). Irritable bowel syndrome and endometriosis: Twins in disguise. *Greenville Health System Proceedings, 2*(1), 43-50. https://hsc.ghs.org/wp-content/uploads/2016/11/GHS-Proc-Ibs-And-Endometriosis.pdf

74   Ervin, S. M., Li, H., Lim, L., Roberts, L. R., Liang, X., Mani, S., & Redinbo, M. R. (2019). Gut microbial β-glucuronidases reactivate estrogens as components of the estrobolome that reactivate estrogens. *The Journal of Biological Chemistry, 294*(49), 18586–18599. https://doi.org/10.1074/jbc.RA119.010950; Kwa, M., Plottel, C. S., Blaser, M. J., & Adams, S. (2016). The intestinal microbiome and estrogen receptor-positive female breast cancer. *Journal of the National Cancer Institute, 108*(8), djw029. https://doi.org/10.1093/jnci/djw029

75   Morris, G., Berk, M., Carvalho, A. F., Caso, J. R., Sanz, Y., & Maes, M. (2016). The role of microbiota and intestinal permeability in the pathophysiology of autoimmune

and neuroimmune processes with an emphasis on inflammatory bowel disease type 1 diabetes and chronic fatigue syndrome. *Current Pharmaceutical Design, 22*(40), 6058–6075. https://doi.org/10.2174/1381612822666160914182822; Buscarinu, M. C., Romano, S., Mechelli, R., Pizzolato Umeton, R., Ferraldeschi, M., Fornasiero, A., Reniè, R., Cerasoli, B., Morena, E., Romano, C., Loizzo, N. D., Umeton, R., Salvetti, M., & Ristori, G. (2018). Intestinal permeability in relapsing-remitting multiple sclerosis. *Neurotherapeutics: The Journal of the American Society for Experimental NeuroTherapeutics, 15*(1), 68–74. https://doi.org/10.1007/s13311-017-0582-3; Mu, Q., Kirby, J., Reilly, C. M., & Luo, X. M. (2017). Leaky gut as a danger signal for autoimmune diseases. *Frontiers in Immunology, 8*, 598. https://doi.org/10.3389/fimmu.2017.00598; Rizzetto, L., Fava, F., Tuohy, K. M., & Selmi, C. (2018). Connecting the immune system, systemic chronic inflammation and the gut microbiome: The role of sex. *Journal of Autoimmunity, 92*, 12–34. https://doi.org/10.1016/j.jaut.2018.05.008

76   Chadchan, S. B., Cheng, M., Parnell, L. A., Yin, Y., Schriefer, A., Mysorekar, I. U., & Kommagani, R. (2019). Antibiotic therapy with metronidazole reduces endometriosis disease progression in mice: A potential role for gut microbiota. *Human Reproduction* (Oxford, England), *34*(6), 1106–1116. https://doi.org/10.1093/humrep/dez041

77   Chadchan, S. B., Popli, P., Ambati, C. R., Tycksen, E., Han, S. J., Bulun, S. E., Putluri, N., Biest, S. W., & Kommagani, R. (2021). Gut microbiota-derived short-chain fatty acids protect against the progression of endometriosis. *Life Science Alliance, 4*(12), e202101224. https://doi.org/10.26508/lsa.202101224

78   Berberine may help due to its ability to help block TLR4, IL-6, IL-8, TGF-β, and VEGF.

79   Liu, L., Chen, L., Jiang, C., Guo, J., Xie, Y., Kang, L., & Cheng, Z. (2017). Berberine inhibits the LPS-induced proliferation and inflammatory response of stromal cells of adenomyosis tissues mediated by the LPS/TLR4 signaling pathway. *Experimental and Therapeutic Medicine, 14*(6), 6125–6130. https://doi.org/10.3892/etm.2017.5316

80   Ciavattini, A., Serri, M., Delli Carpini, G., Morini, S., & Clemente, N. (2017). Ovarian endometriosis and vitamin D serum levels. *Gynecological Endocrinology: The Official Journal of the International Society of Gynecological Endocrinology, 33*(2), 164–167. https://doi.org/10.1080/09513590.2016.1239254; Harris, H. R., Chavarro, J. E., Malspeis, S., Willett, W. C., & Missmer, S. A. (2013). Dairy-food, calcium, magnesium, and vitamin D intake and endometriosis: A prospective cohort study. *American Journal of Epidemiology, 177*(5), 420–430. https://doi.org/10.1093/aje/kws247

81   Horne, A. W., Ahmad, F. S., Carter, R., Simitsidellis, I., Greaves, E., Hogg, C., Morton, N. M., & Saunders, P. T. K. (2019). Repurposing dichloroacetate for the treatment of women with endometriosis. *Proceedings of the National Academy of Sciences, 116*(51), 25389-25391. https://doi.org/10.1073/pnas.1916144116

82   Chen, H., Malentacchi, F., Fambrini, M., Harrath, A. H., Huang, H., & Petraglia, F. (2020). Epigenetics of estrogen and progesterone receptors in endometriosis. *Reproductive Sciences* (Thousand Oaks, Calif.), *27*(11), 1967–1974. https://doi.org/10.1007/s43032-020-00226-2

83   Chen, H., Malentacchi, F., Fambrini, M., Harrath, A. H., Huang, H., & Petraglia, F. (2020). Epigenetics of estrogen and progesterone receptors in endometriosis. *Reproductive Sciences* (Thousand Oaks, Calif.), *27*(11), 1967–1974. https://doi.org/10.1007/s43032-020-00226-2

84   Patel, B. G., Rudnicki, M., Yu, J., Shu, Y., & Taylor, R. N. (2017). Progesterone resistance in endometriosis: Origins, consequences and interventions. *Acta Obstetricia et Gynecologica Scandinavica*, *96*(6), 623–632. https://doi.org/10.1111/aogs.13156

85   Brichant, G., Nervo, P., Albert, A., Munaut, C., Foidart, J. M., & Nisolle, M. (2018). Heterogeneity of estrogen receptor α and progesterone receptor distribution in lesions of deep infiltrating endometriosis of untreated women or during exposure to various hormonal treatments. *Gynecological endocrinology : the official journal of the International Society of Gynecological Endocrinology*, *34*(8), 651–655. https://doi.org/10.1080/09513590.2018.1433160

86   This is due to two factors. One, endometriosis cells make *aromatase*, an enzyme that turns androgens (such as testosterone) into estrogen. Aromatase is not made in the endometrium of a disease-free woman, so it's another epigenetic alteration those of us with endo have been shown to have in both normally placed endometrial cells *and* endometriosis cells. Two, when endometriosis cells are provoked by inflammation, they produce increased levels of both estradiol (the form of estrogen endo cells gobble up). Estradiol (E2) is the strongest and most prominent form of estrogen made during the reproductive years and the one most associated with endometriosis. Estradiol aggravates both the symptoms of endo (such as pain) and the pathology, meaning it directly contributes to the inflammatory scene associated with endo by fueling its growth and spread. Specifically, platelet stimulation can increase production of estradiol in endometriosis cells by 4.5x while prostaglandin-2 can stimulate aromatase production in endo by 19 to 44-fold. Together the amount could be up to 48x more estrogen. Qi, Q., Liu, X., Zhang, Q., & Guo, S. W. (2020). Platelets induce increased estrogen production through NF-κB and TGF-β1 signaling pathways in endometriotic stromal cells. *Scientific Reports*, *10*(1), 1281. https://doi.org/10.1038/s41598-020-57997-6; Noble, L. S., Takayama, K., Zeitoun, K. M., Putman, J. M., Johns, D. A., Hinshelwood, M. M., Agarwal, V. R., Zhao, Y., Carr, B. R., & Bulun, S. E. (1997). Prostaglandin E2 stimulates aromatase expression in endometriosis-derived stromal cells. *The Journal of Clinical Endocrinology and Metabolism*, *82*(2), 600–606. https://doi.org/10.1210/jcem.82.2.3783; Delvoux, B., Groothuis, P., D'Hooghe, T., Kyama, C., Dunselman, G., & Romano, A. (2009). Increased production of 17beta-estradiol in endometriosis lesions is the result of impaired metabolism. *The Journal of Clinical Endocrinology and Metabolism*, *94*(3), 876–883. https://doi.org/10.1210/jc.2008-2218; Bulun, S. E., Monsavais, D., Pavone, M. E., Dyson, M., Xue, Q., Attar, E., Tokunaga, H., & Su, E. J. (2012). Role of estrogen receptor-β in endometriosis. *Seminars in Reproductive Medicine*, *30*(1), 39–45. https://doi.org/10.1055/s-0031-1299596

87   Guo, S. W., Zhang, Q., & Liu, X. (2017). Social psychogenic stress promotes the development of endometriosis in mouse. *Reproductive Biomedicine Online*, *34*(3), 225–239. https://doi.org/10.1016/j.rbmo.2016.11.012

88   Gouin, J.-P. (2011). Chronic stress, immune dysregulation, and health. *American Journal of Lifestyle Medicine, 5*(6), 476–485. https://doi.org/10.1177/1559827610395467

89   Guo, S. W., Zhang, Q., & Liu, X. (2017). Social psychogenic stress promotes the development of endometriosis in mouse. *Reproductive Biomedicine Online, 34*(3), 225–239. https://doi.org/10.1016/j.rbmo.2016.11.012

90   Long, Q., Liu, X., Qi, Q., & Guo, S. W. (2016). Chronic stress accelerates the development of endometriosis in mouse through adrenergic receptor β2. *Human Reproduction* (Oxford, England), *31*(11), 2506–2519. https://doi.org/10.1093/humrep/dew237

91   Brasil, D. L., Montagna, E., Trevisan, C. M., La Rosa, V. L., Laganà, A. S., Barbosa, C. P., Bianco, B., & Zaia, V. (2020). Psychological stress levels in women with endometriosis: systematic review and meta-analysis of observational studies. *Minerva Medica, 111*(1), 90–102. https://doi.org/10.23736/S0026-4806.19.06350-X; Quiñones, M., Urrutia, R., Torres-Reverón, A., Vincent, K., & Flores, I. (2015). Anxiety, coping skills and hypothalamus-pituitary-adrenal (HPA) axis in patients with endometriosis. *Journal of Reproductive Biology and Health, 3*, 2. https://doi.org/10.7243/2054-0841-3-2

92   Quiñones, M., Urrutia, R., Torres-Reverón, A., Vincent, K., & Flores, I. (2015). Anxiety, coping skills and hypothalamus-pituitary-adrenal (HPA) axis in patients with endometriosis. *Journal of Reproductive Biology and Health, 3*, 2. https://doi.org/10.7243/2054-0841-3-2

93   Lima, A. P., Moura, M. D., & Rosa e Silva, A. A. (2006). Prolactin and cortisol levels in women with endometriosis. *Brazilian Journal of Medical and Biological Research = Revista brasileira de pesquisas medicas e biologicas, 39*(8), 1121–1127. https://doi.org/10.1590/s0100-879x2006000800015

94   Akhter, S., Marcus, M., Kerber, R. A., Kong, M., & Taylor, K. C. (2016). The impact of periconceptional maternal stress on fecundability. *Annals of Epidemiology, 26*(10), 710–716.e7. https://doi.org/10.1016/j.annepidem.2016.07.015

95   Chandrasekaran, A., Molparia, B., Akhtar, E., Wang, X., Lewis, J. D., Chang, J. T., Oliveira, G., Torkamani, A., & Konijeti, G. G. (2019). The autoimmune protocol diet modifies intestinal RNA expression in inflammatory bowel disease. *Crohn's & Colitis 360, 1*(3), otz016. https://doi.org/10.1093/crocol/otz016

96   Herzog, R., & Cunningham-Rundles, S. (2015). Malnutrition, immunodeficiency, and Mucosal infection. *Mucosal immunology* (fourth ed.). Retrieved November 2, 2020, from https://www.sciencedirect.com/science/article/pii/B9780124158474000744

97   Santanam, N., Kavtaradze, N., Murphy, A., Dominguez, C., & Parthasarathy, S. (2013). Antioxidant supplementation reduces endometriosis-related pelvic pain in humans. *Translational Research: The Journal of Laboratory and Clinical Medicine, 161*(3), 189–195. https://doi.org/10.1016/j.trsl.2012.05.001

98   Drake, V. J. (2022, April 14). *Micronutrient inadequacies in the US population: An overview.* Linus Pauling Institute. Retrieved April 14, 2022, from https://lpi. oregonstate.edu/mic/micronutrient-inadequacies/overview

99   Guadagni, M., & Biolo, G. (2009). Effects of inflammation and/or inactivity on the need for dietary protein. *Current Opinion in Clinical Nutrition and Metabolic Care, 12*(6), 617–622. https://doi.org/10.1097/MCO.0b013e32833193bd

100   Savaris, A. L., & do Amaral, V. F. (2011). Nutrient intake, anthropometric data and correlations with the systemic antioxidant capacity of women with pelvic endometriosis. *European Journal of Obstetrics, Gynecology, and Reproductive Biology, 158*(2), 314–318. https://doi.org/10.1016/j.ejogrb.2011.05.014

101   Ryle, P. R., & Thomson, A. D. (1984). Nutrition and vitamins in alcoholism. *Contemporary Issues in Clinical Biochemistry, 1*, 188–224; Palmery, M., Saraceno, A., Vaiarelli, A., & Carlomagno, G. (2013). Oral contraceptives and changes in nutritional requirements. *European Review for Medical and Pharmacological Sciences, 17*(13), 1804–1813.

102   de Souza e Silva, A. V., Lacativa, P. G., Russo, L. A., de Gregório, L. H., Pinheiro, R. A., & Marinheiro, L. P. (2013). Association of back pain with hypovitaminosis D in postmenopausal women with low bone mass. *BMC Musculoskeletal Disorders, 14*, 184. https://doi.org/10.1186/1471-2474-14-184; Ciavattini, A., Serri, M., Delli Carpini, G., Morini, S., & Clemente, N. (2017). Ovarian endometriosis and vitamin D serum levels. *Gynecological endocrinology : the official journal of the International Society of Gynecological Endocrinology, 33*(2), 164–167. https://doi.org/10.1080/09513590.2016.1239254

103   Halpern, G., Schor, E., & Kopelman, A. (2015). Nutritional aspects related to endometriosis. *Revista da Associacao Medica Brasileira (1992), 61*(6), 519–523. https://doi.org/10.1590/1806-9282.61.06.519

104   Harris, H. R., Chavarro, J. E., Malspeis, S., Willett, W. C., & Missmer, S. A. (2013). Dairy-food, calcium, magnesium, and vitamin D intake and endometriosis: A prospective cohort study. *American Journal of Epidemiology, 177*(5), 420–430. https://doi.org/10.1093/aje/kws247; Savaris, A. L., & do Amaral, V. F. (2011). Nutrient intake, anthropometric data and correlations with the systemic antioxidant capacity of women with pelvic endometriosis. *European Journal of Obstetrics, Gynecology, and Reproductive Biology, 158*(2), 314–318. https://doi.org/10.1016/j.ejogrb.2011.05.014; Trabert, B., Peters, U., De Roos, A., Scholes, D., & Holt, V. (2011). Diet and risk of endometriosis in a population-based case–control study. *British Journal of Nutrition, 105*(3), 459-467. https://www.doi.org/10.1017/S0007114510003661

105   Heilier, J. F., Donnez, J., Nackers, F., Rousseau, R., Verougstraete, V., Rosenkranz, K., Donnez, O., Grandjean, F., Lison, D., & Tonglet, R. (2007). Environmental and host-associated risk factors in endometriosis and deep endometriotic nodules: A matched case-control study. *Environmental Research, 103*(1), 121–129. https://doi.org/10.1016/j.envres.2006.04.004; Parazzini, F., Chiaffarino, F., Surace, M., Chatenoud, L., Cipriani, S., Chiantera, V., Benzi, G., & Fedele, L. (2004). Selected food intake and risk of endometriosis. *Human Reproduction* (Oxford, England),

19(8), 1755–1759. https://doi.org/10.1093/humrep/deh395; Trabert, B., Peters, U., De Roos, A. J., Scholes, D., & Holt, V. L. (2011). Diet and risk of endometriosis in a population-based case-control study. *The British Journal of Nutrition, 105*(3), 459–467. https://doi.org/10.1017/S0007114510003661

106   Heilier, J. F., Donnez, J., Nackers, F., Rousseau, R., Verougstraete, V., Rosenkranz, K., Donnez, O., Grandjean, F., Lison, D., & Tonglet, R. (2007). Environmental and host-associated risk factors in endometriosis and deep endometriotic nodules: A matched case-control study. *Environmental Research, 103*(1), 121–129. https://doi.org/10.1016/j.envres.2006.04.004; Parazzini, F., Chiaffarino, F., Surace, M., Chatenoud, L., Cipriani, S., Chiantera, V., Benzi, G., & Fedele, L. (2004). Selected food intake and risk of endometriosis. *Human Reproduction* (Oxford, England), *19*(8), 1755–1759. https://doi.org/10.1093/humrep/deh395; Trabert, B., Peters, U., De Roos, A. J., Scholes, D., & Holt, V. L. (2011). Diet and risk of endometriosis in a population-based case-control study. *The British Journal of Nutrition, 105*(3), 459–467. https://doi.org/10.1017/S0007114510003661; Yamamoto, A., Harris, H. R., Vitonis, A. F., Chavarro, J. E., & Missmer, S. A. (2018). A prospective cohort study of meat and fish consumption and endometriosis risk. *American Journal of Obstetrics and Gynecology, 219*(2), 178.e1–178.e10. https://doi.org/10.1016/j.ajog.2018.05.034

107   Parazzini, F. Chiaffarino, M. Surace, L. Chatenoud, S. Cipriani, V. Chiantera, G. Benzi, L. Fedele. (2004). Selected food intake and risk of endometriosis. *Human Reproduction,* 19(8), 1755–9. https://doi.org/10.1093/humrep/deh395; Trabert, B., Peters, U., De Roos, A., Scholes, D., & Holt, V. (2011). Diet and risk of endometriosis in a population-based case-control study. *British Journal of Nutrition, 105*(3), 459-467. https://doi.org/10.1017/S0007114510003661

108   Harris, H., Chavarro, J., Malspeis, S., Willett, W., Missmer, S. (2013). Dairy-food, calcium, magnesium, and vitamin D intake and endometriosis: A prospective cohort study. *American Journal of Epidemiology, 177*(5), 420–30. https://doi.org/10.1093/aje/kws247

109   Maier, J. A., Castiglioni, S., Locatelli, L., Zocchi, M., & Mazur, A. (2021). Magnesium and inflammation: Advances and perspectives. *Seminars in Cell & Developmental Biology, 115*, 37–44. https://doi.org/10.1016/j.semcdb.2020.11.002

110   Zheltova, A. A., Kharitonova, M. V., Iezhitsa, I. N., & Spasov, A. A. (2016). Magnesium deficiency and oxidative stress: An update. *BioMedicine, 6*(4), 20. https://doi.org/10.7603/s40681-016-0020-6

111   Chhabra, S., Gokhale, S., & Yadav, S. (2017). Primary dysmenorrhea and serum magnesium in young girls a pilot study. *Nessa J Gynecology, 1*(3).

112   Ebrahimi, E., Khayati Motlagh, S., Nemati, S., & Tavakoli, Z. (2012). Effects of magnesium and vitamin B6 on the severity of premenstrual syndrome symptoms. *Journal of Caring Sciences, 1*(4), 183–189. https://doi.org/10.5681/jcs.2012.026

113   Seifert, B., Wagler, P., Dartsch, S., Schmidt, U., & Nieder, J. (1989). Magnesium—eine therapeutische Alternative bei der primären Dysmenorrhoe [Magnesium—a new

therapeutic alternative in primary dysmenorrhea]. *Zentralblatt fur Gynakologie*, *111*(11), 755–760.

114   Parazzini, F., Di Martino, M., & Pellegrino, P. (2017). Magnesium in the gyneco-logical practice: A literature review. *Magnesium Research, 30*(1), 1–7. https://doi.org/10.1684/mrh.2017.0419

115   Gröber, U., Schmidt, J., Kisters, K. (2015). Magnesium in prevention and therapy. *Nutrients, 7*, 8199-226. https://doi.org/10.3390/nu7095388

116   Lai, G. L., Yeh, C. C., Yeh, C. Y., Chen, R. Y., Fu, C. L., Chen, C. H., & Tzeng, C. R. (2017). Decreased zinc and increased lead blood levels are associated with endometriosis in Asian women. *Reproductive Toxicology* (Elmsford, NY), *74*, 77–84. https://doi.org/10.1016/j.reprotox.2017.09.001

117   Messalli, E. M., Schettino, M. T., Mainini, G., Ercolano, S., Fuschillo, G., Falcone, F., Esposito, E., Di Donna, M. C., De Franciscis, P., & Torella, M. (2014). The possible role of zinc in the etiopathogenesis of endometriosis. *Clinical and Experimental Obstetrics & Gynecology, 41*(5), 541–546.

118   Tian, X., & Diaz, F. J. (2013). Acute dietary zinc deficiency before conception com-promises oocyte epigenetic programming and disrupts embryonic development. *Developmental Biology, 376*(1), 51–61. https://doi.org/10.1016/j.ydbio.2013.01.015

119   Gammoh, N. Z., & Rink, L. (2017). Zinc in infection and inflammation. *Nutrients, 9*(6), 624. https://doi.org/10.3390/nu9060624

120   Eby, G. A. (2007). Zinc treatment prevents dysmenorrhea. *Medical Hypotheses, 69*(2), 297–301. https://doi.org/10.1016/j.mehy.2006.12.009

121   Foster, M., Chu, A., Petocz, P., & Samman, S. (2013). Effect of vegetarian diets on zinc status: A systematic review and meta-analysis of studies in humans. *Journal of the Sci-ence of Food and Agriculture, 93*(10), 2362–2371. https://doi.org/10.1002/jsfa.6179

122   Chavarro, J. E., Rich-Edwards, J. W., Rosner, B. A., & Willett, W. C. (2006). Iron intake and risk of ovulatory infertility. *Obstetrics and Gynecology, 108*(5), 1145–1152. https://doi.org/10.1097/01.AOG.0000238333.37423.ab; Soyano, A., & Gómez, M. (1999). Participación del hierro en la inmunidad y su relación con las infecciones [Role of iron in immunity and its relation with infections]. *Archivos Latinoamericanos de Nutricion, 49*(3 Suppl 2), 40S–46S.

123   Isler, M., Delibas, N., Guclu, M., Gultekin, F., Sutcu, R., Bahceci, M., & Kosar, A. (2002). Superoxide dismutase and glutathione peroxidase in erythrocytes of patients with iron deficiency anemia: Effects of different treatment modalities. *Croatian Medical Journal, 43*(1), 16–19.

124   Kurtoglu, E., Ugur, A., Baltaci, A. K., & Undar, L. (2003). Effect of iron supplementa-tion on oxidative stress and antioxidant status in iron-deficiency anemia. *Biological Trace Element Research, 96*(1-3), 117–123. https://doi.org/10.1385/BTER:96:1-3:117

125   Atkins, H. M., Appt, S. E., Taylor, R. N., Torres-Mendoza, Y., Lenk, E. E., Rosenthal, N. S., & Caudell, D. L. (2018). Systemic iron deficiency in a nonhuman primate model of endometriosis. *Comparative Medicine*, *68*(4), 298–307. https://doi.org/10.30802/AALAS-CM-17-000082

126   Haider, L. M., Schwingshackl, L., Hoffmann, G., & Ekmekcioglu, C. (2018). The effect of vegetarian diets on iron status in adults: A systematic review and meta-analysis. *Critical Reviews in Food Science and Nutrition*, *58*(8), 1359–1374. https://doi.org/10.1080/10408398.2016.1259210

127   Zijp, I. M., Korver, O., & Tijburg, L. B. (2000). Effect of tea and other dietary factors on iron absorption. *Critical Reviews in Food Science and Nutrition*, *40*(5), 371–398. https://doi.org/10.1080/10408690091189194

128   Hallberg, L., & Hulthén, L. (2000). Prediction of dietary iron absorption: An algorithm for calculating absorption and bioavailability of dietary iron. *The American Journal of Clinical Nutrition*, *71*(5), 1147–1160. https://doi.org/10.1093/ajcn/71.5.1147

129   Brittin, H. C., & Nossaman, C. E. (1986). Iron content of food cooked in iron utensils. *Journal of the American Dietetic Association*, *86*(7), 897–901.

130   Huang, Z., Liu, Y., Qi, G., Brand, D., & Zheng, S. G. (2018). Role of vitamin A in the immune system. *Journal of Clinical Medicine*, *7*(9), 258. https://doi.org/10.3390/jcm7090258

131   Shmarakov, I. O., Borschovetska, V. L., & Blaner, W. S. (2017). Hepatic detoxification of bisphenol A is retinoid-dependent. *Toxicological Sciences: An Official Journal of the Society of Toxicology*, *157*(1), 141–155. https://doi.org/10.1093/toxsci/kfx022; Clagett-Dame, M., & Knutson, D. (2011). Vitamin A in reproduction and development. *Nutrients*, *3*(4), 385–428. https://doi.org/10.3390/nu3040385

132   Li, L., Gao, H., Pan, L., Zhao, Y., Liang, Z., Zhang, Q., & Wang, D. (2021). All-trans retinoic acid inhibits epithelial-to-mesenchymal transition (EMT) through the down-regulation of IL-6 in endometriosis. *Annals of Palliative Medicine*, *10*(11), 11348–11361. https://doi.org/10.21037/apm-21-2175

133   Pavone, M. E., Malpani, S. S., Dyson, M., Kim, J. J., & Bulun, S. E. (2016). Fenretinide: A potential treatment for endometriosis. *Reproductive Sciences* (Thousand Oaks, Calif.), *23*(9), 1139–1147. https://doi.org/10.1177/1933719116632920

134   Drake, V. (2021). *Micronutrient inadequacies in the US population: An overview.* Linus Pauling Institute. https://lpi.oregonstate.edu/mic/micronutrient-inadequacies/overview#vitamin-A

135   Tanumihardjo, S. A. (2004). Assessing vitamin A status: Past, present and future. *The Journal of Nutrition*, *134*(1), 290S–293S. https://doi.org/10.1093/jn/134.1.290S; Tanumihardjo, S. A., Russell, R. M., Stephensen, C. B., Gannon, B. M., Craft, N. E., Haskell, M. J., Lietz, G., Schulze, K., & Raiten, D. J. (2016). Biomarkers of nutrition for development (BOND)—vitamin A review. *The Journal of Nutrition*, *146*(9), 1816S–48S. https://doi.org/10.3945/jn.115.229708

136   Simonne, A.H., Green, N.R., Bransby, D.I. (1996). Consumer acceptability and p-carotene content of beef as related to cattle finishing diets. *Food Sci, 61*(6), 1254-1257. https://doi.org/10.1111/j.1365-2621.1996.tb10973.x

137   Tang, G. (2010). Bioconversion of dietary provitamin A carotenoids to vitamin A in humans. *The American Journal of Clinical Nutrition, 91*(5), 1468S–1473S. https://doi.org/10.3945/ajcn.2010.28674G

138   Ciavattini, A., Serri, M., Delli Carpini, G., Morini, S., & Clemente, N. (2017). Ovarian endometriosis and vitamin D serum levels. *Gynecological Endocrinology: The Official Journal of the International Society of Gynecological Endocrinology, 33*(2), 164–167. https://doi.org/10.1080/09513590.2016.1239254

139   Harris, H. R., Chavarro, J. E., Malspeis, S., Willett, W. C., & Missmer, S. A. (2013). Dairy-food, calcium, magnesium, and vitamin D intake and endometriosis: A prospective cohort study. *American Journal of Epidemiology, 177*(5), 420–430. https://doi.org/10.1093/aje/kws247

140   Miyashita, M., Koga, K., Izumi, G., Sue, F., Makabe, T., Taguchi, A., Nagai, M., Urata, Y., Takamura, M., Harada, M., Hirata, T., Hirota, Y., Wada-Hiraike, O., Fujii, T., & Osuga, Y. (2016). Effects of 1,25-dihydroxy vitamin D3 on endometriosis. *The Journal of Clinical Endocrinology and Metabolism, 101*(6), 2371–2379. https://doi.org/10.1210/jc.2016-1515

141   Paffoni, A., Ferrari, S., Viganò, P., Pagliardini, L., Papaleo, E., Candiani, M., Tirelli, A., Fedele, L., & Somigliana, E. (2014). Vitamin D deficiency and infertility: Insights from in vitro fertilization cycles. *The Journal of Clinical Endocrinology and Metabolism, 99*(11), E2372–E2376. https://doi.org/10.1210/jc.2014-1802

142   Ozkan, S., Jindal, S., Greenseid, K., Shu, J., Zeitlian, G., Hickmon, C., & Pal, L. (2010). Replete vitamin D stores predict reproductive success following in vitro fertilization. *Fertility and Sterility, 94*(4), 1314–1319. https://doi.org/10.1016/j.fertnstert.2009.05.019

143   Santanam, N., Kavtaradze, N., Murphy, A., Dominguez, C., & Parthasarathy, S. (2013). Antioxidant supplementation reduces endometriosis-related pelvic pain in humans. *Translational Research: The Journal of Laboratory and Clinical Medicine, 161*(3), 189–195. https://doi.org/10.1016/j.trsl.2012.05.001

144   Mier-Cabrera, J., Aburto-Soto, T., Burrola-Méndez, S., Jiménez-Zamudio, L., Tolentino, M. C., Casanueva, E., & Hernández-Guerrero, C. (2009). Women with endometriosis improved their peripheral antioxidant markers after the application of a high antioxidant diet. *Reproductive Biology and Endocrinology: RB&E, 7*, 54. https://doi.org/10.1186/1477-7827-7-54

145   Henmi, H., Endo, T., Kitajima, Y., Manase, K., Hata, H., & Kudo, R. (2003). Effects of ascorbic acid supplementation on serum progesterone levels in patients with a luteal phase defect. *Fertility and Sterility, 80*(2), 459–461. https://doi.org/10.1016/s0015-0282(03)00657-5

146 Vural, P., Akgül, C., Yildirim, A., & Canbaz, M. (2000). Antioxidant defence in recurrent abortion. *Clinica Chimica Acta: International Journal of Clinical Chemistry*, *295*(1-2), 169–177. https://doi.org/10.1016/s0009-8981(99)00255-7

147 Cohen, S. P., & Mao, J. (2014). Neuropathic pain: Mechanisms and their clinical implications. *BMJ (Clinical Research Ed.)*, *348*, f7656. https://doi.org/10.1136/bmj.f7656

148 Erten, O. U., Ensari, T. A., Dilbaz, B., Cakiroglu, H., Altinbas, S. K., Çaydere, M., & Goktolga, U. (2016). Vitamin C is effective for the prevention and regression of endometriotic implants in an experimentally induced rat model of endometriosis. *Taiwanese Journal of Obstetrics & Gynecology*, *55*(2), 251–257. https://doi.org/10.1016/j.tjog.2015.07.004

149 Drake, V. (2021, January 27). *Micronutrient inadequacies in the US population: An overview*. Linus Pauling Institute. https://lpi.oregonstate.edu/mic/micronutrient-inadequacies/overview#vitamin-A

150 Livdans-Forret, A. B., Harvey, P. J., & Larkin-Thier, S. M. (2007). Menorrhagia: A synopsis of management focusing on herbal and nutritional supplements, and chiropractic. *The Journal of the Canadian Chiropractic Association*, *51*(4), 235–246.

151 Carr, A. C., & McCall, C. (2017). The role of vitamin C in the treatment of pain: New insights. *Journal of Translational Medicine*, *15*(1), 77. https://doi.org/10.1186/s12967-017-1179-7; Ellulu, M. S., Rahmat, A., Patimah, I., Khaza'ai, H., & Abed, Y. (2015). Effect of vitamin C on inflammation and metabolic markers in hypertensive and/or diabetic obese adults: A randomized controlled trial. *Drug Design, Development and Therapy*, *9*, 3405–3412. https://doi.org/10.2147/DDDT.S83144; Crha, I., Hrubá, D., Ventruba, P., Fiala, J., Totusek, J., & Visnová, H. (2003). Ascorbic acid and infertility treatment. *Central European Journal of Public Health*, *11*(2), 63–67.

152 Santanam, N., Kavtaradze, N., Murphy, A., Dominguez, C., & Parthasarathy, S. (2013). Antioxidant supplementation reduces endometriosis-related pelvic pain in humans. *Translational Research: The Journal of Laboratory and Clinical Medicine*, *161*(3), 189–195. https://doi.org/10.1016/j.trsl.2012.05.001

153 Barrett, D., Rickman, J., & Bruhn, C. (2007). Nutritional comparison of fresh, frozen, and canned fruits and vegetables II. Vitamin A and carotenoids, vitamin E, minerals and fiber. *Journal of the Science of Food and Agriculture*, *87*, 1185–1196. https://doi.org/10.1002/jsfa.2824

154 Netsu, S., Konno, R., Odagiri, K., Soma, M., Fujiwara, H., & Suzuki, M. (2008). Oral eicosapentaenoic acid supplementation as possible therapy for endometriosis. *Fertility and Sterility*, *90*(4 Suppl), 1496–1502. https://doi.org/10.1016/j.fertnstert.2007.08.014

155 Covens, A. L., Christopher, P., & Casper, R. F. (1988). The effect of dietary supplementation with fish oil fatty acids on surgically induced endometriosis in the rabbit. *Fertility and Sterility*, *49*(4), 698–703. https://doi.org/10.1016/s0015-0282(16)59842-2; Akyol, A., Şimşek, M., İlhan, R., Can, B., Baspinar, M., Akyol, H., Gül, H. F., Gürsu, F., Kavak, B., & Akın, M. (2016). Efficacies of vitamin D and

omega-3 polyunsaturated fatty acids on experimental endometriosis. *Taiwanese Journal of Obstetrics & Gynecology, 55*(6), 835–839. https://doi.org/10.1016/j. tjog.2015.06.018

156   Tomio, K., Kawana, K., Taguchi, A., Isobe, Y., Iwamoto, R., Yamashita, A., Kojima, S., Mori, M., Nagamatsu, T., Arimoto, T., Oda, K., Osuga, Y., Taketani, Y., Kang, J. X., Arai, H., Arita, M., Kozuma, S., & Fujii, T. (2013). Omega-3 polyunsaturated fatty acids suppress the cystic lesion formation of peritoneal endometriosis in transgenic mouse models. *PloS One, 8*(9), e73085. https://doi.org/10.1371/journal. pone.0073085

157   Gazvani, M. R., Smith, L., Haggarty, P., Fowler, P. A., & Templeton, A. (2001). High omega-3:omega-6 fatty acid ratios in culture medium reduce endometrial-cell survival in combined endometrial gland and stromal cell cultures from women with and without endometriosis. *Fertility and Sterility, 76*(4), 717–722. https://doi. org/10.1016/s0015-0282(01)01991-4

158   Wu, M. H., Lu, C. W., Chuang, P. C., & Tsai, S. J. (2010). Prostaglandin E2: The master of endometriosis? *Experimental Biology and Medicine* (Maywood, NJ), *235*(6), 668–677. https://doi.org/10.1258/ebm.2010.009321

159   Weylandt, K. H., Chen, Y. Q., Lim, K., Su, H. M., Cittadini, A., & Calviello, G. (2015). ω-3 PUFAs in the prevention and cure of inflammatory, degenerative, and neoplastic diseases 2014. *BioMed Research International, 2015,* 695875. https://doi. org/10.1155/2015/695875

160   Stark, K. D., Van Elswyk, M. E., Higgins, M. R., Weatherford, C. A., & Salem, N., Jr (2016). Global survey of the omega-3 fatty acids, docosahexaenoic acid and eicosapentaenoic acid in the blood stream of healthy adults. *Progress in Lipid Research, 63,* 132–152. https://doi.org/10.1016/j.plipres.2016.05.001

161   Thuppal, S. V., von Schacky, C., Harris, W. S., Sherif, K. D., Denby, N., Steinbaum, S. R., Haycock, B., & Bailey, R. L. (2017). Discrepancy between knowledge and perceptions of dietary omega-3 fatty acid intake compared with the omega-3 index. *Nutrients, 9*(9), 930. https://doi.org/10.3390/nu9090930

162   Gerster, H. (1998). Can adults adequately convert alpha-linolenic acid (18:3n-3) to eicosapentaenoic acid (20:5n-3) and docosahexaenoic acid (22:6n-3)? *International Journal for Vitamin and Nutrition Research, 68*(3), 159–173.

163   Bruner-Tran, K. L., Osteen, K. G., Taylor, H. S., Sokalska, A., Haines, K., & Duleba, A. J. (2011). Resveratrol inhibits development of experimental endometriosis in vivo and reduces endometrial stromal cell invasiveness in vitro. *Biology of Reproduction, 84*(1), 106–112. https://doi.org/10.1095/biolreprod.110.086744; Ergenoğlu, A. M., Yeniel, A. Ö., Erbaş, O., Aktuğ, H., Yildirim, N., Ulukuş, M., & Taskiran, D. (2013). Regression of endometrial implants by resveratrol in an experimentally induced endometriosis model in rats. *Reproductive Sciences* (Thousand Oaks, Calif.), *20*(10), 1230–1236. https://doi.org/10.1177/1933719113483014; Ricci, A. G., Olivares, C. N., Bilotas, M. A., Bastón, J. I., Singla, J. J., Meresman, G. F., & Barañao, R. I. (2013). Natural therapies assessment for the treatment of endometriosis. *Human Reproduction*

(Oxford, England), *28*(1), 178–188. https://doi.org/10.1093/humrep/des369; Ozcan Cenksoy, P., Oktem, M., Erdem, O., Karakaya, C., Cenksoy, C., Erdem, A., Guner, H., & Karabacak, O. (2015). A potential novel treatment strategy: Inhibition of angiogenesis and inflammation by resveratrol for regression of endometriosis in an experimental rat model. *Gynecological Endocrinology: The Official Journal of the International Society of Gynecological Endocrinology, 31*(3), 219–224. https://doi.org/10.3109/0 9513590.2014.976197; Bayoglu Tekin, Y., Guven, S., Kirbas, A., Kalkan, Y., Tumkaya, L., & Guvendag Guven, E. S. (2015). Is resveratrol a potential substitute for leuprolide acetate in experimental endometriosis? *European Journal of Obstetrics, Gynecology, and Reproductive Biology, 184*, 1–6. https://doi.org/10.1016/j.ejogrb.2014.10.041

164   Yavuz, S., Aydin, N. E., Celik, O., Yilmaz, E., Ozerol, E., & Tanbek, K. (2014). Resveratrol successfully treats experimental endometriosis through modulation of oxidative stress and lipid peroxidation. *Journal of Cancer Research and Therapeutics, 10*(2), 324–329. https://doi.org/10.4103/0973-1482.136619

165   Zhang, Y., Cao, H., Yu, Z., Peng, H. Y., & Zhang, C. J. (2013). Curcumin inhibits endometriosis endometrial cells by reducing estradiol production. *Iranian Journal of Reproductive Medicine, 11*(5), 415–422.

166   Chowdhury, I., Banerjee, S., Driss, A., Xu, W., Mehrabi, S., Nezhat, C., Sidell, N., Taylor, R. N., & Thompson, W. E. (2019). Curcumin attenuates proangiogenic and proinflammatory factors in human eutopic endometrial stromal cells through the NF-κB signaling pathway. *Journal of Cellular Physiology, 234*(5), 6298–6312. https://doi.org/10.1002/jcp.27360

167   Kohama, T., Herai, K., & Inoue, M. (2007). Effect of French maritime pine bark extract on endometriosis as compared with leuprorelin acetate. *The Journal of Reproductive Medicine, 52*(8), 703–708.

168   Maia, H., Jr, Haddad, C., & Casoy, J. (2013). Combining oral contraceptives with a natural nuclear factor-kappa B inhibitor for the treatment of endometriosis-related pain. *International Journal of Women's Health, 6*, 35–39. https://doi.org/10.2147/ IJWH.S55210

169   Xu, H., Lui, W. T., Chu, C. Y., Ng, P. S., Wang, C. C., & Rogers, M. S. (2009). Anti-angiogenic effects of green tea catechin on an experimental endometriosis mouse model. *Human Reproduction* (Oxford, England), *24*(3), 608–618. https://doi.org/10.1093/ humrep/den417

170   Laschke, M. W., Schwender, C., Scheuer, C., Vollmar, B., & Menger, M. D. (2008). Epigallocatechin-3-gallate inhibits estrogen-induced activation of endometrial cells in vitro and causes regression of endometriotic lesions in vivo. *Human Reproduction* (Oxford, England), *23*(10), 2308–2318. https://doi.org/10.1093/humrep/den245

171   Nahari, E., & Razi, M. (2018). Silymarin amplifies apoptosis in ectopic endometrial tissue in rats with endometriosis; implication on growth factor GDNF, ERK1/2 and Bcl-6b expression. *Acta Histochemica, 120*(8), 757–767. https://doi.org/10.1016/j. acthis.2018.08.003

172   Ilhan, M., Ali, Z.. Khan, I.,Taştan, H., & Akkol, E.K. (2020). The regression of endo-metriosis with glycosylated flavonoids isolated from *Melilotus officinalis* (L.) Pall. in an endometriosis rat model. *Taiwanese Journal of Obstetrics and Gynecology*, *59*(2), 211-219. https://doi.org/10.1016/j.tjog.2020.01.008

173   Park, S., Lim, W., Bazer, F. W., Whang, K. Y., & Song, G. (2019). Quercetin inhibits proliferation of endometriosis regulating cyclin D1 and its target microRNAs in vitro and in vivo. *The Journal of Nutritional Biochemistry*, *63*, 87–100. https://doi.org/10.1016/j.jnutbio.2018.09.024

174   Rossi, M., Edefonti, V., Parpinel, M., Lagiou, P., Franchi, M., Ferraroni, M., Decarli, A., Zucchetto, A., Serraino, D., Dal Maso, L., Negri, E., & La Vecchia, C. (2013). Proanthocyanidins and other flavonoids in relation to endometrial cancer risk: A case-control study in Italy. *British Journal of Cancer*, *109*(7), 1914–1920. https://doi.org/10.1038/bjc.2013.447

175   Martínez Steele, E., Baraldi, L. G., Louzada, M. L., Moubarac, J. C., Mozaffarian, D., & Monteiro, C. A. (2016). Ultra-processed foods and added sugars in the US diet: Evidence from a nationally representative cross-sectional study. *BMJ Open*, *6*(3), e009892. https://doi.org/10.1136/bmjopen-2015-009892

176   Ramasamy, R., Vannucci, S. J., Yan, S. S., Herold, K., Yan, S. F., & Schmidt, A. M. (2005). Advanced glycation end products and RAGE: A common thread in aging, diabetes, neurodegeneration, and inflammation. *Glycobiology*, *15*(7), 16R–28R. https://doi.org/10.1093/glycob/cwi053

177   Fujii, E. Y., Nakayama, M., & Nakagawa, A. (2008). Concentrations of receptor for advanced glycation end products, VEGF and CML in plasma, follicular fluid, and peri-toneal fluid in women with and without endometriosis. *Reproductive Sciences* (Thou-sand Oaks, Calif.), *15*(10), 1066–1074. https://doi.org/10.1177/1933719108323445

178   Bloemer, J., Bhattacharya, S., Amin, R., & Suppiramaniam, V. (2014). Impaired insulin signaling and mechanisms of memory loss. *Progress in Molecular Biology and Translational Science*, *121*, 413–449. https://doi.org/10.1016/B978-0-12-800101-1.00013-2

179   Horne, A.W., Ahmad, F.S., Carter, R., Simitsidellis, I., Greaves, E., Hogg, C., Morton, N.M., & Saunders, P.T.K. (2019). Repurposing dichloroacetate for the treatment of women with endometriosis. *Proceedings of the National Academy of Sciences*, *116*(51), 25389-25391. https://doi.org/10.1073/pnas.1916144116

180   Zheng, J., Dai, Y., Lin, X., Huang, Q., Shi, L., Jin, X., Liu, N., Zhou, F., & Zhang, S. (2021). Hypoxia-induced lactate dehydrogenase A protects cells from apoptosis in endometriosis. *Molecular Medicine Reports*, *24*(3), 637. https://doi.org/10.3892/mmr.2021.12276; Choi, S. Y., Collins, C. C., Gout, P. W., & Wang, Y. (2013). Can-cer-generated lactic acid: A regulatory, immunosuppressive metabolite? *The Journal of Pathology*, *230*(4), 350–355. https://doi.org/10.1002/path.4218

181   Hirschhaeuser, F., Sattler, U. G., & Mueller-Klieser, W. (2011). Lactate: A metabolic key player in cancer. *Cancer Research, 71*(22), 6921–6925. https://doi.org/10.1158/0008-5472.CAN-11-1457

182   David, L. A., Maurice, C. F., Carmody, R. N., Gootenberg, D. B., Button, J. E., Wolfe, B. E., Ling, A. V., Devlin, A. S., Varma, Y., Fischbach, M. A., Biddinger, S. B., Dutton, R. J., & Turnbaugh, P. J. (2014). Diet rapidly and reproducibly alters the human gut microbiome. *Nature, 505*(7484), 559–563. https://doi.org/10.1038/nature12820

183   Gupta, R. K., Gangoliya, S. S., & Singh, N. K. (2015). Reduction of phytic acid and enhancement of bioavailable micronutrients in food grains. *Journal of Food Science and Technology, 52*(2), 676–684. https://doi.org/10.1007/s13197-013-0978-y

184   Guadagni, M., & Biolo, G. (2009). Effects of inflammation and/or inactivity on the need for dietary protein. *Current Opinion in Clinical Nutrition and Metabolic Care, 12*(6), 617–622. https://doi.org/10.1097/MCO.0b013e32833193bd

185   Cruzat, V., Macedo Rogero, M., Noel Keane, K., Curi, R., & Newsholme, P. (2018). Glutamine: Metabolism and immune function, supplementation and clinical translation. *Nutrients, 10*(11), 1564. https://doi.org/10.3390/nu10111564

186   Lu, H., Hu, H., Yang, Y., & Li, S. (2020). The inhibition of reactive oxygen species (ROS) by antioxidants inhibits the release of an autophagy marker in ectopic endometrial cells. *Taiwanese Journal of Obstetrics & Gynecology, 59*(2), 256–261. https://doi.org/10.1016/j.tjog.2020.01.014

187   Porpora, M. G., Brunelli, R., Costa, G., Imperiale, L., Krasnowska, E. K., Lundeberg, T., Nofroni, I., Piccioni, M. G., Pittaluga, E., Ticino, A., & Parasassi, T. (2013). A promise in the treatment of endometriosis: An observational cohort study on ovarian endometrioma reduction by N-acetylcysteine. *Evidence-Based Complementary and Alternative Medicine: eCAM, 2013*, 240702. https://doi.org/10.1155/2013/240702

188   Zhong, Z., Wheeler, M. D., Li, X., Froh, M., Schemmer, P., Yin, M., Bunzendaul, H., Bradford, B., & Lemasters, J. J. (2003). L-glycine: A novel antiinflammatory, immunomodulatory, and cytoprotective agent. *Current Opinion in Clinical Nutrition and Metabolic Care, 6*(2), 229–240. https://doi.org/10.1097/00075197-200303000-00013

189   Meléndez-Hevia, E., De Paz-Lugo, P., Cornish-Bowden, A., & Cárdenas, M. L. (2009). A weak link in metabolism: The metabolic capacity for glycine biosynthesis does not satisfy the need for collagen synthesis. *Journal of Biosciences, 34*(6), 853–872. https://doi.org/10.1007/s12038-009-0100-9

190   See: Saturated fat and endometriosis–diet myth debunked at https://www.healendo.com/blog-1/2020/6/16/saturatedfat

191   Deol, P., Fahrmann, J., Yang, J., Evans, J. R., Rizo, A., Grapov, D., Salemi, M., Wanichthanarak, K., Fiehn, O., Phinney, B., Hammock, B. D., & Sladek, F. M. (2017). Omega-6 and omega-3 oxylipins are implicated in soybean oil-induced obesity in mice. *Scientific Reports, 7*(1), 12488. https://doi.org/10.1038/s41598-017-12624-9

192   Blasbalg, T. L., Hibbeln, J. R., Ramsden, C. E., Majchrzak, S. F., & Rawlings, R. R. (2011). Changes in consumption of omega-3 and omega-6 fatty acids in the United States during the 20th century. *The American Journal of Clinical Nutrition, 93*(5), 950–962. https://doi.org/10.3945/ajcn.110.006643

193   *Nutrition data: Know what you eat:* https://nutritiondata.self.com/

194   Cai, F., Dupertuis, Y. M., & Pichard, C. (2012). Role of polyunsaturated fatty acids and lipid peroxidation on colorectal cancer risk and treatments. *Current Opinion in Clinical Nutrition and Metabolic Care, 15*(2), 99–106. https://doi.org/10.1097/MCO.0b013e32834feab4

195   Keshavarzian, A., Farhadi, A., Forsyth, C. B., Rangan, J., Jakate, S., Shaikh, M., Banan, A., & Fields, J. Z. (2009). Evidence that chronic alcohol exposure promotes intestinal oxidative stress, intestinal hyperpermeability and endotoxemia prior to development of alcoholic steatohepatitis in rats. *Journal of Hepatology, 50*(3), 538–547. https://doi.org/10.1016/j.jhep.2008.10.028; Wang, H. J., Zakhari, S., & Jung, M. K. (2010). Alcohol, inflammation, and gut-liver-brain interactions in tissue damage and disease development. *World Journal of Gastroenterology, 16*(11), 1304–1313. https://doi.org/10.3748/wjg.v16.i11.1304

196   Al-Sader, H., Abdul-Jabar, H., Allawi, Z., & Haba, Y. (2009). Alcohol and breast cancer: The mechanisms explained. *Journal of Clinical Medicine Research, 1*(3), 125–131. https://doi.org/10.4021/jocmr2009.07.1246

197   Bold, J., & Rostami, K. (2015). Non-coeliac gluten sensitivity and reproductive disorders. *Gastroenterology and Hepatology from Bed to Bench, 8*(4), 294–297.

198   Marziali, M., Venza, M., Lazzaro, S., Lazzaro, A., Micossi, C., & Stolfi, V. M. (2012). Gluten-free diet: A new strategy for management of painful endometriosis related symptoms? *Minerva Chirurgica, 67*(6), 499–504.

199   Bernardo, D., Garrote, J. A., Fernández-Salazar, L., Riestra, S., & Arranz, E. (2007). Is gliadin really safe for non-coeliac individuals? Production of interleukin 15 in biopsy culture from non-coeliac individuals challenged with gliadin peptides. *Gut, 56*(6), 889–890. https://doi.org/10.1136/gut.2006.118265

200   Stephansson, O., Falconer, H., & Ludvigsson, J. F. (2011). Risk of endometriosis in 11,000 women with celiac disease. *Human Reproduction* (Oxford, England), *26*(10), 2896–2901. https://doi.org/10.1093/humrep/der263

201   Caserta, D., Matteucci, E., Ralli, E., Bordi, G., & Moscarini, M. (2014). Celiac disease and endometriosis: An insidious and worrisome association hard to diagnose: A case report. *Clinical and Experimental Obstetrics & Gynecology, 41*(3), 346–348.

202   Fan, M. S., Zhao, F. J., Fairweather-Tait, S. J., Poulton, P. R., Dunham, S. J., & McGrath, S. P. (2008). Evidence of decreasing mineral density in wheat grain over the last 160 years. *Journal of Trace Elements in Medicine and Biology: Organ of the Society for Minerals and Trace Elements (GMS), 22*(4), 315–324. https://doi.org/10.1016/j.jtemb.2008.07.002; Temkin, A., & Naidenko, O. (2021). *Glyphosate contamination*

in food goes far beyond oat products. Environmental Working Group. https://www.ewg.org/news-insights/news/glyphosate-contamination-food-goes-far-beyond-oat-products

203   Read the extensive research here: https://www.healendo.com/blog-1/redmeat

204   Afrin, S., AlAshqar, A., El Sabeh, M., Miyashita-Ishiwata, M., Reschke, L., Brennan, J. T., Fader, A., & Borahay, M. A. (2021). Diet and nutrition in gynecological disorders: A focus on clinical studies. *Nutrients, 13*(6), 1747. https://doi.org/10.3390/nu13061747; Helbig, M., Vesper, A. S., Beyer, I., & Fehm, T. (2021). Does nutrition affect endometriosis? *Geburtshilfe und Frauenheilkunde, 81*(2), 191–199. https://doi.org/10.1055/a-1207-0557

205   Rohrmann, S., Overvad, K., Bueno-de-Mesquita, H. B., Jakobsen, M. U., Egeberg, R., Tjønneland, A., Nailler, L., Boutron-Ruault, M. C., Clavel-Chapelon, F., Krogh, V., Palli, D., Panico, S., Tumino, R., Ricceri, F., Bergmann, M. M., Boeing, H., Li, K., Kaaks, R., Khaw, K. T., Wareham, N. J., … Linseisen, J. (2013). Meat consumption and mortality—results from the European Prospective Investigation into cancer and nutrition. *BMC Medicine, 11*, 63. https://doi.org/10.1186/1741-7015-11-63

206   Van Elswyk, M. E., & McNeill, S. H. (2014). Impact of grass/forage feeding versus grain finishing on beef nutrients and sensory quality: The U.S. experience. *Meat Science, 96*(1), 535–540. https://doi.org/10.1016/j.meatsci.2013.08.010; Daley, C. A., Abbott, A., Doyle, P. S., Nader, G. A., & Larson, S. (2010). A review of fatty acid profiles and antioxidant content in grass-fed and grain-fed beef. *Nutrition Journal, 9*, 10. https://doi.org/10.1186/1475-2891-9-10

207   Ribas-Agustí, A., Díaz, I., Sárraga, C., García-Regueiro, J. A., & Castellari, M. (2019). Nutritional properties of organic and conventional beef meat at retail. *Journal of the Science of Food and Agriculture, 99*(9), 4218–4225. https://doi.org/10.1002/jsfa.9652

208   *Food Safety and Inspection Service: Safe and suitable ingredients used in the production of meat, poultry and egg products—revision 55.* United States Department of Agriculture. https://www.fsis.usda.gov/policy/fsis-directives/7120.1; *Glyphosate; tolerances for residues.* Electronic Code of Federal Regulations (eCFR). https://www.ecfr.gov/cgi-bin/text-idx?SID=2c85909360c7c5aff63ddd1447545d6a&mc=true&node=se40.24.180_1364&rgn=div8

209   Meat Eater's Guide. (2011). *Meat Eater's Guide to Climate Change + Health.* Environmental Working Group. https://www.ewg.org/meateatersguide/a-meat-eaters-guide-to-climate-change-health-what-you-eat-matters/climate-and-environmental-impacts/

210   O'Callaghan, T. F., Faulkner, H., McAuliffe, S., O'Sullivan, M. G., Hennessy, D., Dillon, P., Kilcawley, K. N., Stanton, C., & Ross, R. P. (2016). Quality characteristics, chemical composition, and sensory properties of butter from cows on pasture versus indoor feeding systems. *Journal of Dairy Science, 99*(12), 9441–9460. https://doi.org/10.3168/jds.2016-11271; Pustjens, A. M., Boerrigter-Eenling, R., Koot, A. H., Rozijn, M., & van Ruth, S. M. (2017). Characterization of retail conventional,

organic, and grass full-fat butters by their fat contents, free fatty acid contents, and triglyceride and fatty acid profiling. *Foods* (Basel, Switzerland), *6*(4), 26. https://doi. org/10.3390/foods6040026

211   González, S., Fernández-Navarro, T., Arboleya, S., de Los Reyes-Gavilán, C. G., Salazar, N., & Gueimonde, M. (2019). Fermented dairy foods: Impact on intestinal microbiota and health-linked biomarkers. *Frontiers in Microbiology, 10*, 1046. https://doi.org/10.3389/fmicb.2019.01046

212   Kuellenberg de Gaudry, D., Lohner, S., Bischoff, K., Schmucker, C., Hoerrlein, S., Roeger, C., Schwingshackl, L., & Meerpohl, J. J. (2022). A1- and A2 beta-casein on health-related outcomes: a scoping review of animal studies. *European journal of nutrition, 61*(1), 1–21. https://doi.org/10.1007/s00394-021-02551-x

213   Ul Haq, M. R., Kapila, R., Sharma, R., Saliganti, V., & Kapila, S. (2014). Comparative evaluation of cow β-casein variants (A1/A2) consumption on Th2-mediated inflammatory response in mouse gut. *European Journal of Nutrition, 53*(4), 1039–1049. https://doi.org/10.1007/s00394-013-0606-7

214   Deth, R., Clarke, A., Ni, J., & Trivedi, M. (2016). Clinical evaluation of glutathione concentrations after consumption of milk containing different subtypes of β-casein: Results from a randomized, cross-over clinical trial. *Nutrition Journal, 15*(1), 82. https://doi.org/10.1186/s12937-016-0201-x

215   Welsh, J., Braun, H., Brown, N., Um, C., Ehret, K., Figueroa, J., & Boyd Barr, D. (2019). Production-related contaminants (pesticides, antibiotics and hormones) in organic and conventionally produced milk samples sold in the USA. *Public Health Nutrition, 22*(16), 2972-2980. https://www.doi.org/10.1017/S136898001900106X

216   Pugeat, M., Nader, N., Hogeveen, K., Raverot, G., Déchaud, H., & Grenot, C. (2010). Sex hormone-binding globulin gene expression in the liver: Drugs and the metabolic syndrome. *Molecular and Cellular Endocrinology, 316*(1), 53–59. https://doi. org/10.1016/j.mce.2009.09.020

217   Tsuchiya, M., Miura, T., Hanaoka, T., Iwasaki, M., Sasaki, H., Tanaka, T., Nakao, H., Katoh, T., Ikenoue, T., Kabuto, M., & Tsugane, S. (2007). Effect of soy isoflavones on endometriosis: Interaction with estrogen receptor 2 gene polymorphism. *Epidemiology* (Cambridge, Mass.), *18*(3), 402–408. https://doi.org/10.1097/01. ede.0000257571.01358.f9

218   Chen, K. I., Chiang, C. Y., Ko, C. Y., Huang, H. Y., & Cheng, K. C. (2018). Reduction of phytic acid in soymilk by immobilized phytase system. *Journal of Food Science, 83*(12), 2963–2969. https://doi.org/10.1111/1750-3841.14394

219   Bøhn, T., Cuhra, M., Traavik, T., Sanden, M., Fagan, J., & Primicerio, R. (2014). Compositional differences in soybeans on the market: Glyphosate accumulates in Roundup Ready GM soybeans. *Food Chemistry, 153*, 207–215. https://doi.org/10.1016/j. foodchem.2013.12.054

220   Hashida, S., Ishikawa, E., Nakamichi, N., & Sekino, H. (2002). Concentration of egg white lysozyme in the serum of healthy subjects after oral administration. *Clinical and Experimental Pharmacology & Physiology, 29*(1-2), 79–83. https://doi.org/10.1046/j.1440-1681.2002.03605.x

221   Lovallo, W. R., Farag, N. H., Vincent, A. S., Thomas, T. L., & Wilson, M. F. (2006). Cortisol responses to mental stress, exercise, and meals following caffeine intake in men and women. *Pharmacology, Biochemistry, and Behavior, 83*(3), 441–447. https://doi.org/10.1016/j.pbb.2006.03.005

222   Schliep, K. C., Schisterman, E. F., Mumford, S. L., Pollack, A. Z., Zhang, C., Ye, A., Stanford, J. B., Hammoud, A. O., Porucznik, C. A., & Wactawski-Wende, J. (2012). Caffeinated beverage intake and reproductive hormones among premenopausal women in the BioCycle Study. *The American Journal of Clinical Nutrition, 95*(2), 488–497. https://doi.org/10.3945/ajcn.111.021287

223   O'Callaghan, F., Muurlink, O., & Reid, N. (2018). Effects of caffeine on sleep quality and daytime functioning. *Risk Management and Healthcare Policy, 11*, 263–271. https://doi.org/10.2147/RMHP.S156404

224   Awad, E., Ahmed, H., Yousef, A., & Abbas, R. (2017). Efficacy of exercise on pelvic pain and posture associated with endometriosis: Within subject design. *Journal of Physical Therapy Science, 29*(12), 2112–2115. https://doi.org/10.1589/jpts.29.2112

225   Koppan, A., Hamori, J., Vranics, I., Garai, J., Kriszbacher, I., Bodis, J., Rebek-Nagy, G., & Koppan, M. (2010). Pelvic pain in endometriosis: painkillers or sport to alleviate symptoms? *Acta Physiologica Hungarica, 97*(2), 234–239. https://doi.org/10.1556/APhysiol.97.2010.2.10

226   Merino, J. J., Roncero, C., Oset-Gasque, M. J., Naddaf, A., & González, M. P. (2014). Antioxidant and protective mechanisms against hypoxia and hypoglycaemia in cortical neurons in vitro. *International Journal of Molecular Sciences, 15*(2), 2475–2493. https://doi.org/10.3390/ijms15022475

227   *Aching for an answer*. Nutritious Movement. Accessed February 12, 2022, from: https://www.nutritiousmovement.com/aching-for-an-answer/

228   Blackwell, D. L., & Clarke, T. C. (2018). State variation in meeting the 2008 federal guidelines for both aerobic and muscle-strengthening activities through leisure-time physical activity among adults aged 18–64: United States, 2010–2015. *National Health Statistics Reports*, (112), 1–22.

229   Abraham, P., Picquet, J., Vielle, B., Sigaudo-Roussel, D., Paisant-Thouveny, F., Enon, B., & Saumet, J. L. (2003). Transcutaneous oxygen pressure measurements on the buttocks during exercise to detect proximal arterial ischemia: Comparison with arteriography. *Circulation, 107*(14), 1896–1900. https://doi.org/10.1161/01.CIR.0000060500.60646.E0

230   Krishnasamy, K., Limbourg, A., Kapanadze, T., Gamrekelashvili, J., Beger, C., Häger, C., Lozanovski, V. J., Falk, C. S., Napp, L. C., Bauersachs, J., Mack, M., Haller, H.,

Weber, C., Adams, R. H., & Limbourg, F. P. (2017). Blood vessel control of macrophage maturation promotes arteriogenesis in ischemia. *Nature Communications*, *8*(1), 952. https://doi.org/10.1038/s41467-017-00953-2

231   Regan, M. A., Teasell, R. W., Wolfe, D. L., Keast, D., Mortenson, W. B., Aubut, J. A., & Spinal Cord Injury Rehabilitation Evidence Research Team. (2009). A systematic review of therapeutic interventions for pressure ulcers after spinal cord injury. *Archives of Physical Medicine and Rehabilitation*, *90*(2), 213–231. https://doi.org/10.1016/j.apmr.2008.08.212

232   Moore, J. S., Gibson, P. R., Perry, R. E., & Burgell, R. E. (2017). Endometriosis in patients with irritable bowel syndrome: Specific symptomatic and demographic profile, and response to the low FODMAP diet. *The Australian & New Zealand Journal of Obstetrics & Gynaecology*, *57*(2), 201–205. https://doi.org/10.1111/ajo.12594

233   McIntosh, K., Reed, D. E., Schneider, T., Dang, F., Keshteli, A. H., De Palma, G., Madsen, K., Bercik, P., & Vanner, S. (2017). FODMAPs alter symptoms and the metabolome of patients with IBS: A randomised controlled trial. *Gut*, *66*(7), 1241–1251. https://doi.org/10.1136/gutjnl-2015-311339

234   Konijeti, G. G., Kim, N., Lewis, J. D., Groven, S., Chandrasekaran, A., Grandhe, S., Diamant, C., Singh, E., Oliveira, G., Wang, X., Molparia, B., & Torkamani, A. (2017). Efficacy of the autoimmune protocol diet for inflammatory bowel disease. *Inflammatory Bowel Diseases*, *23*(11), 2054–2060. https://doi.org/10.1097/MIB.0000000000001221

235   Abbott, R. D., Sadowski, A., & Alt, A. G. (2019). Efficacy of the autoimmune protocol diet as part of a multi-disciplinary, supported lifestyle intervention for Hashimoto's thyroiditis. *Cureus*, *11*(4), e4556. https://doi.org/10.7759/cureus.4556

236   Etxeberria, U., Fernández-Quintela, A., Milagro, F. I., Aguirre, L., Martínez, J. A., & Portillo, M. P. (2013). Impact of polyphenols and polyphenol-rich dietary sources on gut microbiota composition. *Journal of Agricultural and Food Chemistry*, *61*(40), 9517–9533. https://doi.org/10.1021/jf402506c; Evensen, N. A., & Braun, P. C. (2009). The effects of tea polyphenols on *Candida albicans*: Inhibition of biofilm formation and proteasome inactivation. *Canadian Journal of Microbiology*, *55*(9), 1033–1039. https://doi.org/10.1139/w09-058

237   Costantini, L., Molinari, R., Farinon, B., & Merendino, N. (2017). Impact of omega-3 fatty acids on the gut microbiota. *International Journal of Molecular Sciences*, *18*(12), 2645. https://doi.org/10.3390/ijms18122645

238   Costantini, L., Molinari, R., Farinon, B., & Merendino, N. (2017). Impact of omega-3 fatty acids on the gut microbiota. *International Journal of Molecular Sciences*, *18*(12), 2645. https://doi.org/10.3390/ijms18122645

239   Auchtung, T. A., Fofanova, T. Y., Stewart, C. J., Nash, A. K., Wong, M. C., Gesell, J. R., Auchtung, J. M., Ajami, N. J., & Petrosino, J. F. (2018). Investigating colonization of the healthy adult gastrointestinal tract by fungi. *mSphere*, *3*(2), e00092-18. https://doi.org/10.1128/mSphere.00092-18

240 Khaleque Newaz Khan, Akira Fujishita, Michio Kitajima, Koichi Hiraki, Masahiro Nakashima, Hideaki Masuzaki. (2014). Intra-uterine microbial colonization and occurrence of endometritis in women with endometriosis. *Human Reproduction, 29*(11), 2446–56. https://doi.org/10.1093/humrep/deu222

241 Reid, G., Charbonneau, D., Erb, J., Kochanowski, B., Beuerman, D., Poehner, R., & Bruce, A. W. (2003). Oral use of *Lactobacillus rhamnosus* GR-1 and L. fermentum RC-14 significantly alters vaginal flora: Randomized, placebo-controlled trial in 64 healthy women. *FEMS Immunology and Medical Microbiology, 35*(2), 131–134. https://doi.org/10.1016/S0928-8244(02)00465-0

242 Besedovsky, L., Lange, T., & Haack, M. (2019). The sleep-immune crosstalk in health and disease. *Physiological Reviews, 99*(3), 1325–1380. https://doi.org/10.1152/physrev.00010.2018

243 Joo, E. Y., Yoon, C. W., Koo, D. L., Kim, D., & Hong, S. B. (2012). Adverse effects of 24 hours of sleep deprivation on cognition and stress hormones. *Journal of Clinical Neurology* (Seoul, Korea), *8*(2), 146–150. https://doi.org/10.3988/jcn.2012.8.2.146

244 Arion, K., Orr, N. L., Noga, H., Allaire, C., Williams, C., Bedaiwy, M. A., & Yong, P. J. (2020). A quantitative analysis of sleep quality in women with endometriosis. *Journal of Women's Health, 29*(9), 1209–1215. https://doi.org/10.1089/jwh.2019.8008

245 Elsevier. (2008). Loss of sleep, even for a single night, increases inflammation in the body. *ScienceDaily.* Retrieved from www.sciencedaily.com/releases/2008/09/080902075211.htm

246 Van Niekerk, L., Johnstone, L., & Matthewson, M. (2022). Predictors of self-compassion in endometriosis: The role of psychological health and endometriosis symptom burden. *Human Reproduction* (Oxford, England), *37*(2), 264–273. https://doi.org/10.1093/humrep/deab257

247 Taylor, S. E., Klein, L. C., Lewis, B. P., Gruenewald, T. L., Gurung, R. A., & Updegraff, J. A. (2000). Biobehavioral responses to stress in females: Tend-and-befriend, not fight-or-flight. *Psychological Review, 107*(3), 411–429. https://doi.org/10.1037/0033-295x.107.3.411

248 Qi, Q., Liu, X., Zhang, Q., & Guo, S. W. (2020). Platelets induce increased estrogen production through NF-κB and TGF-β1 signaling pathways in endometriotic stromal cells. *Scientific Reports, 10*(1), 1281. https://doi.org/10.1038/s41598-020-57997-6; Noble, L. S., Takayama, K., Zeitoun, K. M., Putman, J. M., Johns, D. A., Hinshelwood, M. M., Agarwal, V. R., Zhao, Y., Carr, B. R., & Bulun, S. E. (1997). Prostaglandin E2 stimulates aromatase expression in endometriosis-derived stromal cells. *The Journal of Clinical Endocrinology and Metabolism, 82*(2), 600–606. https://doi.org/10.1210/jcem.82.2.3783; Delvoux, B., Groothuis, P., D'Hooghe, T., Kyama, C., Dunselman, G., & Romano, A. (2009). Increased production of 17beta-estradiol in endometriosis lesions is the result of impaired metabolism. *The Journal of Clinical Endocrinology and Metabolism, 94*(3), 876–883. https://doi.org/10.1210/jc.2008-2218; Bulun, S. E., Monsavais, D., Pavone, M. E., Dyson, M., Xue, Q., Attar, E., Tokun-

aga, H., & Su, E. J. (2012). Role of estrogen receptor-β in endometriosis. *Seminars in Reproductive Medicine, 30*(1), 39–45. https://doi.org/10.1055/s-0031-1299596

249 Lessey, B. A., & Kim, J. J. (2017). Endometrial receptivity in the eutopic endometrium of women with endometriosis: It is affected, and let me show you why. *Fertility and Sterility, 108*(1), 19–27. https://doi.org/10.1016/j.fertnstert.2017.05.031

250 Campbell, K. L., Foster-Schubert, K. E., Alfano, C. M., Wang, C. C., Wang, C. Y., Duggan, C. R., Mason, C., Imayama, I., Kong, A., Xiao, L., Bain, C. E., Blackburn, G. L., Stanczyk, F. Z., & McTiernan, A. (2012). Reduced-calorie dietary weight loss, exercise, and sex hormones in postmenopausal women: randomized controlled trial. *Journal of Clinical Oncology: Official Journal of the American Society of Clinical Oncology, 30*(19), 2314–2326. https://doi.org/10.1200/JCO.2011.37.9792

251 Thompson, P. A., Khatami, M., Baglole, C. J., Sun, J., Harris, S. A., Moon, E. Y., Al-Mulla, F., Al-Temaimi, R., Brown, D. G., Colacci, A., Mondello, C., Raju, J., Ryan, E. P., Woodrick, J., Scovassi, A. I., Singh, N., Vaccari, M., Roy, R., Forte, S., Memeo, L., … Bisson, W. H. (2015). Environmental immune disruptors, inflammation and cancer risk. *Carcinogenesis, 36 Suppl 1*(Suppl 1), S232–S253. https://doi.org/10.1093/carcin/bgv038

252 Peinado, F. M., Ocón-Hernández, O., Iribarne-Durán, L. M., Vela-Soria, F., Ubiña, A., Padilla, C., Mora, J. C., Cardona, J., León, J., Fernández, M. F., Olea, N., & Artacho-Cordón, F. (2021). Cosmetic and personal care product use, urinary levels of parabens and benzophenones, and risk of endometriosis: results from the EndEA study. *Environmental Research, 196*, 110342. https://doi.org/10.1016/j.envres.2020.110342; Louis, G. M., Peterson, C. M., Chen, Z., Hediger, M. L., Croughan, M. S., Sundaram, R., Stanford, J. B., Fujimoto, V. Y., Varner, M. W., Giudice, L. C., Kennedy, A., Sun, L., Wu, Q., & Kannan, K. (2012). Perfluorochemicals and endometriosis: The ENDO study. *Epidemiology* (Cambridge, Mass.), *23*(6), 799–805. https://doi.org/10.1097/EDE.0b013e31826ccocf

253 Avinash Kar, Anna Reade, Susan Lee, Daniel Raichel, Jennifer Sass, Anna Reade, Susan Lee, Daniel Rosenberg ,Veena Singla, Darby Hoover, Miriam Rotkin-Ellman, & Tom Hucker. (2021). *Toxic chemicals*. NRDC. https://www.nrdc.org/issues/toxic-chemicals

254 Smith, R., Lourie, B., & Dopp, S. (2009). *Slow death by rubber duck: The secret danger of everyday things*. Berkeley, CA: Counterpoint.

255 Braun, J. M., Just, A. C., Williams, P. L., Smith, K. W., Calafat, A. M., & Hauser, R. (2014). Personal care product use and urinary phthalate metabolite and paraben concentrations during pregnancy among women from a fertility clinic. *Journal of Exposure Science & Environmental Epidemiology, 24*(5), 459–466. https://doi.org/10.1038/jes.2013.69

256 Duty, S. M., Ackerman, R. M., Calafat, A. M., & Hauser, R. (2005). Personal care product use predicts urinary concentrations of some phthalate monoesters. *Environmental Health perspectives, 113*(11), 1530–1535. https://doi.org/10.1289/ehp.8083

257   Upson, K., De Roos, A. J., Thompson, M. L., Sathyanarayana, S., Scholes, D., Barr, D. B., & Holt, V. L. (2013). Organochlorine pesticides and risk of endometriosis: Findings from a population-based case-control study. *Environmental Health Perspectives, 121*(11-12), 1319–1324. https://doi.org/10.1289/ehp.1306648

258   Kolakowski, B. M., Miller, L., Murray, A., Leclair, A., Bietlot, H., & van de Riet, J. M. (2020). Analysis of glyphosate residues in foods from the Canadian retail markets between 2015 and 2017. *Journal of Agricultural and Food Chemistry, 68*(18), 5201–5211. https://doi.org/10.1021/acs.jafc.9b07819

259   Fagan, J., Bohlen, L., Patton, S., & Klein, K. (2020). Organic diet intervention significantly reduces urinary glyphosate levels in U.S. children and adults. *Environmental Research, 189*, 109898. https://doi.org/10.1016/j.envres.2020.109898

260   Hori, T., Nakagawa, R., Tobiishi, K., Iida, T., Tsutsumi, T., Sasaki, K., & Toyoda, M. (2005). Effects of cooking on concentrations of polychlorinated dibenzo-p-dioxins and related compounds in fish and meat. *Journal of Agricultural and Food Chemistry, 53*(22), 8820–8828. https://doi.org/10.1021/jf050978l

261   Morita, K., Ogata, M., & Hasegawa, T. (2001). Chlorophyll derived from chlorella inhibits dioxin absorption from the gastrointestinal tract and accelerates dioxin excretion in rats. *Environmental Health Perspectives, 109*(3), 289–294. https://doi.org/10.1289/ehp.01109289

262   Takekoshi, H., Suzuki, G., Chubachi, H., & Nakano, M. (2005). Effect of chlorella pyrenoidosa on fecal excretion and liver accumulation of polychlorinated dibenzo-p-dioxin in mice. *Chemosphere, 59*(2), 297–304. https://doi.org/10.1016/j.chemosphere.2004.11.026

263   Çolak, D. A., & Uysal, H. (2017). Protective effects of coenzyme Q10 and resveratrol on oxidative stress induced by various dioxins on transheterozigot larvae of *Drosophila melanogaster. Toxicology Research, 6*(4), 521–525. https://doi.org/10.1039/c7tx00027h

264   Pérez, F., Nadal, M., Navarro-Ortega, A., Fàbrega, F., Domingo, J. L., Barceló, D., & Farré, M. (2013). Accumulation of perfluoroalkyl substances in human tissues. *Environment International, 59*, 354–362. https://doi.org/10.1016/j.envint.2013.06.004

265   Huang, M., Liu, S., Fu, L., Jiang, X., & Yang, M. (2020). Bisphenol A and its analogues bisphenol S, bisphenol F and bisphenol AF induce oxidative stress and biomacromolecular damage in human granulosa KGN cells. *Chemosphere, 253*, 126707. https://doi.org/10.1016/j.chemosphere.2020.126707

266   Genuis, S. J., Beesoon, S., Birkholz, D., & Lobo, R. A. (2012). Human excretion of bisphenol A: Blood, urine, and sweat (BUS) study. *Journal of Environmental and Public Health, 2012*, 185731. https://doi.org/10.1155/2012/185731; Genuis, S. J., Beesoon, S., & Birkholz, D. (2013). Biomonitoring and elimination of perfluorinated compounds and polychlorinated biphenyls through perspiration: Blood, urine, and sweat study. *ISRN Toxicology, 2013*, 483832. https://doi.org/10.1155/2013/483832; Genuis, S. J., Beesoon, S., Lobo, R. A., & Birkholz, D. (2012). Human elimination of

phthalate compounds: Blood, urine, and sweat (BUS) study. *The Scientific World Journal, 2012,* 615068. https://doi.org/10.1100/2012/615068

267 Palmery, M., Saraceno, A., Vaiarelli, A., & Carlomagno, G. (2013). Oral contraceptives and changes in nutritional requirements. *European Review for Medical and Pharmacological Sciences, 17*(13), 1804–1813.

268 Williams, W. V. (2017). Hormonal contraception and the development of autoimmunity: A review of the literature. *The Linacre Quarterly, 84*(3), 275–295. https://doi.org/10.1080/00243639.2017.1360065

269 Jess, T., Frisch, M., Jørgensen, K. T., Pedersen, B. V., & Nielsen, N. M. (2012). Increased risk of inflammatory bowel disease in women with endometriosis: A nationwide Danish cohort study. *Gut, 61*(9), 1279–1283. https://doi.org/10.1136/gutjnl-2011-301095

270 Chung, M. K., Chung, R. P., & Gordon, D. (2005). Interstitial cystitis and endometriosis in patients with chronic pelvic pain: The "evil twins" syndrome. *JSLS: Journal of the Society of Laparoendoscopic Surgeons, 9*(1), 25–29; U.S. Department of Health and Human Services. (2002). *Women with endometriosis have higher rates of some diseases.* Eunice Kennedy Shriver National Institute of Child Health and Human Development. https://www.nichd.nih.gov/newsroom/releases/endometriosis

271 Wallace, J. L. (2000). How do NSAIDs cause ulcer disease? *Bailliere's Best Practice & Research. Clinical Gastroenterology, 14*(1), 147–159. https://doi.org/10.1053/bega.1999.0065

272 Sigthorsson, G., Tibble, J., Hayllar, J., Menzies, I., Macpherson, A., Moots, R., Scott, D., Gumpel, M. J., & Bjarnason, I. (1998). Intestinal permeability and inflammation in patients on NSAIDs. *Gut, 43*(4), 506–511. https://doi.org/10.1136/gut.43.4.506

273 Park, S. C., Chun, H. J., Kang, C. D., & Sul, D. (2011). Prevention and management of non-steroidal anti-inflammatory drugs-induced small intestinal injury. *World Journal of Gastroenterology, 17*(42), 4647–4653. https://doi.org/10.3748/wjg.v17.i42.4647

274 Li, D. K., Ferber, J. R., Odouli, R., & Quesenberry, C. (2018). Use of nonsteroidal anti-inflammatory drugs during pregnancy and the risk of miscarriage. *American Journal of Obstetrics and Gynecology, 219*(3), 275.e1–275.e8. https://doi.org/10.1016/j.ajog.2018.06.002

275 Vowles, K. E., McEntee, M. L., Julnes, P. S., Frohe, T., Ney, J. P., & van der Goes, D. N. (2015). Rates of opioid misuse, abuse, and addiction in chronic pain: A systematic review and data synthesis. *Pain, 156*(4), 569–576. https://doi.org/10.1097/01.j.pain.0000460357.01998.f1

276 Lee, M., Silverman, S. M., Hansen, H., Patel, V. B., & Manchikanti, L. (2011). A comprehensive review of opioid-induced hyperalgesia. *Pain Physician, 14*(2), 145–161.

277   Berger, A. (1999). Researchers discover how opiates cause immunosuppression. *BMJ (Clinical research ed.)*, *318*(7179), 280B. https://doi.org/10.1136/bmj.318.7179.280b

278   Donaldson, C., Mefford, B. (2020) Opioids and the immune system. *US Pharm.* Retrieved from: https://www.uspharmacist.com/article/opioids-and-the-immune-system

279   Wang, J., Barke, R. A., Ma, J., Charboneau, R., & Roy, S. (2008). Opiate abuse, innate immunity, and bacterial infectious diseases. *Archivum Immunologiae et Therapiae Experimentalis*, *56*(5), 299–309. https://doi.org/10.1007/s00005-008-0035-0

280   Kim, P. S., & Fishman, M. A. (2020). Low-dose naltrexone for chronic pain: Update and systemic review. *Current Pain and Headache Reports*, *24*(10), 64. https://doi.org/10.1007/s11916-020-00898-0

281   Bouaziz, J., Bar On, A., Seidman, D. S., & Soriano, D. (2017). The clinical significance of endocannabinoids in endometriosis pain management. *Cannabis and Cannabinoid Research*, *2*(1), 72–80. https://doi.org/10.1089/can.2016.0035

282   Glace, E. (2019, February 19). The importance of the pelvic floor for endometriosis. *Endometriosis.net*. https://endometriosis.net/clinical/pelvic-floor-matters

283   Weir, K. (2020). Nurtured by nature. *Monitor on Psychology*. Retrieved April 19, 2022, from https://www.apa.org/monitor/2020/04/nurtured-nature

284   Chen, H., Malentacchi, F., Fambrini, M., Harrath, A. H., Huang, H., & Petraglia, F. (2020). Epigenetics of estrogen and progesterone receptors in endometriosis. *Reproductive Sciences* (Thousand Oaks, Calif.), *27*(11), 1967–1974. https://doi.org/10.1007/s43032-020-00226-2

285   Chen, H., Malentacchi, F., Fambrini, M., Harrath, A. H., Huang, H., & Petraglia, F. (2020). Epigenetics of estrogen and progesterone receptors in endometriosis. *Reproductive Sciences* (Thousand Oaks, Calif.), *27*(11), 1967–1974. https://doi.org/10.1007/s43032-020-00226-2

286   Wen, X., Xiong, Y., Jin, L., Ming, Z., Huang, L., Mao, Y., Zhou, C., Qiao, Y., & Zhang, Y. (2020). Bisphenol A exposure enhances endometrial stromal cell invasion and has a positive association with peritoneal endometriosis. *Reproductive Sciences, 27*, 704–712. https://doi.org/10.1007/s43032-019-00076-7

287   Kalluri, R., & Weinberg, R. A. (2009). The basics of epithelial-mesenchymal transition. *The Journal of Clinical Investigation*, *119*(6), 1420–1428. https://doi.org/10.1172/JCI39104

288   Bruner-Tran, K. L., Ding, T., & Osteen, K. G. (2010). Dioxin and endometrial progesterone resistance. *Seminars in Reproductive Medicine*, *28*(1), 59–68. https://doi.org/10.1055/s-0029-1242995; Koukoura, O., Sifakis, S., & Spandidos, D. A. (2016). DNA methylation in endometriosis. *Molecular Medicine Reports*, *13*(4), 2939–2948. https://doi.org/10.3892/mmr.2016.4925

289 Shmarakov, I. O. (2015). Retinoid-xenobiotic interactions: The ying and the yang. *Hepatobiliary Surgery and Nutrition, 4*(4), 243–267. https://doi.org/10.3978/j.issn.2304-3881.2015.05.05

290 Pierzchalski, K., Taylor, R. N., Nezhat, C., Jones, J. W., Napoli, J. L., Yang, G., Kane, M. A., & Sidell, N. (2014). Retinoic acid biosynthesis is impaired in human and murine endometriosis. *Biology of Reproduction, 91*(4), 84. https://doi.org/10.1095/biolreprod.114.119677

291 Capobianco, A., & Rovere-Querini, P. (2013). Endometriosis, a disease of the macrophage. *Frontiers in Immunology, 4*, 9. https://doi.org/10.3389/fimmu.2013.00009; Hogg, C., Horne, A. W., & Greaves, E. (2020). Endometriosis-associated macrophages: Origin, phenotype, and function. *Frontiers in Endocrinology, 11*, 7. https://doi.org/10.3389/fendo.2020.00007

292 Bacci, M., Capobianco, A., Monno, A., Cottone, L., Di Puppo, F., Camisa, B., Mariani, M., Brignole, C., Ponzoni, M., Ferrari, S., Panina-Bordignon, P., Manfredi, A. A., & Rovere-Querini, P. (2009). Macrophages are alternatively activated in patients with endometriosis and required for growth and vascularization of lesions in a mouse model of disease. *The American Journal of Pathology, 175*(2), 547–556. https://doi.org/10.2353/ajpath.2009.081011

293 291 Dmowski, W. P., & Braun, D. P. (2004). Immunology of endometriosis. *Best Practice & Research Clinical Obstetrics & Gynaecology, 18*(2), 245–263. https://doi.org/10.1016/j.bpobgyn.2004.02.001; Zhou, W. J., Yang, H. L., Shao, J., Mei, J., Chang, K. K., Zhu, R., & Li, M. Q. (2019). Anti-inflammatory cytokines in endometriosis. *Cellular and Molecular Life Sciences: CMLS, 76*(11), 2111–2132. https://doi.org/10.1007/s00018-019-03056-x

294 Qi, Q., Liu, X., Zhang, Q., & Guo, S. W. (2020). Platelets induce increased estrogen production through NF-κB and TGF-β1 signaling pathways in endometriotic stromal cells. *Scientific Reports, 10*(1), 1281. https://doi.org/10.1038/s41598-020-57997-6

295 Symons, L. K., Miller, J. E., Tyryshkin, K., Monsanto, S. P., Marks, R. M., Lingegowda, H., Vanderbeck, K., Childs, T., Young, S. L., Lessey, B. A., Koti, M., & Tayade, C. (2020). Neutrophil recruitment and function in endometriosis patients and a syngeneic murine model. *FASEB Journal: Official Publication of the Federation of American Societies for Experimental Biology, 34*(1), 1558–1575. https://doi.org/10.1096/fj.201902272R

296 Malutan, A. M., Drugan, T., Costin, N., Ciortea, R., Bucuri, C., Rada, M. P., & Mihu, D. (2015). Pro-inflammatory cytokines for evaluation of inflammatory status in endometriosis. *Central-European Journal of Immunology, 40*(1), 96–102. https://doi.org/10.5114/ceji.2015.50840

297 Malutan, A. M., Drugan, T., Costin, N., Ciortea, R., Bucuri, C., Rada, M. P., & Mihu, D. (2015). Pro-inflammatory cytokines for evaluation of inflammatory status in endometriosis. *Central-European Journal of Immunology, 40*(1), 96–102. https://doi.org/10.5114/ceji.2015.50840

298   Dmowski, W. P., & Braun, D. P. (2004). Immunology of endometriosis. *Best Practice & Research Clinical Obstetrics & Gynaecology, 18*(2), 245–263. https://doi.org/10.1016/j.bpobgyn.2004.02.001

299   Wu, M. H., Wang, C. A., Lin, C. C., Chen, L. C., Chang, W. C., & Tsai, S. J. (2005). Distinct regulation of cyclooxygenase-2 by interleukin-1beta in normal and endometriotic stromal cells. *The Journal of Clinical Endocrinology and Metabolism, 90*(1), 286–295. https://doi.org/10.1210/jc.2004-1612

300   Chegini, N. (2008). TGF-beta system: The principal profibrotic mediator of peritoneal adhesion formation. *Seminars in Reproductive Medicine, 26*(4), 298–312. https://doi.org/10.1055/s-0028-1082388

301   Thiruchelvam, U., Wingfield, M., & O'Farrelly, C. (2015). Natural killer cells: Key players in endometriosis. *American Journal of Reproductive Immunology, 74*(4), 291–301. https://doi.org/10.1111/aji.12408; Xu, H. (2019). Expressions of natural cytotoxicity receptor, NKG2D and NKG2D ligands in endometriosis. *Journal of Reproductive Immunology, 136*, 102615. https://doi.org/10.1016/j.jri.2019.102615

302   Hogg, C., Horne, A. W., & Greaves, E. (2020). Endometriosis-associated macrophages: Origin, phenotype, and function. *Frontiers in Endocrinology, 11*, 7. https://doi.org/10.3389/fendo.2020.00007

303   Wu, M. H., Shoji, Y., Wu, M. C., Chuang, P. C., Lin, C. C., Huang, M. F., & Tsai, S. J. (2005). Suppression of matrix metalloproteinase-9 by prostaglandin E(2) in peritoneal macrophage is associated with severity of endometriosis. *The American Journal of Pathology, 167*(4), 1061–1069. https://doi.org/10.1016/S0002-9440(10)61195-9

304   Bacci, M., Capobianco, A., Monno, A., Cottone, L., Di Puppo, F., Camisa, B., Mariani, M., Brignole, C., Ponzoni, M., Ferrari, S., Panina-Bordignon, P., Manfredi, A. A., & Rovere-Querini, P. (2009). Macrophages are alternatively activated in patients with endometriosis and required for growth and vascularization of lesions in a mouse model of disease. *The American Journal of Pathology, 175*(2), 547–556. https://doi.org/10.2353/ajpath.2009.081011

305   Laganà, A. S., Garzon, S., Götte, M., Viganò, P., Franchi, M., Ghezzi, F., & Martin, D. C. (2019). The pathogenesis of endometriosis: Molecular and cell biology insights. *International Journal of Molecular Sciences, 20*(22), 5615. https://doi.org/10.3390/ijms20225615

306   Riccio, L., Santulli, P., Marcellin, L., Abrão, M. S., Batteux, F., & Chapron, C. (2018). Immunology of endometriosis. *Best Practice & Research Clinical Obstetrics & Gynaecology, 50*, 39–49. https://doi.org/10.1016/j.bpobgyn.2018.01.010

307   Dmowski, W. P., & Braun, D. P. (2004). Immunology of endometriosis. *Best Practice & Research Clinical Obstetrics & Gynaecology, 18*(2), 245–263. https://doi.org/10.1016/j.bpobgyn.2004.02.001

308   Malutan, A. M., Drugan, T., Costin, N., Ciortea, R., Bucuri, C., Rada, M. P., & Mihu, D. (2015). Pro-inflammatory cytokines for evaluation of inflammatory status in

endometriosis. *Central-European Journal of Immunology, 40*(1), 96–102. https://doi.org/10.5114/ceji.2015.50840

309   Dmowski, W. P., & Braun, D. P. (2004). Immunology of endometriosis. *Best Practice & Research Clinical Obstetrics & Gynaecology, 18*(2), 245–263. https://doi.org/10.1016/j.bpobgyn.2004.02.001

310   Laganà, A. S., Garzon, S., Götte, M., Viganò, P., Franchi, M., Ghezzi, F., & Martin, D. C. (2019). The pathogenesis of endometriosis: Molecular and cell biology insights. *International Journal of Molecular Sciences, 20*(22), 5615. https://doi.org/10.3390/ijms20225615; Symons, L. K., Miller, J. E., Tyryshkin, K., Monsanto, S. P., Marks, R. M., Lingegowda, H., Vanderbeck, K., Childs, T., Young, S. L., Lessey, B. A., Koti, M., & Tayade, C. (2020). Neutrophil recruitment and function in endometriosis patients and a syngeneic murine model. *FASEB Journal: Official Publication of the Federation of American Societies for Experimental Biology, 34*(1), 1558–1575. https://doi.org/10.1096/fj.201902272R

311   Zhou, W. J., Yang, H. L., Shao, J., Mei, J., Chang, K. K., Zhu, R., & Li, M. Q. (2019). Anti-inflammatory cytokines in endometriosis. *Cellular and Molecular Life Sciences: CMLS, 76*(11), 2111–2132. https://doi.org/10.1007/s00018-019-03056-x

312   Kikuchi, Y., Ishikawa, N., Hirata, J., Imaizumi, E., Sasa, H., & Nagata, I. (1993). Changes of peripheral blood lymphocyte subsets before and after operation of patients with endometriosis. *Acta Obstetricia et Gynecologica Scandinavica, 72*(3), 157–161. https://doi.org/10.3109/00016349309013364

313   Brenhouse, H. C., & Schwarz, J. M. (2016). Immunoadolescence: Neuroimmune development and adolescent behavior. *Neuroscience and Biobehavioral Reviews, 70*, 288–299. https://doi.org/10.1016/j.neubiorev.2016.05.035; Martin, D. C. (2021). *Trust these teens: Early detection is the prevention.* EndoFound & ISGE Patient Day, https://www.youtube.com/watch?v=D7lI_10AnK4, accessed 3/23/2021

314   Emani, R., Alam, C., Pekkala, S., Zafar, S., Emani, M. R., & Hänninen, A. (2015). Peritoneal cavity is a route for gut-derived microbial signals to promote autoimmunity in non-obese diabetic mice. *Scandinavian Journal of Immunology, 81*(2), 102–109. https://doi.org/10.1111/sji.12253

315   Laschke, M. W., & Menger, M. D. (2016). The gut microbiota: A puppet master in the pathogenesis of endometriosis? *American Journal of Obstetrics and Gynecology, 215*(1), 68.e1–68.e4. https://doi.org/10.1016/j.ajog.2016.02.036

316   Emani, R., Alam, C., Pekkala, S., Zafar, S., Emani, M. R., & Hänninen, A. (2015). Peritoneal cavity is a route for gut-derived microbial signals to promote autoimmunity in non-obese diabetic mice. *Scandinavian Journal of Immunology, 81*(2), 102–109. https://doi.org/10.1111/sji.12253

317   United States Department of Agriculture. (2015). *DIOXIN FY2013 Survey: Dioxins and dioxin-like compounds in the U.S. domestic meat and poultry supply.* Food Safety and Inspection Service. https://www.fsis.usda.gov/sites/default/files/media_file/2020-07/Dioxin-Report-FY2013.pdf

318   Papadopoulos, A., Vassiliadou, I., Costopoulou, D., Papanicolaou, C., & Leondiadis, L. (2004). Levels of dioxins and dioxin-like PCBs in food samples on the Greek market. *Chemosphere, 57*(5), 413–419. https://doi.org/10.1016/j.chemosphere.2004.07.006

319   Baars, A. J., Bakker, M. I., Baumann, R. A., Boon, P. E., Freijer, J. I., Hoogenboom, L. A., Hoogerbrugge, R., van Klaveren, J. D., Liem, A. K., Traag, W. A., & de Vries, J. (2004). Dioxins, dioxin-like PCBs and non-dioxin-like PCBs in foodstuffs: Occurrence and dietary intake in The Netherlands. *Toxicology Letters, 151*(1), 51–61. https://doi. org/10.1016/j.toxlet.2004.01.028

320   Diletti, G., Scortichini, G., Abete, M. C., Binato, G., Candeloro, L., Ceci, R., Chessa, G., Conte, A., Di Sandro, A., Esposito, M., Fedrizzi, G., Ferrantelli, V., Ferretti, E., Menotta, S., Nardelli, V., Neri, B., Piersanti, A., Roberti, F., Ubaldi, A., & Brambilla, G. (2018). Intake estimates of dioxins and dioxin-like polychlorobiphenyls in the Italian general population from the 2013–2016 results of official monitoring plans in food. *The Science of the Total Environment, 627,* 11–19. https://doi.org/10.1016/j. scitotenv.2018.01.181

321   U.S. Department of Health and Human Services. (n.d.). Dioxins. National Institute of Environmental Health Sciences. https://www.niehs.nih.gov/health/topics/agents/ dioxins/index.cfm